AF541610

MEDICAL WORLD OF THE TRIBALS

MEDICAL WORLD OF THE TRIBALS

Explorations in illness Ideology, Body Symbolism and Ritual Healing

By

Robin D.Tribhuwan

Ma., Msc., Ph.d.

1998

Discovery Publishing House

New Delhi-110002 (India)

First Published-1998
Reprinted-2010

ISBN 81-7141-408-7

Published by:

Discovery Publishing House
4831/24, Ansari Road, Prahlad Street,
Daryaganj, New Delhi-110002 (*INDIA*)
Phone: 327 9245
Fax: 91-11-3253457

Printed at:

Sachin Printers Delhi

Dedicated to :-

My Dearest Friend,
Ms. Joan Dutli
(Canada)

PREFACE

During the last three decades Anthropologists have increasingly turned their attention towards the problems health & disease of people they studied. As a consequence a specialization known as Medical Anthropology came into being. Anthropological interest in Medicine stems from the fact that health and disease though scientifically understood as biological in nature, are related to people's belief system. The theoretical concern of Anthropology in Medicine is made explicit by Lieban (1973: 1034) by stating that "Medical Anthropology encompasses the study of Medical phenomena as they are influenced by social and cultural phenomena and social and cultural phenomena as they are illuminated by their medical aspects.

Throughout the ages, man has been devising ways and means of caring for the sick in the community (Newell 1975 : 55). Every culture, has its own beliefs and practices regarding health and diseases. It is to such beliefs and practices related to health and disease. Which are products of indigenous cultural development and not explicitly derived from the conceptual framework of modern medicine, the term "Ethnomedicine" is applied (Hughes 1968: 99).

Ethnomedical accounts have highlighted studies on illness ideology, body symbolism, nature and role of ethnomedical specialists, various forms of therapies, ritual healing, ethnophysiology, preventive medicine, witchcraft & sorcery and so on. (Foster G.M. 1976, 1981 Fabrega 1977; Hughes 1968, Douglas 1970; 1975 Lieban Richard 1973; Turner 1967, Nitcher & Nitcher 1981) Studies conducted on health related beliefs and practices of various groups assume significance in view of developing and implementing appropriate and culturally acceptable health care system and programmes for the tribal and rural masses. Anthropological studies related to health behaviour are fast gaining importance due to the introduction of modern health care programmes in rural & tribal areas. Health care policy planners and health administers often have faced stiff resistance in tribal and rural areas when trying to introduce modern medicine. This is due to the ignorance and lack of indepth understanding on the part of these health workers of the people's (tribal & rural) belief system.

Next to Africa, India has a considerable size of tribal population. In comparison to the numerous studies carried out on Africa and Latin American tribes in the field of ethnomedicine, few such studies are conducted on some Indian tribes. Thus a study of ethnomedicine from a symbolic and meaningful perspective will definitely lend great insight into the medical beliefs and practices of the tribals and be of great use in developing and shaping health care and health education programmes.

The current research is aimed at treating the domain of ethnomedicine as a symbolic system. Ethnomedicine is conceptually defined as a culturally ordered interrelationship of medical symbols and meanings that are associated with a community's notions of illness ideology, body image and the entire set of preventive, promotive, curative and destructive health rituals and/or therapeutic actions performed by the participant actors in various healing contexts, as a symbolic system there by representing the cultural whole.

Chapter 1: Introduction / Theoretical framework and Aims and objectives.

Aims and Objectives:

The major aims and objectives of the research are:

1. To understand the illness ideology of the natives as defined and experienced by them (from an emic perspective) and more specifically.

a) To document their perception regarding the origin and cause of illness and disease as revealed in their system of disease classification and their etiological categories.

b) To record the various pathogenic agents which cause illness and understand their role in Thakur culture.

c) To explore the various cultural factors or criteria, symptoms and situations where disease is defined as illness by those participating in healing processes; which seek to alter or restore the patient's health.

d) To uncover the symbolic elements and their meanings that shape illness experience.

2. To explore the tribals concepts/s regarding body physiology and about the various symbolic elements which find expression through the body during a patients ill-health.

a) Recording the Thakurs perception about the elements constituting the human body, by studying their notions regarding the morphology, anatomy and physiology of the body.

b) Studying the symbolic elements (social, cosmological, spiritual, natural and supernatural) that find expression through the physical form, i.e. in the form of body during ill-health.

3. To understand the symbolic and meaningful aspects of ritual healing including.

a) All the actions (rituals or otherwise) performed in collection preparation and administration of potions, drugs or any other substance perceived to be medicinal in nature.

b) All actions (rituals or otherwise) performed during diagnosis & interpretation of the cause of illness.

c) The entire set of ritual which is perceived as an instrument which reconstructs the disrupted cultural order (ill-health) and disharmony and attempts to bring back cultural order (health) & harmony.

d) All actions and rituals involved in thanks giving ceremonies which involve the originator and / or curer of illness.

4. To understand from a meaningful perspective the set processes wherein those involved in (which include family members elders the village and medical specialists) initiate a purposive alteration in the health of the patient.

Chapter II. Research Methodology

The research population selected are the Thakurs, tribal community residing in Pathraj and Kashale Grampanchayat in the Karjat Tehsil, Raigad district in Maharastra. Traditional Anthropological tools and techniques such as Participant observation, Indepth-Informal. Interviews of 77 heads of house holds above 45 years of age were documented from six Thakur Hamlets. 50 patients and fifty-one medical practitioners including shamans, bone setters, herbalists, midwives and other therapists were recorded in the form illness Episodes and Case Studies respectively. Both males and females are included in the study. On certain occasion group interviews were also conducted.

To support the data slides and photographs were also taken. The researcher underwent training as a Shaman so as to be able to comprehend an indepth understanding of medical symbols as defined by the Thakurs. The data was collected over a period of two years. It was data was analyzed manually since it was qualitative in nature.

Chapter III. Ethnography

This Chapter briefly highlights the ethnography of the Thakur community with special emphasis on maternal and child health care beliefs and practices.

Chapter IV. Illness Ideology

This chapter gives comprehensive details of what the Thakurs perceive to be the origin and cause of illness. The various contexts and situations wherein disease is defined as illness and more significantly how illness etiology reflects the Thakurs conception of cultural disorder and/ or disharmony of man with social, spiritual, cosmological, natural and supernatural entities/ forces. Besides this a detailed account of the manner in which meanings shape illness experience is presented in the form of fifty illness episodes.

Chapter V: Body Symbolism

This chapter throws light on the Thakurs concept of Body Physiology and more importantly on the various symbols and symbolic forms expressed through the body during the state of ill- health. The study has also pointed out how human body during the process of ritual healing gets a natural, social, spiritual, cosmological and supernatural status.

Chapter VI: Ethnomedical Specialists

This chapter gives a comprehensive picture of the nature and role of seven types of traditional medical practitioners existing in the Thakur culture in the form of case studies. It covers the symbolic aspects of apprenticeship, taboos associated, rituals associated with collection, preparation and administration of drugs, diagnosis, healing and thanks giving rituals and their meanings and other therapeutic actions.

Chapter VII: Ritual Healing

This chapter focuses on the Thakurs concepts regarding intrinsic (Healing) qualities of medicine used by them. The entire set of action, objects, songs, words, chants, gestures and utterances etc. in a ritual healing context are explored so as to understand their meaning as perceived by the natives. Besides this a conceptual model has been evolved which aptly describes the entire process of culturally designed clinically meaningful reality through which a sick person passes.

Chapter VII : Summary and Conclusion

This study has pointed out how illness experience is a symbolic expression of the society's (Thakurs) disrupted relationship with social, spiritual, cosmological, supernatural and natural agents and/ or forces. That the human body as physical form of selfhood is the symbolic frame in which these social, spiritual, cosmological, supernatural and natural paradoxes of existence are most powerfully expressed. That all actions, objects, gestures, songs, utterances, chants, words etc. exist in structural relationship with each other and that these structural relationships are built around a centrally organized meaning system. That ethnomedicine is a symbolic system, not merely in its own right but a representation of the whole culture.

Contribution to the Knowledge and Hints in Application

The heuristic value of this approach lies on two distinct levels:

i) On the theoretical level the study intends to demonstrate that it is possible for anthropologists to unravel the organizing structure of the complex cultures by restricting themselves to the study of a single area or domain of social life.

ii) At a more practical level this research aims to show that the marked resistance by alien cultures to the government health care and health education programmes as well to programmes in other spheres of social life do not stem out of ignorance, illiteracy and superstitions as erroneously thought.

The study emphasizes that deep and radically different categorization which arise from the meaning systems prevent the meshing of forms, other than their own into their meaning structures.

Such indepth studies have tremendous potential in the field of application as they provide symbolic information on indigenous health beliefs and more specifically on illness ideology, body symbolism, ritual healing, maternal & child health care beliefs & practices, ethnomedical specialists, food habits and health behaviour. This information serves the purpose of planning and implementing culturally acceptable and appropriate health care & health education programmes for the tribal & rural areas such knowledge also contributes to a general understanding of human behaviour in relation to culture change.

Dr. Robin. D. Tribhuwan
MA, MSc, Ph.D.

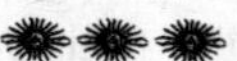

ACKNOWLEDGEMENTS

It gives me great delight to place on record the unstinting support and help gives to me by certain individuals and organizations so as to enable me to complete this work. My first word of thanks goes to my teacher and my guide Prof. R.K. Mutatkar. He helped me present papers at National and International Conferences in the field of Traditional Medicine. His constant inspiration and valuable suggestions and criticisms have enabled me to complete my work. Next, I wish to thank Ms. Joan Dutli from Canada who will always be a treasured friend of mine. Had it not been for her moral and financial support right from my high school upto my Ph. D. I would have not been able to sail smoothly right upto the end. It is very difficult to repay her.

Thirdly I would like to thank Dr. J.C. Kurian who is not only my teacher but also friends, philosopher and guide. He contributed his valuable suggestions right from planning, through data collection upto discussing the data. A special thanks for preparing the slides and photographs.

I further extend my thanks to Dr. Padam Singh, Director, Medical Statistics, ICMR for his valuable comments on Research Methodology. Mr. Darshan Shanker, Chairman and Founder member of Academy of Development Science and his colleagues Mr. R.P. Palekar, Dr. Sanjay Dakhore, Mr. Mathpaty, Mr. Padekar for introducing me to the tribals and to their beliefs on health and disease. I also thank them for their co-operation and excellent lodging and boarding facilities in Karjat during the periods of data collection. Dr. Horst Rolly, Head of Dept. of Social Service for partly sponsoring my data collection. Dr. R.D. Gambhir for discussing and contributing towards the model of Ethnomedical pathway. Dr. Merry Wood, Dr. B.V. Bhanu, Dr. K.S. Nair, Dr. Rajendra Vora and Dr. Meena Kelkar for discussing the data and giving their valuable suggestions. Mr. N. Chandrashekhar for his help from time to time. Mr. Earl Rosario for making comfortable arrangements for lodging and boarding in the field. Darius Kothawala, a good friend who inspired me to deal with this challenging subject of symbolism in Ethnomedicine. John Gaikwad, of Tribal Research Institute who actively discussed my data with me. My Guru Walku Thorad (Bhagat/ Shaman) who was kind enough to accept me as his pupil and give me valuable reality and secrets of Shamanism. My key informants and respondents who patiently answered my questions.

Dr. M. Daniels, from England, Mrs. Rita P. Shaw and Dr. Madhukar Ohal from U.S.A., and my mother-in-law Mrs. S.D. Peters who searched for material pertaining to my subject and took the trouble to xerox them and send them from U.K. and U.S.A. My father-in-law Mr. D.R. Peters for typing my work and brother-in-law Mr. Gaurav Peters who patiently and artistically draw diagrams related to the chapters.

Mrs. Lalita Bhat from A.F.K., Shefali Mehta, Bharat Phalak. of Datum Services, Mrs. Mrunalini & Mrs. Suvarna, of NIN for typing. Mr. S.D. Diwane of NIN for printing the work. Ms. Aarti Kelkar for helping in the writing of few drafts. The Spicer College Press for binding the thesis. My parents Mr. and Mrs. D.J. Tribhuwan for their moral support. Tribal Research and Training Institute for the Scholarship which helped lighten the financial burden. And my wife Preeti who with a lot of patience edited the chapters, wrote the drafts. I also thank her for her continuous patience and moral support. My heartiest thanks to my friend Shri Tilak Wasan, the publisher of this book for seeing it through. Lastly, I am most grateful to the Thakurs (my respondents) for their co-operation in giving valuable information on the symbolic aspects of their Ethnomedical System.

Robin David Tribhuwan

CONTENTS

CHAPTER I

INTRODUCTION

During the last threedecades Anthropologists have increasingly turned their attention towards the problems of health & disease of the people they studied. As a consequence a specialization known as Medical Anthropology came into being. This sub-discipline is engaged in carrying out researches in the field of a health, drug abuse, definition of health & disease, ethnomedicine, nutritional concepts, ethnophysiology, doctor-patient relationship, body symbolism, preventive medicine & so on.

Some researchers like Weaver (1968) have given importance to applied dimensions of Medical Anthropology. In his paper, "Medical Anthropology : Trends in research & Medical Education", has stated that "Medical Anthropology is that branch of applied Anthropology which deals with various aspects of health & disease".

Others view Medical Anthropology as a combination of two approaches. Foster & Anderson (1978) following the model of Sociologist Straus speak of Anthropology of Medicine (the theoretical side) and Anthropology in Medicine (the applied side).

Yet another definition suggests that, "Medical Anthropology is that branch of the "Science of Man, which studies biological & cultural (including historical) aspects of man from the point of view of understanding the medical, medico-historical, medico-legal, medico-social and public health problems of human beings" (Hasan & Prasad 1959:21-22). Hochstrasser and tap (1975:24) emphasize the bio-cultural dimension of the field. "Medical Anthropology according to them is concerned with bio-cultural understanding of man and his work in relation to health and medicine".

Fabrega (1972) says, "A Medical Anthropology is one that : (a) elucidates the factors, mechanisms, and processes that play a role in or influence the way in which individual and groups are affected by and respond to illness and disease; and(b) examines their problems with an emphasis on patterns of behaviour" (cited in Foster & Anderson,1978).

The data on traditional medical beliefs and practices that had been gathered by Anthropologists is earlier years, their information on cultural values & Social forms and their knowledge about the dynamics of social stability and change provided the needed key to many of the problems encountered in public health programmes.

On the basis of their studies, the Anthropologists were in a position to explain to the health personnel and Administrations that how traditional beliefs and practices conflicted with modern/western medical assumptions; how socio-cultural factors influenced health and disease; how socio-cultural factors took care of health and cured illness; and how health & disease are similarly aspects of total cultural patterns, which also change in the company of broader and more comprehensive socio-cultural changes in the society (Rizvi 1991:5).

Statement of the Problem

During the last few decades there has been considerable amount of literature published both by Medical and Social Scientists on Biological and Socio-Cultural aspects of health and decease. Anthropological interest in medicine stems from the fact that though health and disease as understood scientifically as biological in nature they are related to people's belief system.

The theoretical concern of Anthropology in Medicine is explained by Lieban Richard (1973 : 1034) by stating that "Medical Anthropology encompasses the study of Medical phenomena as they are influenced by social and cultural phenomena and social & cultural phenomena as they are illuminated by their Medical aspects".

At a more practical level the study of medically related beliefs and practices of various groups assumes significance in developing and implementing culturally acceptable health care systems and health education programmes for the tribal and rural masses.

Disease in some or the other form is one of the fundamental problems facing every human society. Every known Society has developed methods for coping with disease and has thus created Medicine (Caudil William 1955:772).

Through out the ages man has been devising ways and means to care for the sick in the community (Newell 1975:55) It is to such beliefs and practices which are indigenous of culture and are not derived from the conceptual framework of modern medicine the term ethnomedicine is applied (Hughes 1968:99). Fabrega (1977:201-228) pointed out more specifically that "Ethnomedicine deals with information pertaining to social adaption, deviance, folkmedical knowledge and systems medical care".

Some of the problems inherent in studying ethnomedical issues as highlighted by Fabrega include

(1) What is ill vs what is not ill.

(2) The role of sick person.

(3) Interpretation of illness by social group.
(4) Interpretation of illness symptoms.
(5) Institution used for treatment.
(6) Organizations and Quality of Medical System.

Similarly (Lieban 1973: 1042:47 and Foster 1983:17-24) have highlighted the various areas of ethnomedicine which have been dealt descriptively. Some of these areas are disease classification, causality concepts, the nature and role of therapists, forms of therapies and preventive medicine.

Excellent studies have been carried out by anthropologists since 1935 on the ethnography of Medicine and health related beliefs and practices. Some examples are Field (1937) among the Ga people, Evans Pritchard (1937) the Azande, Harley (1941) the Mana in Africa, Warner (1957) the Murngin in Australia, Opler (1936, 1941) the Apathi, Hallowell (1934, 1942,1950) Oplcr (1936, 1941) thc Apathi; Hallowcll (1934, 1942, 1950) the Ojiba; Kluckhon (1944) & Leighton & Leighton (1941, 1944, 1949) the Navaho; Kluckhon & Spencer the Navaho; Redfield and Redfield (1940); Gillion (1948), Adams (1951) the Maya in North America. These works have highlighted descriptively the ethnographic contents of medicine. But mere documentation and description of any phenomenon is not sufficient. In order to understand from a holistic aspect, health behaviour it becomes imperative to know why people behave in a certain manner and thus try to find the cause and reason for their behaviour. Attempts must be made to understand the described phenomena and find out how the various happenings are inter related and how they are interpreted by the native himself. Hence an emic perspective is what the anthropologist should be concerned with foremost.

In a developing country like India, where major portion of its population is residing in rural and tribal areas and which have their own culture specific medical heritage, it is necessary to document and understand this medical heritage from an emic perspective. Despite frequent efforts made by the Health Policy makers and Health Care Planners, many health care programmes have met with stiff resistance. The main reason contributing to the failure of the programmes is ignorance of the Health Providers towards understanding the people beliefs practices and the meaning they attach to their health behaviour.

A number of anthropological questions come into being some of them are :

1. How do meanings and symbolic forms shape illness experiences?
2. What are the processes and phases associated with ritual healing wherein participant actors such as the medical specialists, family and

village elders and others participate with the sick person in order to alter the patients health ?

3. What is the meaning and the aim of the various ritual symbols ? (acts, objects, words, chants, prayers, songs, utterances, gestures ideas, relationships etc.)
4. How do the tribals construct a meaningful world with reference to etiological categories and the human body ?
5. How do other social spheres of life such as religion, cosmic objects, social groups kinship etc influence illness career?
6. How does the domain of ethnomedicine represent the cultural whole and all the actions associated with ritual healing, body symbolism and illness ideology into a system of culturally aroused meanings and symbols ?

As Turner (1967) is justified in saying that the task of an anthropologist is to uncover the hidden meanings. Schneider David (1976:204) adds that meaning is simply not attributed to reality, but reality itself is constructed by the beliefs, understandings and comprehensions entailed in cultural meanings.

It is therefore very necessary for anthropologists to discover the symbols and meanings associated with the illness ideology and illness experience, human body, and all ritualistic actions, objects, words, prayers, utterances, gestures, songs etc which are performed while attending the sick person/s by the participant actors who include family members, village elders, friends, medical specialists and others in order to restore the health of the patient, thereby creating a culturally accepted and clinically meaningful reality, which in a true sense has been constructed from beliefs, understandings and culturally held perceptions.

In India the health administrators, policy makers, health educators and the health care providers need to understand that the beliefs and practices associated with health are prevalent because people attach cultural meanings, values & emotions to them.

Their health behaviour cannot and should not be underestimated by categorizing them as illiterate, ignorant, uncivilized or superstitious. There has been resistance from the tribals and even the rural folk in accepting modern health care and educational programmes. The programmes do not give any room or facility to understand people's cultural values, meanings, emotions and behaviour associated with health and disease. The basic question which needs to be given a thought is why do people behave the way they do in a given socio-cultural context ?

Aims and Objectives of the Study

The major aims of the research are :

1. To understand the illness ideology of the natives as defined and experienced by them (from an emic perspective) and more specifically,

a) To document their perception regarding the origin and cause of illness and disease as revealed in their system of disease-classification and their etiological categories.

b) To record the different types of pathogenic agents which cause illness and to understand the role played by these agents in Thakur culture.

c) To explore the various cultural factors or criteria, symptoms and situations where disease is defined as illness by those participating in the healing processes, which seek to alter or restore the patient's health.

d) To uncover the symbolic elements and their meanings that shape illness experience.

2. To explore the native's concept/s regarding body physiology and about the various symbolic elements which find expression through the body during a patient's ill- health by,

a) Recording the native's perceptions about the elements constituting the human body, by studying their notions regarding the morphology, anatomy and physiology of the body.

b) Studying the symbolic elements (social, cosmological, spiritual, natural and supernatural) that find expression through the physical form i.e. in the form of the body during ill-health.

3. To understand the symbolic and meaningful aspects of ritual healing including,

a) all the actions (rituals or otherwise) performed in the collection, preparation and administration of potions, drugs or any other substance perceived to be medicinal in nature.

b) All the actions (rituals or otherwise) performed during diagnosis and interpretation of the cause of illness.

c) The entire process of ritual healing which is perceived as an instrument which reconstructs the disrupted cultural order (ill-health) and disharmony and attempts to bring back cultural order (health) and harmony.

d) All actions and rituals involved in thanks giving ceremonies which involve the originator or/ and curer of illness.

4. To understand from a meaningful perspective the entire set of

processes wherein those involved (which include family members, elders of the village and medical specialists) initiate a purposive alteration in the health of the patient. This research is based on two theoretical postulates:

i) that any domain of social life (which includes ethnomedicine as well) is built on a frame work of implicit meanings.

ii) that these meanings are not confined to a single area/sphere of social life but that the same pervade the whole social system. (Lee 1950; Hallowell 1955; Schneider 1969, 1976; Turner 1972).

The purpose of the study will be to demonstrate how the set/s of actions (normative, symbolic and meaningful behaviour) performed during the healing process emerge out of a basic central meaning system which ungirds the entire social system. In doing so this study intends to highlight;

i that the healing processes entail articulation of cultural thought regarding origin and cause of illness, the natives perception of body symbolism as expressed through illness experience and ritual actions performed to restore the health of the patient.

ii that no act, object, song, prayer, chant, gesture, utterance ideas, etc in the healing process is arbitrary.

iii that consequently all these acts objects and ideas exist ina meaningfully structured inter-relationship.

iv that these structured relationships are built around a centrally organized meaning system.

v that the whole ritual healing process is perceived as a meaning system's not merely in its own right but as a representation of the whole culture which according to Schneider is the system of symbols and meanings.

Justification of the Study

A number of studies have directly proved that when scientific/ allopathic medicine and measures are introduced for the first time in tribal and rural communities, they have been met with stiff resistance particularly when the scientific medicine/measures are in direct conflict with their (tribal/rural) traditional medicine systems, their beliefs and practices. Kark and Kark (1962) in their study and social medicine among the Zulus of South Africa have shown the reluctance on the part of the Zulus to accept the pit latrine programmes. This programme met with stiff resistance as the Zulus believe that their excreta and other bodily wastes may be used as objects of witchcraft to harm them.

Richard Adams (1955 : 466-67) also cites an example in his study in a Gautemalan Indian village. The people here consider blood as a finite substance which is "non-renewable" and/or " non-regenerative". They believe that when a person loses blood due to an injury or in a disease his resistance lessens permanently. The doctors who were collecting blood samples from children for a health survey could not succeed in their programme. The people failed to understand how the blood lost (during collection) could improve the health of the children.

The study carried out by McCracken (1971) in Gautemalan and Columbian villages show that the population view milk, which is considered to be essential for proper nutrition by technologically advanced societies) with indifference and it is accorded a status comparable to blood or urine. Hence the programme which supplied them milk powder to enhance their nutritional status met with little/no success. The population took the milk powder supplied to them and instead of consuming it, used it to whitewash their huts. Thus merely supplying any tribal/rural community with imported food is not sufficient, but the acceptance of this by the population is the key to the improvement of their nutritional status.

The study of indigenous beliefs and practices regarding health and disease in different cultures is of great significance in understanding human behaviour. Kurian J.C. & Tribhuwan Robin (1990:225) in their study of the Medical Practitioners of Sahyadri have pointed out that over 99% of the deliveries among the Thakurs, Kathkaris and Mahadev Kolis take place at home. Home is the place preferred because there are a number of rituals to be performed like burial of the umbilical chord outside the western wall of the hut, the ritual of bathing the mother and child for five days and the direction symbolism associated with it, the ritual of offering the child to Goddess Satvai and many others. The participation of women, the midwife (suine), the new-mother and other family members participate in these rituals and the completion and participation in these rituals have deep significance in their culture.

Health Educators often fail to understand the cultural meanings which people associate with health behaviour. Attempts must be made to understand why people behave the way they do .An indepth study of folk medicine from an emic perspective will help in understanding the cultural symbols & meanings and their integration with the culture. Such a study will also help in understanding the reasons for the resistance encountered or refusal to accept the modern medical programmes. Also one is able to understand the native's view point and his concept of health and disease and the role played by culture in maintaining health and treating disease Ethnographic documentation of anthropological data on ethnomedicine is instrumental in understanding the people's health related beliefs.

It is imperative that the educatorsmust have a thorough understanding of the indigenous medical system so as to bring about the necessary changes in their values, habits, beliefs and practices rather than to change their therapeutic practices. A chinese proverb is certainly justified and it says "Go in search of people, Begin with what they know, Build on what they have". This should be the guideline for health educators. As Foster George (1962) and Paul (1955) have pointed out that incompatibilities in the culture of those receiving and rendering help create hurdles to meaningful and effective communication and education.

It has been realized that health is not merely a bio-medical problem but is influenced by various social, cultural, psychological and political factors. The study of ethnomedicine helps us in identifying these factors and the accompanying behavioural patterns.

The present study will help in emphasizing certain aspects which will boost the health of the people while framing health care programmes. The study unravels the various meanings and symbolic forms that the Thakurs associate with disease etiology, body symbolism, ethnophysiology, ethnomedical therapies and ritual healing from an emic perspective. It gives a comprehensive picture of the socio-cultural beliefs and practices regarding health and disease which will be useful at two levels.

On the theoretical level it aims to show that it will be possible for anthropologists to unravel the organizing structure of the complex symbolic elements and meanings of a culture by restricting their study to a single area or domain of social life.

At a practical level this research aims to show that the resistance offered by the target population/culture to health care, education and development programmes in social life does not stem from "ignorance" or superstitious as supposedly thought.

The study seeks to emphasize that deep and at times radically different concepts of the tribals regarding the universe they live in arise from the meaning system which prevent the meshing of forms, other than their own into their meaning structures. Such a qualitative piece of work will certainly help in the formulation of appropriate health policies for the tribal and rural masses. It will help health administration and policy makers to plan, implement and follow health education and health care programmes which will be culturally acceptable to the tribal and rural masses to improve the quality of their health so as to achieve the goal of the W.H.O "Health for all" in future.

Realizing the value of and usefulness of ethnomedicine serious consideration is being given by the W.H.O. and the Agency for International Development to induct the non-western curers as well as parts of non-western therapies (Foster 1978).

REVIEW OF LITERATURE

Concept of Medicine

The Oxford dictionary defines "Medicine" as an art of restoring and preserving health. The institution of medicine is as old as mankind. Disease has been one of the fundamental problems faced by every human society, every known human society has developed ways and means to cope up with it, thereby creating a system of medicine (Caudil William 1955:721).

The institution of medicine thus has been a part and parcel of human society since the evolution of disease., Medicine can be interpreted from two aspects.

a) Biomedical which interpret disease on the germ theory line.
b) Socio-cultural which interprets disease in terms of Spiritual, cosmic, ancestral,supernatural social, etc., pathogenic agents/forces that intervene the human body and are either driven out or pleased ritually with the help of socio-cultural procedures or ritually with the help of a Shaman and/ or medicine man.

According to the second interpretation the reaction of an ill person may express his world views and important cultural values of his society (Clark 1959).

The relationship between medicine and the rest of culture has been noted by Ackernecht (1942) who said "Medicine is no where independent and followings its own motivations. Its character and dynamism depend on the place it takes in every cultural pattern, they depend on the pattern itself.

The studies made by early pioneering social scientists in the field of medicine did give new theoretical dimensions to ethnomedical studies. Some of these studies are as follows :

Mead and Henry (1949) have discussed the general relationship of Anthropology with psycho-somatic medicine Hall (1951) has outlined the progress of sociological research in the field of medicine; outstanding over the years is the classic statement by Rivers (1924) which gives the relationship between Religion, magic Medicine and Clement's work tracing the world-wide distribution of five basic categories of disease attributable to sorcery, breach of taboo, object intrusion, spirit intrusion loss of soul (Clements 1932).

Since 1935 a few really good studies have been published for example the work of Field (1937) on religion and medicine of the Ga people, spencer (1941) on Disease, Religion and Society in Fiji Islands; (1941) and on the Mano of Liberia which includes the analysis of African Medicine in general.

In broader terms Sigerist (1951) has reviewed in his first volume of the projected history of medicine of the primitive and archaic medicine' simultaneously there is excellent work both in Medicine and Ethnography for example Field (1937) the Ga people; Evans Pritchard (1937) the Azande; Harley (1941) the Mana in Africa; Warner (1957) the Murngin in Australia, Opler (1936,1941) the Apathi; Hallowell (1934,1942, 1950) the Ojiba Kluckhon (1944) and Leighton and Leighton (1941,1944,1949) the Navaho, Kluckhon & Spencer the Navaho; Redfield & Redfield (1940) Gillin (1948) Adams (1951) the Maya in North America.

Definition of Ethnomedicine

Most studies carried out by the early pioneering ethnographer are concentrated on the native inhabitants of Africa, Latin, America and Australia, but a very few studies on Medicine were conducted in India. The publisned accounts of world's medical systems have made possible the new discipline of "Ethnomedicine" i.e. those belief and practices relating to Health and Disease, which are products of indigenous cultural development and not explicitly derived from the conceptual framework of modern medicine (Hughes Charles 1968:99).

In addition to "ethnomedicine" various other terms have been used to refer to the domain under discussion or part of it, "Folk Medicine" Popular medicine", "Popular Health Culture " ethnoiatry (Scarpa 1967) ethnoiatric (Haurd 1969).

Areas of Ethnomedicine

The subject of ethnomedicine focuses on the nature and illness as it is conceived by the natives, their own methods and criteria for classifying disease, the causes and cures, types of therapists and healers who seek to alleviate illness and their skills and social roles, preventive measures, the relationship between medicine and religion, cultural aspects of medicine. (Hughes 1968) and Foster (1978).

In his paper on "the scope of Ethnomedical Science", Fabrega (1977: 201-228) has stated that the Ethnomedicine deals with information pertaining to social adaption, deviant behaviour, illness, disease, medical taxonomy, folk medical knowledge & systems of medical care. Some of the problems inherent in studying these issues include : (i) What is illness what is not (ii) the role of sick person (iii) the interpretation of Symptoms (iv) treatment of illness by social group (v) Institutions used for treatment (vi) organization & quality of medical systems.

The subject of ethnomedicine began to get a strong theoretical base with the studies of George Foster (1981:17-24) & Lieban Richard (1973: 1042-48) who reviewed the major areas of ethnomedicine namely disease classification: causality concepts: nature & role of ethnomedical specialists: the various forms of ethnomedical therapies including chemo, mechanical & magico-religious , the hot & cold concept & preventive medicine.

The phenomenon of ethnomedicine has been also studied from Symbolic & meaningful angle by Turner (1967), Murray David (1977), Munn Nancy (1973), Camaroff Jean (1981) on the Symbolic & communicational aspects of ritual healing by Douglas Mary (1966, 1970, 1957), Sutherland (1976), Camaroff Jean (1981). While other Anthropologists studied different aspects of medicine such as illness ideology, Body Symbolism, ritual healing, hot & cold concepts, ethnophysiology etc. Separately or singly isolating its relevance, medicine in its cultural context. One has to understand every aspect of medicine is associated by natives from an emic perspective. As to how do the natives define disease & categorize their etiological experiences: what is their image about human body: how does body symbolize various aspects of human culture during ill-health, what are the various objects: rituals, chants, etc. used in ritual healing by the participant actors (family members, elders, medical practitioners) what do they mean ? How are the medical symbols inter-related to each other and are organized into a central meaning system (culture).

Illness Ideology

The etiology of disease is the central to any discussion of the connection between medical phenomenon & their cultural setting. (Lieban 1973: 1048) To begin with, in most indigenous medical systems the primary consideration in the diagnosis of disease is its cause (Glick 1967: see also Adams 1953, Alland 1964). And causality in these systems is sought in relationship between the victims of illness and his surroundings This relationship is culturally interpreted. While traditional etiologies may attribute illness to mechanical and emotional as well as surgical & religious causes. (Polgar 1962) and since etiology is so in extricable from its socio-cultural context, Explanation of the occurrence of illness are at the same time representation of the world as it is experienced & comprehended by members of the Society.

Analysis of the representative "causes" of illness listed in the world's ethnomedical accounts according Foster George (1981: 18-19) are as follows:

i) Angry deities who punish wrong doers, for example those who violate taboos.
ii) Ancestors & Ghosts who feel that they have been soon forgotten or otherwise not recognized.

iii) Sorcerers or Witches, working for hire or for personal reasons.
iv) Loss of Soul, following a bad fright that jars it loose from the body or as the consequence of the work of a Sorcerer or Supernatural Spirit.
v) Spirit possession or intrusion of an object into the body.
vi) Loss of the basic body equilibrium, usually because of the entry of excessive heat or cold in the body
vii) The evil eye.

In ethnomedical accounts causes such as these are commonly described as "magical" or "Supernatural", in contrast or "natural". Illness caused due to angry deities, ghosts ancestors, & witches fall in the first category, while those due to an upset in body humours & consequent loss of bodily equilibrium fall into the second. (Foster 1981: 19), Tribhuwan Robin & Gambhir R.D (1990) in their paper of Ethnomedical pathway:a conceptual Model,pointed out the third category which combines the supernatural as well as natural elements in the etiology of the disease.

Illness as Social Sanction

The belief that illness is a punishment for wrong doing is wide spread in human society. Where it occurs, the social order is identified with the moral order of a universe in which Health depends on virtue (Lieban 1973: 1049).

The attribution of illness as misconduct may have been a very early from of social control in the development of human society (Hallowell 1963), and in Paul's view perhaps, the most important purpose of indigenous concepts of etiology & curing is to provide sanction & support for moral & social systems. (Paul 1963). The idea of punitive sickness is, of course, no stranger to Western traditions.

It has been a feature of Judeo -Christian beliefs concerning the consequences of sin (Polgar 1968,Crombie 1969) and today in many non-western societies illness is a major social sanction.

Illness as Deviance

Illness is considered a social sanction, its occurrence is a sign that some one has deviated from the social norms. But illness can also be seen as a form of deviance in its own right. The position that in certain respects illness may be viewed as a type of deviance subject to Social Control especially associated with the work of Parsons. (1951, 1953, 1958, 1964) Parsons & Fox 1952). He points out that a high incidence of illness is dys functional for a social system. Therefore society has a functional interest in exercising whatever controls it to minimize illness. Parson's approach to illness as a form of deviance has been the subject to criticism. However, he provides a valuable theoretical frame work for the analysis of facts of the relationship between illness & social control, and his thesis appears to be constant with behaviour that occur in certain kinds of medical situations.

Illness as an Indication of Social System Performance

Illness & responses to it can be related to the structure & maintenance of a Social system, a system of interactions among the members of a society & a systems that is linked to its environments. But medical phenomena also can be indicative of the performance of social system. (Lieban Richard 1973: 1055)

Illness as Disruption of the Cultural Order

Writers like Jean Camaroff (1981: 369) & Fortes (1976) have stressed that illness is an expression of social conflict or cosmic disorder, revealed in disruptions in the normal relations of men, spirit & nature. Illness is caused due to the disruption of cultural order. Every culture has its own explanation for illness. Clifford Geertz is of the view that culture's provide people with ways of thinking that are simultaneously models of and models for reality. These models simultaneously create order & meaning, give plans for purposive actions & help to produce the conditions required for their own perpetuation or revision.

Ethnomedical Therapy

Therapy in ethnomedicine is an important area & a vast subject. It includes both magico-religious and mechanical & Chemical procedure (Lieban 1973: 1044), studies conducted on practices regarding therapeutic knowledge both in indigenous and non-literate societies have shown an impressive array of practices that demonstrate empirical therapeutic knowledge including trepheniry, bonesetting, removal of ovaries, obstetrics including caesarean sanction, laprotomy, Unulectomy, comparative anatomy, autopsy, cautery, inoculations, baths, poultices, inhalations, laxatives, enemas, ointments & cupping (Ackernecht 1942, Simmons 1955, Laughlin 1963, & Huard 1969).

The pharmacopoeia of ethnomedicine is copious and includes such proven drugs as quinine, opium, cocoa, cinchona, copaiba, curare, chaulmoorga oil, ephedrine & rauwolfia etc.(Lieban 1973: 1045)

Quisumbing (1951) lists more than eight hundred known medicinal plants in the Philippines alone. Merely listing down the medicinal plants and their efficacy to heal disease is not enough for an anthropologist or even describing a therapeutic procedure in a given society does not help. An Anthropologist's job is to search for meanings that are associated with therapeutic practices and health behaviour. How these symbols and meanings are inter related to the cultural whole.

Nature & Role of Ethnomedical Specialists

When illness occurs, it may be ignored or treated without the help of a specialist (Polgar 1962). If treatment is sought from a medical practitioner, various types of specialists may be available, including herbals diviners, shamans, midwives, masseurs. (Nurge 1958, Lieban 1962, Maclean 1969). Kurian J.C. and Tribhuwan Robin (1990 : 251-57) have reported seven different types of medical specialists in the Thakur Society, namely Bhagat (male shaman), Bhagatin (female shaman) Vaidu (Herbalists) Had Vaidu (Bone-setter). Mantrik (specialized herbalist in snake and scorpion bites) Suine (mid-Wife) & potdhari (assistant mid-wife).

Therapists may specialize in only one type of skill or calling, or they may combine several in their practice (Lieban 1962). Qualifications for folk medical roles vary considerably. In some cases, no formal training may be required for the practitioners. (Metzer and Williams 1963): in other, along apprenticeship may be required for the practitioners. (Maclean 1969).

Thus, there are two major classes of cures from the data of traditional medicine: those with supernatural or magical powers who diagnose (i.e identify the efficient cause) who also may administer therapy, & those who accept the patient's self-diagnosis and administer the appropriate remedies. Anthropological studies just do not stop by documenting the different types of medical practitioners in a given society & therapeutic procedures they employ. What is necessary to understand is their emic interpretation about the status & role they have in their society and analyze all the therapeutic rituals. chants, objects, prayers, songs, actions that are used during the healing rites). Why do they perform healing rituals? What kind of chants (Mantras) are used & what do they mean? These aspects have remained unexplored or have been not brought into light.

Glick (1967) has pointed out that in many cultures medical practices are often fused with religious, and even when mechanical therapy is employed, magico-religious elements, may also be as essential part of the prescription, or treatment may be regarded as incomplete without attention to mystical factors involved in etiology of the illness.

Shiloh (1961) describes indigenous Middle Eastern medical beliefs that attribute a burn or a fall from a high place, such as a house-top or a tree, to an evil spirit or the evil eye. In such cases the bruised or torn flesh is dressed with curative preparations and bandaged, and broken bones are set but concurrent with such straight forward mechanical treatment there will be a search for the evil spirit or evil eye responsible for the accident.

Herbalist- Surgeons in Ethiopia employ pragmatic means to treat illness, including an elaborate pharmacopoeia, but mysticism is mixed with materia medica; the name of a curative plant may not be said aloud, for instance, because this would enable the spirit causing disease to defend itself against the therapy (Messing 1968).

In the Philippines, healers may prescribe a simple decoction of certain plants for illness- but the leaves will have been picked from the east side of the plant, because that is the directions in which sun rises, and the healer may have learned the prescription itself from a spiritual benefactor who conveyed it to him in a dream or vision, (Lieban 1967).

Turner's (1967:360) own observation suggests, whenever rites to propitiate or exorcise the shades as distinct from private treatment by Herbalists- are performed, there is a factor of social conflict present. Therapy then becomes a matter of sealing up the breaches in social relationship simultaneously riding the patient of his pathological symptoms. He further points that the medicines employed from the leaves,barks, scrapings & roots of the forest trees & bushes have a principle underlying their use. They are not derived from the experiments but from a part of the Ndembu magical system. (Turner 1967 : 369).

The above studies have clearly indicated that ethnomedical therapies may it be mechanical, Herbal or magico-religious are not employed simply they are often combined with religious, magical or mystical elements. Secondly as Turner states that therapies are employed to breach social relationship. Thirdly the herbal medicines as defined by the Ndembu have magical factors associated with them Tribhuwan Robin (1989: 66) has pointed out that the medical practitioners of the Thakur society have special rites of collection, preparation & administration of herbs & potion drugs, which are very meaningful to them.

Ritual Healing

Ritual healing is another term used for the concept of ethnomedical therapy by some symbolic & Medical Anthropologists. Before getting into the theoretical explanation of what Ritual Healing is it is necessary to understand what a ritual means & what are the divorce opinions of Anthropologists about rituals & the social cultural functions of rituals as highlighted theoretically.

Diverse Opinions of What a Ritual is ?

The life of an individual in any society "wrote van Gennep is series of passages from one stage to another." (1908: 3) In majority of human communities the primary transitions, or what has been termed as the life crises-birth, puberty, marriage, death etc. are the focus of elaborate rites. In preliterate communities such rites constitute an important aspect of cultural life.

The term " ritual" although seems to be a simpler matter, few terms in the study of religions have been explained in more confusing ways for example Edmund Leach (1968 : 524) a contemporary cultural anthropologist after noting the general disagreement among the anthropological theories suggested that the term, " ritual" should be applied to all cultural sets of behaviour that is the symbolic dimensions of human behaviour such regardless of its explicit religious, social or other context.

Ritual

A ritual is a set of activities which encompasses basic rules to accomplish given tasks or goals in any social sphere. Nancy Mun (1973: 580) has stated that a ritual is a generalized medium of social interactions which becomes a vehicle for constructing messages through iconic symbols (acts, words and other things) that convert the load of significance of complex Socio-cultural meanings embedded in and generated by the on going process of social existence into common currency. In other words, shared socio-cultural meanings constituted, which are symbolically transacted through the medium of ritual action.

According to David Lotz (1987 : 405) a ritual is referred to as those conscious and voluntary repetitious and stylized bodily actions that are centered on cosmic structures or sacred presence, he includes verbal behaviour such as chants, songs and prayers in the category or bodily actions.

Kartz and Kirkland (1988: 1179) are if a view that " Rituals are stylized, repetitive arbitrary and exaggerated forms of behaviour Firth Raymond (1973: 76) states that a ritual is a symbolic mode of communication of saying. Something in a formal way not to be said in an ordinary language or informal behaviour. Victor Turner (1976: 183) uses the term ritual to refer to "prescribed formal behaviour for occasions not given over to technological routine, having reference to beliefs in mystical (or non empirical) being of power".

"Rituals are thus a set of voluntary, conscious and stylized bodily actions (which include iconic symbols such as acts, words, gestures, prayers chants, songs and other things) performed in a defined place, situation or context by particular actor/s only, encompassing basic rules to accomplish given task or goal in any social sphere with in a particular cultural frame of reference."

Socio Cultural Functions of Rituals

A number of social scientists interested in ritual's socio-cultural functions have pointed out varied functions of rituals. Anthropologists such as Clifford Geertz and Victor Turner who are interested in the explicit religious meaning of ritual symbolism and pointed out that ritual acts do endow culturally important cosmological conceptions and values with persuasive emotive force, thus unifying individual participants into a genuine community.

Here ritual is viewed sociologically to be sure, but in terms of its existential important and explicit meanings rather than its purely cognitive grammar, its psychological dynamics or its merely social reference.

However, other anthropologists are of view that rituals have a number socio-cultural functions These are as follows.

1. Rituals encourage cohesion (Gluckman 1970).
2. Rituals facilitate transition (Van Gennep 1960).
3. Rituals define conceptual categories (Mary Douglas 1966).
4. Help resolve conflict (Gluckman 1970 : Turner Victor 1967).
5. Enhance individual and group autonomy (Kartz P 1981: 325-350).
6. Help achieve actors goals (Turner 1977).
7. Ritual actions express and communicate shared socio- cultural meanings which are symbolically transacted through the medium of ritual action (Munn 1073: 589).
8. They reveal the knowledge of meanings of symbols involved in them (Honingman 1959-506).
9. Firth raymond (1973: 176) states that rituals function as symbolic modes of communication.
10. Ritual acts endow culturally important cosmological conceptions (Geertz: 1970 Turner 1967: Douglas 1975).

Symbolism in Ritual Healing

Symbolization is a universal human process. It is the most important human trait that man can create symbols. Through symbols ideas and meanings are represented. As Richard Cavendish (1985 : 258-75) states that a symbol by definition is not what it represents. It stands for suggests and reveals a mind reality other than itself. He further states that the function of symbols is to act as a "rallying point for meaning" through it the mind connects several meanings.

Symbols have been analyzed by logicians, metaphysicians, linguists, psychologists, theologicians, historians and Folklorists. But the anthropological approach is expected to be comparative, observationist, functionalists and relative neutralists. It links the occurrence in a society and interpretation of symbols to social structure and social events in specific conditions.

Anthropologists observe symbols, study them and their meanings. Understand the inter-relationship of these symbols in their cultural context as a system of the whole. Their explanation of how people derive meanings out of symbols? How they co-relate them and how these symbols and meanings are finally organized into a system, helps to understand the process of social life as a meaningful system.

In the case of ritual healing it becomes necessary to understand how the meanings of ritual symbols are interpreted and how ideas are ordered and organized into a system with in the cultural frame of reference are some questions to be analyzed through this study.

Ritual symbol according to Turner (1967: 48) is the smallest unit of behaviour. Rituals whether associated with birth, puberty, marriage or death reveals a meaningful reality to the participant actors performing and participating in it. Rituals are performed to achieve certain goals or ends. Secondly in ritual situations symbols (actions, words, prayer, gesture, objects, utterances, etc.) are vehicles for constructing and communicating messages that convert the load of significance of complex socio-cultural meanings constituted in the rituals performed are symbolically transacted through the medium of ritual action (Munn 1973: Turner 1967: Murray 1977).

Thus the ritual symbols do not remain in isolation but they are ordered through an inter-relationship with other symbols and meanings in a self enclosed system which ultimately represents the whole culture.

Fritjof Carpa (1991: 3) has stated that " The outstanding characteristics of shamanistic conceptions of illness is the belief that human beings are integral parts of an ordered system and that illness is the consequence of some disharmony with the cosmic order. Accordingly shamanistic rites emphasize the restoration of harmony or balance with in the nature, in human relationships and in relationships with the spirit world.

He further pointed out that shamanistic healing rituals often have the function of raising unconscious conflicts and resistances to conscious level, where they can develop freely and find resolutions. The shaman does not work with the patient's individual conscious; from which these problem arise, but rather with collective and social unconscious which is shared by the whole. Therapies according to (Turner 1967: 360) became a matter of sealing up breaches in social relationships.

Body Symbolism

Yet another area of interest in the study of ethnomedicine is Body Symbolism or in other words the body image as perceived by the natives in different social contexts. The use of human body as basic symbolic material has been discussed by a number of anthropologists. As a symbolic instrument, a person may use his body as a means of communication, to indicate by bodily actions to represent a cultural phenomena (Joshi 1992:9).

Mary Douglas (1975:65) has stated that "the social body constrains the way the physical body is perceived. The physical experience of the body is always modified by the social categories through which it is known and sustains a particular view of society". There is a continual exchange of meanings between the two kinds of bodily experience so that each reinforces categories of other.

Both Turner (1966) and Douglas (1970) have discussed the use of the body and bodily emissions as non-verbal categories in society. Following the interest sparked by Levistrauss in dual organization and the work of Robert Hertz on the natural proclivity of the body to other spheres of social behaviour (See Needhab 1973). Anne Sutherland's (1976: 375-389) study among the Rom, has pointed out that the Romany conceptions of purity and pollution, are based on an ideal of separating the upper and lower halves of the body, including in certain instances male/female adult/child and food and non-food separation is a metaphor for expressing various levels of social behaviour, relations with outsiders, internal political divisions, age status, ritual arrangements and furnishing of the house hold, clothing and washing, cooking eating and the most personal activities and the functions of the body.

She has compared elsewhere the upper/lower and inside/outside boundaries among the Rom and English Gypsies (Sutherland Anne 1976).

Devisch, Renaat (1985: PP693-700) has shown how the northern yak, construct a meaningful world by reference to the human body. They understand the socio-cultural domains in terms of bodily exchanges such as ingestion and excretion, sexual process or, listening and speech. The physical body as the tangible form the selfhood is the symbolic frame through which social spiritual, cosmological procedures are expressed through the body during the ill health of the patient.

Preventive Medicine

Preventive medicine is one of the important area in the study of a ethnomedicine, which has been seen as last important than modern medicine. Foster George (1962) studies such as that of Colson (1969) indicates how significant preventive measure can be in a traditional medical system, and the literature shows that prophylactic practices are widely prevalent in indigenous Medicine.

These include both mechanical and magico-religious measures, such as bathing, massage, and rapid rewarming to prevent hypothermia, dietary restrictions, surgery, inoculation, incantation, and prayers at shrines (Laughlin 1963, Hughes 1963). Thus in many areas of the , including Latin America and South and South East Asia, Africa one finds prevalent notions, derived from Hippocratic humeral theory of comparable ideas of Indian medicine, that health depends in part on a proper balance between "hot" and "cold" (Foster 1953,1967) Jellifee 1956, Polgar 1962, Nash 1965, Hart 1969)

Associated with this theory is the prescription of detailed precautions to maintain the equilibrium of health, such as measures to prevent chilling in a Gautemalan Mayan Community, keeping oneself covered, avoiding cold water and foods that are classified as "cool" & not getting caught in the rain. (Adams 1953). The idea that the evil eye is drawn to what is attractive is demonstrated by a study in Turkish villages where villagers protect their children by hanging unattractive objects in their clothings (Ozturk 1964).

Not many studies have been conducted on the preventive medical aspects of ethnomedicine. It is therefore imperative that the meanings and symbolic forms attributed to preventive medicine by the Thakurs, be covered under the study of preventive medicine.

Theoretical Considerations

People every act on the basis of knowledge ane beliefs, about the world, about themselves about action itself. Beliefs form among every people a system: This system can be seen as a group of propositions about the world, which on further examination, reveal themselves to be ordered in their relationships with one another (Dolgin & others 1976: 3).

In every belief system there are, for example propositions of a very specific nature nature, about one or another aspect of the world, or of action, or of people, these sets are termed as domains (Ibid 1976 : 3). There are also in every belief system propositions about the distinctions between the domains, the manner in which boundaries are drawn and the inter-relationship between the domains.

Anthropologists have been studying cultural domains either separately or as integrated parts of the cultural hole. Schneider States (1976: 197) The significance of studying culture is to contribute to an understanding of social action as a meaningful activity of human beings. He further states that social action requires commonalty of understandings it implies common codes of communication, it entails generalized relationships among its parts mediated by human understanding.

That one act can have consequence for another is not only a function of the efforts of that act it is also a function of the meaning that act has for the persons involved. (Schneider, 1976 : 198). Thus the study of culture is concerned with the study of social action as a meaningful system of actions and is therefore by definition concerned with the action of meaning in action.

Hallowell I.A (1942) has rightly pointed out that human beings live in a meaningful universe not a world of bare physical objects. Social life thus has meaning. the things people do are communicable and this entails a system of signs and symbols in which meaning is expressed and embedded.

To develop this point, it is helpful to distinguish between a sign and a symbol. Susan Langer (1956: 45-49) has defined a symbol as something that serves as a vehicle for a conception, the conception being the symbols meaning, a sign is seen as indicating the existence-past present or future of a thing, event or condition.

Symbols in different spheres or domains of life have different meanings and functions (Joshi 1992: 5) Turner (1967:50) has emphasized the polysemic nature of ritual symbols, with different meanings of the same symbol becoming paramount in different context. Citing an example of polysemy as an obvious quality of symbols used in healing rituals of the manambal. Lieban(1977:60) states that one of the most frequently and widely used symbols "the cross" has various referents used by the manambals, including divine lone, sacrifice, martydom, hope, protection and salvation.

Symbols are used for conveying values and meaning of ideas and conceptions which are recognized within the cultural frame of reference. Cavendish (1985 : 258) defines a symbol as something that stands for suggests it reveals the mind reality other than itself. He further states that the function of symbols is to act as a rallying point for meaning and through it the mind connects together several meanings, which are not outwardly or immediately connected. Schneider (1976: 204) is certainly justified in saying that meaning is not simply attributed to reality. Reality itself is constructed by beliefs, understandings and comprehensions entailed in cultural meanings.

Meanings of symbols of any domain of social life (which includes ethnomedicine as well) do not exist independently or they are isolated but are inter related and meaningfully ordered into the cultural system. Further on these domains of social life are inter-related to each other with their cultural frame of references through a system of symbols and meanings.

Schneider has rightly pointed out that pure cultural domains cross cut institutional structures. He further states that the only way to study symbols and meanings is by studying all into occurrences in context, it is only through an indepth study of all possible kinds of context that the full array of difference meanings associated with a given symbol, or a cluster of symbols, is possible / (Schneider 1976: 212).

It is not only the study of the occurrences of symbols in contexts, but their inter relationship with other symbols of a domain that need to be studied and also the manner in which the meanings finally emerge in the cultural system is also very essential, while studying symbols and their meanings. As indicated by cavendish symbols reveal a perspective in which diverse realities can be fitted together or even integrated into a system.

In a similar way this study focuses on the "ethnomedicine" and should provide a methodological device which will help penetrate into the entire meaning system.

Anthropological studies have pointed out that any domain of social life is built on implicit frame work of meanings and that these meanings are not confined to a single area of social sphere but cross cut different institutional structures and provide the whole social system (Lee 1950: Hallowell 1955, Schneider 1969, 1976, Turner 1972, Douglas 1975, 1976).

Ethnomedicine : A Symbolic System

The purpose of studying ethnomedicine was to understand the concrete normative health behaviour from the symbolic point of view. This study expresses the community's assumptions and perceptions about the nature and universe and man's place in it, by studying the various symbols and meanings associated with Thakur illness ideology, body symbolism, ethnophysiology and preventive, promotive, curative and destructive rituals of health and their inter-relationship into a symbolic system as a representation of the cultural whole.

Implicit in this approach is that all normative behaviour (which includes health behaviour also) requires commonalty of understanding (Schneider 1976) because the meaning which a normative or social act has for the people is context defined or context determined (Schneider 1976: Douglas 1975) This meaning is not explicit but is based on shared, unspoken assumptions derived from the actor's perception about the nature of universe. (Douglas 1975, Schneider 1976) It is this body of perception which is embedded in all normative behaviour Consequently all social acts become vehicles for conceptions (Schneider 1976: 206) a representation or a 'Symbol' for the community's perceptions and beliefs.

"Culture" and "Norms" are two different entities. Culture consists of the whole body of definitions, postulates and premises of the nature of world (Schneider 1976: 203) It is these concepts which are "embedded" in norms. Norms are comprised of detailed instructions of how to act in relatively in specific situations. (Schneider 1976: 202) where norms guide the actor as to how to behave, culture tells the actor how to scene is set and what it means. Where norms tell the actor how to behave in presence of Gods, Ghosts and human beings, culture tells the actors what ghosts, gods and human beings are.

Since culture and norms are contrasted, the cultural aspects embedded in the norm may be separated in order to derive meaning. This meaning relates to certain assumptions and presumptions of the universe that are represented in certain symbols or vehicles for conception (Schneider 1976: 202) The normative act may itself stand as a 'symbol' or one of the 'forms' of another symbol. The full meaning of a symbol can only be established by showing its (the symbols) occurrence in all kinds of contexts. Following the theoretical understanding of Schneider D.M.(1976) Turner Victor (1967), Wilson Monica 1957) & Munn Nancy (1973) the symbols in this study were empirically observed & documented through indepth interviews and interpreted using an emic approach, to study Objects, actions, gestures, words, utterances, prayers, chants, songs, human body, spatial units, diseases, pathogenic agents and forces, plants, animals and personnels which are associated with the preventive promotive, curative and destructive aspects of Thakur health behaviour within their cultural frame of reference.

The current research is aimed at treating the domain of ethnomedicine as a symbolic system. Ethnomedicine is conceptually defined as a culturally ordered inter-relationship of medical symbols and meanings that are associated with a community's notions of illness ideology, body image and the entire set of preventive, promotive and destructive health rituals and/or actions performed by the participant actors in various healing context, as a symbolic system, and which represents the cultural whole.

Research Postulates

Given this theoretical background and overview of literature, this study intends to test the following research postulates empirically.

1. That the domain of ethnomedicine is built on implicit frame work of meanings.
2. That these meanings, are not confined to the single area of social life (in this context, ethnomedicine)but they pervade the whole social system (Lee 1950, Hallowell 1942, 1955, Schneider 1976, 1969, Douglas 1970, Turner 1972).

The theoretical purpose of the study will be to show how the set of normative actions (symbols and meanings) performed during the healing process works out of a basic central meaning system and it will be possible for the anthropologists to ungird the organizing structure of the complex symbols and meanings of a culture by restricting themselves to a single area of social life (in this context ethnomedicine).

In doing so this study intends to demonstrate the following ideas :

1. That the native's concept of ill-health reflectsthe disruption and/or the disharmony of man's relationship with the natural, cosmological, social, spiritual, ancestral and supernatural beings and/or forces.
2. Thatthe human body as a physical form of selfhood in the symbolic frame through which social natural spiritual, ancestral cosmological and supernatural paradoxes of existence are most powerfully expressed
3. That no act, object, gesture, chant, song,conception, personnel, pathogenic agents etc in the healing process is arbitrary.
4. That consequently all the acts, objects, gestures, chants songs, conceptions, personnels, pathogenic agents, spatial units etc. co-exist in a structural relationship with each other.
5. That these structural relationships are built around a centrally organized meaning system.
6. That the whole ritual healing process is perceived as a meaning system, not in it's own right but as a representation of the whole culture.
7. That the entire set of healing rituals and actions are geared towards bringing about harmony and patching up the disrupted relationship between man and social, spiritual, natural, ancestral, supernatural and cosmological entities/forces in order to restore the patient's health.

CHAPTER II

RESEARCH METHODOLOGY

Research Setting

The present research fieldwork was conducted in six Thakur hamlets namely Thakurwadi, Lobhiewadi, Khondewadi, Borwadi, Naldewadi & Kautewadi in the Grampanchayats of Pathraj & Kashale villages of Karjat. Tehsil in Raigarh district in the state of Maharashtra, India.

Pathraj & Kashale are two rural caste villages with areas of 1400 hectares and 761 hectares respectively. The villages are situated on the western flanks of the Sahyadri mountain ranges. These villages can be approached by road, and are situated at a distance of 17-24 Km from the tehsil headquarters. (Karjat) Karjat is a railway junction on the Pune-Bombay rail route.

The six Thakur Settlements selected come under the jurisdiction of Pathraj and Kashale grampanchayat. These hamlets are in close proximity to each other. The other hamlets of communities like the Mahars, Marathas, Kathkaris, Agris, Mahadev Kolis etc. are aloof from these Thakur settlements. Most of these Thakur hamlets do not have a metalled approach road.

Karjat tehsil is located in the north east of Raigarh district. Karjat has 175 villages which include both multicaste and multi tribal communities. It is predominantly inhabited by three tribal communities viz. The Thakur, Kathkaris and the Mahadev Kolis.

Karjat is a part of one the most forested districts of Maharashtra viz. Raigarh. Raigarh is situated on the extreme west of Maharashtra state, bounded by the Arabian Sea. Raigarh stretches 100 miles from North to South and 15-30 miles from East to West. It has an area of 2,715 square miles with a total Tribal population of 47,970 of which 24,576 are males and 23,494 are females, as per 1981 census.

On the east, the district's boundary runs partly along the foothill zones and partly along the watershed of the major Sahyadrian scrap. On the southern side the Savitri river runs as a boundary over a stretch of 20 miles.

Though Raigarh forms an important part of the Konkan plain, raggedness and an uneven topography form the governing theme in its physical features. Prominent on the Eastern horizon stands the main Sahyadrian scarp with a crystalline of peaks and saddles. Nearly one fifth of the total area of Raigarh is forested.

The northern tehsils including Karjat have thick forests. Higher slopes associated with high rainfall are two factors responsible for the development of forests in these areas. Among the various species found in the district are teak (Tectona, grandis) Palas (Butea frondosa), Mauha (Bacia latifolia) Karavanda (Carissa carandis) silk cotton (Salmalia malbaricum) and many others. Since Raigarh is forested a number of wild animals are found in the area. The tribals to a great extent depend on the local forest resources for their livelihood.

The People

The Thakurs are hunters, agricultural labourers and small scale agriculturists. The total Thakur population of Maharashtra state is 3,24,181 with 1,66, 571 males and 1,57,610 female (1981 Census of Maharashtra) They live in small groups of 100-800 in small hamlets popularly known as Thakurwadis. The members of the Thakur tribe today, are distributed in five districts of Maharashtra viz, Thane, Raigarh, Pune, Nasik, Ahmednagar.

The Thakurs are divided into two divisions the "Ma" and the "Ka" Thakurs, that do not inter marry and live in separate hamlets. Each of these divisions are further sub divided into patrilineal clans in which polygyny is the norm. This Ph.D study is conducted among the "Ma" Thakurs which are predominantly found in Raigarh. If one travels towards Thane and Nasik. One comes across a large number of "Ka" Thakurs. More detailed information about the Thakur lifestyle, and the various aspects of their culture are briefly highlighted in the Chapter "Ethnography of the Thakurs".

Justification for Selecting the Thakurs

Of the three tribal communities residing in Karjat tehsil, Raigarh district in the state of Maharashtra, the Thakurs were selected for the present study for reasons.

1) The study aims at studying all the medical symbols and the meanings associated with the healing process. It further aims to show how these symbolic actions performed during the healing blossoms into a basic central meaning system which ungirds the social system. The study further attempts to show that the domain of ethnomedicine, may therefore be seen as a meaning system, not only in its own right, but as a representation of the whole culture. As Schneider D.M. (1976: 212) points that pure cultural domains cross cut different institutional structures, what he calls that system of symbols and meanings, permeate the total society and its institutions and are not confined to religion, to ritual, to magic or to myth alone. The system of meanings symbols intertwine every other

system in a society be it Kinship political technological economic etc. In order to get a comprehensive understanding of the symbols and meanings associated with tribal medicine and the significance of these in other social spheres, as well as to uncover how these symbols are ordered it was imperative to establish its meanings in a variety of cultural contexts. These symbols would enable me to perceive and understand the depth of these culturally held perceptions and beliefs of their universe their conceptions of meaningful reality.

In the context of the present study the symbols and meanings associated with illness ideology, body symbolism, and healing rituals (all actions, words, gestures, utterances, chants, objects, ideas etc involved in healing) which are symbolically interrelated to each other into a meaning system, not restricting itself to the domain of ethnomedicine but representing the whole culture.

Thus probing indepth or deeply into the symbolic aspect of medicine as a representation of culture, it was necessary to choose the Thakurs (a tribal community) as the target population rather than going in for a comparative study of two communities.

2) The second reason for selecting the Thakurs is as follows :

To get a symbolic understanding of tribal medicine it is necessary that a research has personal and first hand contact with his respondents. This was possible as the researcher had close rapport with the Thakurs of Kashale and knew them personally as he has done work on them from time to time during last seven years. The researcher was more familiar and shares better relationship with the Thakurs than the Kathkaris and Mahadev Kolis (other tribes residing in Karjat tehsil). Therefore the Thakurs were given the first preference.

3) Thirdly the Thakur tribe was favourable for study as their hamlets are in close proximity to each other and are more in number. These two factors do not hold true for the Kathkaris and Mahadev Kolis. Thus in brief,

a) Kathkaris and Mahadev kolis tribal settlements are far away from each other.
b) Thakur settlements/hamlets in closer proximity to each other.
c) Thakur reside nearer to the Academy of Development Science, where the researcher lived during his field work.
d) Thakurs are more in number.

4) Fourthly the researcher had already conducted a study on the Ethnomedicine of the Thakurs as a part of Master's programme Course

(fieldwork) in the year 1989. Hence the Thakur community was ideal to carry out an extended and deeper study on the same topic. Thus due to the,

a) social work done by the researcher in the Thakur community for the last seven years led to the establishment of the personal and close rapport.
b) the fieldwork conducted among them prior to this Ph.D study.
c) participation in the cultural events and activities of the Thakurs.

The researcher was able to collect relevant and qualitative data over a period of 2 years.

Pelto & Pelto (1978: 275) are justified in aptly stating that the essence of successful ethnography is a form of behaviour that makes the field worker a "friend" of the community he studies and a friend of a number of persons in it.

All the above factors were greatly instrumental in helping me choose the Thakur community as the target population for this study.

Method of Data Collection

Use of anthropological tools and techniques such as a participant observation indepth interviews, using of interview guide, recording of illness episodes or therapeutic narratives, use of genealogical methods were used effectively to elicit, information from the village and family elders, various medical specialists patients and key informants.

Participant observation method was used to cross check the validity of the data collected through indepth interviews, illness episodes and case studies. The researcher also participated in the rituals of diagnosis and interpretation of the cause of illness, the healing rituals, the rituals associated with collections, preparation and administration of medicinal herbs and animal extracts, the ritual associated with thanks giving to the originator and curer of illness.

Besides these many other ceremonies and rituals of birth, puberty, marriage, death, dance, harvesting etc. were participated in order to understand and comprehend the meanings and symbolic elements associated with them.

The present research work also included the traditional anthropological techniques of living in close contact with the target (research) population in the hamlets for over a period of 2 years in order to document and observe their daily routine, rituals, social acts, economic activities and other aspects of cultural behaviour.

During data collection the main emphasis was on the meanings of all objects, actions, words, utterances, gestures (symbols) which are associated with the domain of ethnomedicine. The only method of collecting information of this nature was to follow the meanings right through, wherever they led. This was done through free ranging unstructured interviews.

Most questions related to ethnomedicine as a symbolic system were framed in the field itself as and when relevant things regarding the Ph.D topic stemmed out through unstructured interviews. Since their conceptual reality was different from that of the researcher, to have formulated questions before hand would have been to enter the field with preconceived views about the nature of their reality. This would have been methodologically incorrect, as this study aims to define the conceptual medical reality of the Thakurs as they define it from an emic perspective.

Each interview session with a respondent was guided by only one factor what Schneider (1976: 220) called a fundamental methodological mencures (which is) to as the natives not once or even twice but in many different ways and therefore at many different times, with every possible eliciting device what cultural symbols are and what they mean. Responses had to consequently cross checked to establish whether the views expressed were generally held ideas or/ and when they were in contradiction with the observation of the researcher.

Research Tools and Techniques

A) Indepth Interviews

It was decided to take a sample of the household heads above 45 years of age in all the six Thakur settlements of Thakurwadi, Lobhiewadi, Borwadi, Naldewadi, Kautewadi and Khondewadi. In order to carry out this exercise a list of all the household heads from the above mentioned six settlements was prepared. A second list was prepared from the original to select the heads or the household above 45 years of age. Thus the total number of respondents for indepth interviews were i.e. 65 males and 12 females above 45 years all six villages.

The main purpose behind selecting this group ie. household heads above 45 years of age was that they are well versed with the cultural meanings, the various symbolic elements and the normative behaviour. Secondly it was observed that these heads perform and participate in most culturally recognized rituals and ceremonies. Thirdly they are the decision makers regarding family life as well as everyday activities. Fourthly they are well informed about the symbols and meanings associated with every domain or sphere of their social life. which has been passed down through generations by what is known as oral tradition.

These household heads were interviewed at various locations like their residence, on farms and even on the river banks. Frequently an interview stretched on to 8-10 sessions due to frequent interruptions by family members and friends. Some times the mood of the informant would prove a hindrance in the progression of the interview. It was also noted that a free and easy talk with informants fetched qualitative and correct data. Many a times (it was noted) a pen and paper in hand discouraged the informants and a frank discussion was not possible. At such the main points were taken and later elaborated upon by reorganizing the (heard) information which was heard keenly and attentively by the researcher. Another way to elicit information (at times highly confidential in nature) was to take a short break by changing the topic of conversation. At such times the researcher gave some information about the urban way of life. Thus this type of barter system of exchanging tribal and urban information was useful in eliciting confidential and relevant information.

The elderly members i.e. the 77 head of the families above 45 years of age were interviewed to gain an understanding of their culturally governed perceptions of disease and illness. The various concepts associated with the origins and cause of illness, the characteristics of the various pathogenic agents and their significant role played in the Thakur culture. The researcher was also keen to comprehend the Thakur's definition of ill health and normal health, the various social, spiritual, symbolic and cosmological elements expressed through body symbolism during ill health and the various meanings associated with healing rituals as well as the objects and actions that befall the ritual healing processes. Besides the researcher strove to understand the different therapeutic procedures involved in restoring the health of a patient.

Both, the elderly members and the key informants were greatly instrumental in giving information related to the above mentioned points/ facts. Thus keeping in mind the scope and limitations of this study informal indepth interviews by using an interview guide helped the researcher collect relevant information.

B) Case Studies of Medical Practitioners

Among the Thakurs there are different types of Medical specialists who are classified into seven different categories depending upon the specific medical functions, the different therapies they employ depending on the perceived cause and origin of illness and disease. These practitioners are :

(i) Bhagats (ii) Bhagatins (iii) Mantriks (iv) Had Vaidus
(v) Suines (vi) Potdhari and (vii) Vaidus
(Kurian J.C. & Tribhuwan Robin 1990: 251-58)

All the medical practitioners of about 15 Thakur settlements of Pathraj, Kashale, Khandus, Kotimbe and Shillar villages were interviewed. The following chart depicts the different types of practitioners interviewed.

SR.NO.	PRACTITIONER	NUMBER INTERVIEWED
1.	BHAGATS (SHAMANS)	4
2.	BHAGATINS (FEMALE SHAMANS)	2
3.	MANTRIKS (SNAKE BITE AND SCORPION BITE SPECIALIST)	2
4.	HAD VAIDU(BONE SETTERS)	4
5.	SUINES (MID WIVES)	20
6.	POTDHARIS (ASST. MID WIVES)	5
7.	VAIDU (HERBALISTS)	14

Case Studies of all the above mentioned types of practitioners were recorded in order to understand their Traditional methods of training and apprenticeship, their perceptions regarding the origin and cause of illness, their understanding of what forces of elements constitute a human body, the various methods of diagnosis of illness, the rituals associated with divining the identity of a Bhagat and other practitioners, the various types of therapies employed by them.

Depending on the perceived origin and cause of illness, the rituals associated with collection, preparation and administration of medicinal herbs and animal extracts. More emphasis were paid to the meanings associated with every medical action of theirs which sought to bring about an alteration in the health of their patients.

To cross check the data collected through careful studies participant observation method was used by participating in rituals associated with collection, preparation and administration of medicinal herbs and animal extracts, rituals of diagnosing illness, the rituals associated with the rituals of thanks giving performed to thank the originator and curer of the cause of illness.

Most confidential data on the symbolic meaningful aspects of Thakur medicine was collected when the researcher himself experienced the apprenticeship of being a Bhagat (Shaman) by participating as a trainee in the rituals of divining the identity of new Bhagat.

The training period was during the nav ratra period October 9-17-

1991 under the guidance of Walku Thorad, a Bhagat of Nagyachiwadi Pathraj Village Panchayat Training session lasted 9 complete days and nights and took 3-4 months in order to understand the symbolic and meaningful elements of Shamanism.

During this training period data on the symbolic and meaningful aspects of pathogenic agents, their characteristics, the hierarchy of spirits and their power capacity, the mantras (chants) of diagnosis and healing were gathered. The training did not stop with nine days but continued over a period of 3 to 4 months during which other chants were studied and some secrets about medicinal plants and animals were discovered. To cross check the information (learnt during apprenticeship period) related to diagnosis, healing and the meanings associated with it, other Bhagats were interviewed. The researcher also participated by observing the healing rituals performed by these Bhagats.

Indepth interviews of the Bhagatins (female shamans) were also conducted using participant and non participant techniques. Similarly to understand the medical knowledge from symbolic and meaningful perspective indepth interviews of the vaidus (herbalists), Had Vaidus (bone setters), Suines (Mid wives), the Potdharis (assistant mid wives) and the Mantriks (Snake and scorpion specialists) were conducted by holding 8-10 sessions which were supported by participant observation.

Other than the Thakur medical practitioners other tribe and caste practitioners were also interviewed as it was observed that the Thakurs also got treatment from these practitioners. Thus practitioners of Mahar and Maratha caste, Kathkarisand Mahadev Kolis tribe were also interviewed, along with the Thakur Key informants.

C) Illness Episodes

Besides interviewing the village elders, key informants and medical practitioners of the Thakur tribe, 50 illness episodes of non randomly selected patients from 15 Thakur settlements were recorded in detail. This exercise was conducted to comprehend the etiological categories regarding the origin and cause of illness, the various pathogenic agents that cause illness, the clinically meaningful reality through which a sick person passes to get cured, as well as to understand all culturally defined actions and rituals performed by the participant actors such as family and village elders, friends and relatives and finally the medical specialists in order to restore the health of the patient.

"An illness episode or therapeutic narrative is one to which Evelyn Early (1982:1481) refers to as a commentary on illness progression, curative actions and surrounding events both relevant and irrelevant fragments embedded in the conversation, which are framed by stylistic shifts that are evidently codified into elaborate accounts and which are reference of years of experience after the illness episode. The illness episodes and therapeutic narratives present a system of medical knowledge which mediates between everyday experience of diagnosis and curative actions which are meaningful within the cultural context. Illness episodes in this context helped gather information about the various processes/ stages of treatment, which start right from defining disease as illness, performing diagnostic rituals, healing rituals and finally performing ceremonies and rituals in which the patients family offers in kind and/or cash to the originator and/or the curer of the cause of illness, as a token of gratefulness for restoring the patient's health.

It was also observed that the Thakurs believe, that people die as a result of becoming victims of witchcraft, sorcery, wrath of gods and goddesses, intervention of evil forces etc. To prevent this certain rituals are performed to please these malevolent folks that take away life. To prevent the soul (atma) of the dead from troubling thc Thakur community the dead bodies are treated in a strange manner.

Genealogical Method

Genealogies of medical specialists were documented in order to understand, to whom was the medical skill/art transferred to and to find out who (individual) in every generation is equipped with the medical skill or art.

Besides the genealogies of medical practitioner families in which albinos and congenitally deformed children were born (and later put to death) were also documented so as to trace the occurrence of albino and congenitally deformed cases in every generation. On observation it was found that the genealogical method supported the validity of the data gathered and contributed to a great extent in the analysis.

Documentation Method

Finally to support the data collected through illness episodes, indepth interviews and participant observation, photographs, slides and a video film were made on the ethnomedical aspects of Thakur culture. This was done to empirically support and validate the data.

A tape recorder was used to record the songs sung during healing rituals. This was done so as to understand the purpose, meanings and the symbolic aspects of performing a particular health ritual.

Often these songs were written by the researcher in Marathi while the natives sang them.

Maximum efforts were made to document every belief, action, objects and the meaningful and symbolic aspects of Thakur ethnomedical system.

It was also experienced that, that which initially appeared irrational, irrelevant became of much significance in the later stage after having documented the meanings associated with it.

Participant Observation

Participant observation was one of the most reliable methods to cross check the validity of the data obtained through in depth interviews, illness episodes and case studies. It was also observed that the information collected from the respondents through indepth interviews and illness episodes at times contradicted with what they (Thakurs) did during a ritual of diagnosis, healing, thanksgiving, or a ritual of collecting medicinal herbs.

The researcher thus participated in the rituals associated with collection preparation and administration of medicinal herbs, the rituals associated with the collection, preparation, and administration of medicinal herbs, the rituals associated with the diagnosis and interpretation of the cause of illness, the healing rituals and ceremonies concerned with the thanksgiving to the originator of the cause and the curer (medical specialist) of the cause of illness. Besides the above mentioned rituals the researcher also observed other ceremonies and rituals related to birth, death, puberty and the ceremonies associated with festivals and traditional dances in order to understand and comprehend the meanings and symbolic elements associated with them.

Participant observation was thus very useful in cross checking the data gathered through interviews and witnessing the natural actions (rituals) performed with a given medical situation or context. This helped the researcher to comprehend and understand the meanings associated with the ethnomedical situations in which the actors behave or act in particular way and are aware of their actions.

On Becoming a Shaman (Bhagat)

The gateways to understanding the meanings and symbols associated with Thakur medical system, were opened when the researcher decided to undergo the training of a Shaman. Thus, this decision was followed a long formal training/apprenticeship period under a guru (teacher) Walku Thorad and Senior and experienced Bhagat of Nagyachiwadi.

The training started on 8th October 1991 till 17th Oct. 1991 (during the Navratra Occasion) There were several rules and restrictions which the researcher had to adhere to some of these being staying the village for nine days and nine nights, abstaining from the consumption of turmeric, in the food, avoid the touch of a menstruating woman, to refrain from eating anymore if the burning lamp goes off (while eating) to avoid sweeping the dwelling place etc. At times the researcher had to spend the night on a tree (Bauhinia recemosa) and chant mantras. At other times the same mantras had to be chanted by standing in the river at night facing the east.

During this nine day training period the researcher learnt and became conversant with methods of diagnosis, the various pathogenic agents (deities, spirits, ghosts, ancestors, witches and sorcerers) which cause illness, the hierarchy of their power, the mantras (chants) associated with diagnosis and healing, the various objects and their meanings which are associated with ritual healing, the symbolic elements associated with the human body.

Finally on 6th Nov. 1991 the researcher was publicly ordained a Shaman by his Guru and a ritual was performed, which declared the researcher a shaman. Thus this was the beginning of learning many things associated with the cultural aspects, their symbols, and meanings associated with health and disease as perceived by the natives.

Later the researcher accompanied his teacher when he had to diagnose, interpret the cause and in the healing rituals Often he accompanied his teacher on long hikes/walks in the forest. The teacher showed him certain medicinal plants which (used by him) were administered to the patients. The teacher also shared with him a number of healing experiences which greatly enhanced the quality of the data.

Doing Away with Religious Biasness

Having firmly decided that he (researcher) would become a shaman, the researcher put behind him all christian ethics and accepted all practices of being a shaman practices such as idol worship, worshipping the Bhagat were done though they were against Christian ethics.

Thus, living among the Thakurs by socializing with them in different situations helped the researcher considerably and thus was instrumental in getting qualitative data on the ethnomedical beliefs and practices of the Thakurs from a holistic view.

Hence being more of an anthropologist and less of an individual (with own religion and ethics) helped the researcher mingle and gather data about the Thakurs.

Sampling Plan

Six Thakur hamlets of Pathraj and Kashale grampanchayat were selected for this study. These Thakur settlements were Thakurwadi, Lobhiewadi, Borwadi, Nalde wadi, Khondewadi and Kaute wadi. These villages are in close proximity to each other. Both Kashale and Pathraj gram panchayat to gather has 12 Thakur hamlets. Kashale has two and

Pathraj has 10 hamlets respectively. Since Kashale has only two thakur hamlets both were selected. From the ten Thakur hamlets of Pathraj four were selected randomly using the lottery method. Thus two hamlets from Kashale four from Pathraj were selected to represent 50% the total number of villages (six) that fall under both the village gram panchayat.

An initial survey of all the finally selected six villages was made to prepare a list of heads of the house holds. From the main list a second list was prepared of households above 45 years of age. The table given below explains number of household heads (above 45 years) of each village who were selected as respondents for indepth interviews.

SR.NO.	THAKUR SETTLEMENTS	MALE	FEMALE	TOTAL
1.	THAKURWADI	08	02	10
2.	LOBHIE WADI	15	02	17
3.	BORWADI	11	01	12
4.	NALDE WADI	13	04	17
5.	KHONDE WADI	08	01	09
6.	KAUTE WADI	10	02	12
		65	**12**	**77**

Thus the total number of respondents selected for indepth interviews were 77. It was very necessary to select heads above 45 years as they were well versed with meanings & symbols associated with their ethnomedicine and also it was these heads who performed and participated in all culturally recognized rituals and knew their meanings.

Since the study demanded a probe into the meaning system of medicine and the healing processes, qualitative information about their conceptual reality about illness ideology, body symbolism, ethnomedical therapy, nature and role of medical specialists, various forms of preventive medicine, their perception about body physiology and so on was collected through indepth informal interviews using a interview guide.

Besides the indepth interviews of house hold heads above 45 the key informants (medical specialists) were selected purposively from15 villages. The operational difficulty faced in this situation was that one does not find all the medical practitioners in one village,hence it was necessary for the researcher to visit the near by 15 villages to interview medical practitioner.

These practitioners come under the panchayat (geographical

jurisdiction) of Kashale, Pathraj, Nalde and Khandus gram panchayat. The table given below depicts the difficult types of medical practitioners belonging to the Thakur community. They were purposively selected to conduct their detailed case studies about their profession.

SR.NO.	MEDICAL SPECIALIST	NO. OF SPECIALIST INTERVIEWED
1.	BHAGATS (MALE SHAMANS)	04
2.	BHAGATINS (FEMALE SHAMANS)	02
3.	MANTRIKS (SNAKE & SCORPION SPECIALISTS)	02
4.	HAD VAIDUS (BONE SETTERS)	04
5.	VAIDUS (HERBALISTS)	20
6.	SUINES (MIDWIVES)	05
7.	POTDHARIS (ASST.MIDWIVES)	14

Other than the 77 indepth interview of heads of the house hold above 45 years age, the case studies of medical specialists of the Thakur tribe, 50 illness episodes of purposively selected patients from fifteen villages were recorded in detail to comprehensively understand the system of medical knowledge that mediates between everyday experience of diagnosis, curative actions and the symbolic elements which are associated with ritual healing and which are meaningful within the cultural frame of reference.

In this book only 7 cases studies are incorporated that is one case study of each type of medical practitioner thus the key informants (medical practitioners) were purposively for recording case studies.

Bernard Russel (1988:97) is certainly justified in stating that life history research and qualitative on special populations (drug addicts, trial layers, shamans etc) rely on purposive sampling. The present study being qualitative in nature demanded a probe into the case studies of all the seven types of medical practitioners prevalent in the Thakur Society.

Besides recording the case studies of the medical specialists, the data was also supported by participants, observation, photographs, slides video and audio recording thus making the data more empirical and authentic.

Variables of the Study

The main objective of this research was to understand the hidden meanings of all the symbols and symbolic forms (including actions, words, objects, gestures, utterances, colour etc) associated with the ethnomedical practices and beliefs of the Thakurs. To understand why the natives acted or performed certain actions during healing and why they behave the way they did?

While doing this, the study intended to explore the culturally held perceptions and conceptions about the clinically meaningful reality as defined by the natives themselves. Schneider (1976 :204) is certainly justified in stating that "Meaning is simply not attributed to reality Reality itself is constructed by beliefs understandings and comprehensions entailed in cultural meanings."

The conceptual reality of the researcher was different from that of his target population so to have entered the field with preformulated questions would have been to enter the field with preconceived, notions about the nature of their reality. This would have been methodically wrong. Thus the only way to collecting information was to follow the meanings right through by conducting free-ranging unstructured interviews.

Each interview session with a respondent was guided by only one factor what Schneider (1976:220) called a fundamental methodological maneuver (which is) to ask the natives not once or even twice but in many different ways and therefore at many different times, with every possible eliciting device what the cultural symbols are and what they mean ? Answers had to be consequently cross checked to establish whether the views expressed were generally held ideas and/or whether they were in contradiction with the researcher's observations.

Although, in most situations questions were formulated in the field itself during the interview sessions. An interview was used in order to collect relevant information on subjects which the study demanded. Thus based on earlier works in ethnomedicine data was collected separate interview guides were used for patients, village and family elders, medical practitioners and key informants Data relevant to the following areas was collected (refer appendix).

Thus the main focus was to record in detail the concepts of Thakur medicine which they associated with illness ideology, body symbolism, and ritual healing. The data incorporated in the theories it self is an evidence of what variables were selected in order to obtain qualitative data.

Data Processing and Analysis

The data collected on the ethnomedical beliefs and practices, the symbols and meanings associated with ritual healing were analyzed manually since the nature of the data was descriptive and qualitative. Thus, the analysis of the data has been descriptive and more importantly interpretive.

The analysis is descriptive, in the sense that the complicated symbols, symbolic forms and they are ordered as a meaning system that represents the cultural whole were understood and reduced to their component parts. In doing so an attempt has been made to demonstrate Schneider's view that all normative behaviour emerges from the underlying assumptions of the nature of the world in which the natives live.

The data collected by using separate interview guides for patients, family heads, village elders, the case studies seven different types of medical specialists and for those family heads where albino children and congenitally deformed children were born and killed as described in detail keeping in mind the scope and limitations of the study.

Meanings of all the actions, objects, words, prayers, songs, gestures, utterances etc that were part of the healing processes and procedures ere analyzed and classified or ordered as defined by the natives. The relationships between these symbols, symbolic forms and their meanings were analyzed to understand the conceptual reality of the world in which the natives live.

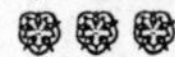

CHAPTER III

ETHNOGRAPHY OF THE THAKURS

The Population, Distribution & Its Origin

The target population selected for the present research is a tribal community namely "The Thakurs" - a major tribe of Western Maharashtra. In Maharashtra, the ka and the Ma Thakurs are declared as a Scheduled tribe in 26 tehsils spread over five districts namely - Thane, Raigarh, Nasik, Poona and Ahmednagar as given below :

1.	AHMED NAGAR	AKOLA RAHURI & SANGAMNER TEHSILS.
2.	RAIGARH	KARJAT, KHALA, PEN, PANVEL & MATHERAN
3.	NASIK	IGATPURI, NASIK & SINNER TEHSILS.
4.	POONA	AMBEGAON, JUNNAR, KHED & MAVAL.
5.	THANA	THANA, KALYAN, MURBAD, BHIVANDI BASSIEN, WADA, SHAHAPUR, PALGHAR, MOKHADA, JAWHAR, & TEHSILS.

According to the1981census, the total Thakur population in Maharashtra State is 3,23,191 with 1,65,571 males and 1,57,620 females residing both in urban and rural areas of Maharashtra State. The Thakur informants selected for the present study are from three panchayat villages of Karjat Tehsil, Raigarh district namely Pathraj and Kashale.

The Thakurs are divided into two endogamous sections, the Ma and the Ka. The Ma are often called Ma probably due to their peculiar way of speech marked by the elongated "ma" pronunciation. There are other explanations regarding the origin of these two sect names. The Ma Thakurs claim their origin from Mahaldesh, a province in Nasik district, while the Ka say that they were from the Konkan plains of the state of Maharashtra. There is yet another explanation given by the Ma Thakurs. They equate their social status with a local Kshatriya caste group namely the marathas and hence call themselves as Maratha Thakurs, while the Ka are categorized as Kadu Thakurs (bitter in nature). Chaphekar (1961 :7), has pointed out that the recurrence of the two letters of the alphabets Ma and Ka in their respective modes of speech have earned their names for these two communities.

The standard Marathi lexicon describes a Thakur as (i) a deity, (ii) an idol, (iii) god, (iv) the names of a hill tribe and its members (in northern Konkan), (v) the leader of a Rajpur or Bhil tribe, (vi) a patel, (vii) a sardar or a nobleman, (viii) a lord, (ix) a title or honour, (x) a priest officiating for some the the Shudra castes, The lexicon however does not give the derivations of the term.

Rajwade (1924:84) derives the name from taksara; taskar,thakkar-thakara-thakura. Taskara means a thief and the term probably denoted a criminal tribe. Rajwade says that the Thakurs were known to Katyana as Taskaras. Although logically the derivation seems sound, it is unreasonable to attribute the origin of the name of a timid god fearing community noted for its honesty to a criminal propensity.

It is the opinion of the contributors to Jnyankash that there is a strain of rajput blood in the Thakurs. The statement however has little validity as no evidence in support of it has been offered. The Nasik, Thana and Poona gazetteer records this theory which seems to have originated with Dr. John Wilson (1876: 20). He thinks that the Thakurs are barons and Gujarat, who fled to the jungles as a result of Sultan Mohammed begada's persecution, induced Hindus of different tribes to join their ranks. Thus this mixed multitude in the north Konkan in known as the Thakur Tribe.

Chaphekar (1960 : 2) states that the original habitat of the Thakurs was in the hilly western parts of Nasik district of the State of Maharashtra, is particularly certain. He supports his statement by saying that the Thakurs from other districts of Maharashtra state namely Ahmednagar, Poona, Raigarh and Thana claim that their vatnas or original places are situated in these parts. In marriage songs, prayers offered to deities are from the very places such as Nasik, Trimbakeshwar, Talegaon and Ajneri. All these places are in Nasik District.

It means that the emigrants walked down from thal Pass from Borli, where a big Thakur fair is held annually even today on the new moon day of paush (Dec-Jan). It is just possible that the emigrants might have left Borli on that day centuries ago. A legend exists in Borli that the emigrants before a starting on their historic march, threw their weapons into a tank. This shows that the Thakur is conscious of emigrants and perhaps of the change of life from that of a fighter to one of a hunter or a cultivator.

How long the Thakur has been occupying the western parts of Nasik district, when he immigrated into Konkan and whether the assimilation of Gujarat Barons into Konkan is a fact, and if so, the date of the Gujarat barons' migration to Nasik and their routes are questions which cannot be discussed to want of reliable data. In the present stage of our knowledge, therefore Chaphekar (1960) has taken the Thakurs to be a hill tribe of Maharashtra State.

Their Physical Features

The Thakurs are a small squat tribe, certainly better looking than their neighbours, the Kathkaris (neighbouring tribe). Most Thakurs are medium height, their general complexion is brown best described as chocolate. Hair is generally straight or wavy, curly being an exception. They have large, though not very prominent cheek bones, rather full lips and deep sunken eyes.

A diminish of marginal type of epicanthic fold may be observed. They are strong people, this may be due the hardy life on the hill. The Thakur women are noted for their bulging stomachs. They tie their saris very tightly below their naval. This is one of the reasons why most Thakur women suffer from fungal rash on their abdominal parts.

Dress Pattern

The men wear a loin-cloth ad occasionally a waist cloth and a blanket draped on the shoulder and a piece of cloth tied around their heads. They wear a traditional type of sleeves shirt known as "bandi", made out of cotton cloth and looks almost like a banyan. The women wear " lugade" (robe) very tightly wound around their waist so as to leave their legs bare. The end of which is always tucked at the waist and never drawn over the head. While the Ka women have a separate lugade piece tucked at their waist, which is drawn over their heads. The only covering for the upper part of the body is a garment which resembles a blouse and a heavy necklace of several rounds of white and blue glass beads is worn by the women.

Earrings are worn both in the lobe and pinna by men, women and children. Bangles are worn in abundance but nose rings are rear. The married women wear a black beaded necklace known as mangalsutra, which is a symbol of their marital status, also the rings which are worn in the second

toe of the feet known as "Jodve" which again is a symbol of their marital status. On the death of the husband, these rings (Jodve) are removed and buried along with the dead body of the husband. A widow always ears a rupee coin in her chain. The rupee coin symbolizes a single status as a widow.

Settlement Pattern

The Thakur lives or rather seems to live aloof. His preference for jungle life is the cause. As a result, there have to come to existence exclusive Thakur hamlets popularly known as the Thakurwadis. In most cases one finds the Thakurwadis situated on the outskirts of the main panchayat Village. The central portion of the village is occupied by the "Marathas" an economically ad politically powerful dominant caste group in this area.

The generic term for each Thakurwadi or village is often called by the most prominent clan residing in it, Kautewadi, Lobhiewadi, Bangarwadi, Bhagatachiwadi, etc.are few instances. Some wadis are known by the names of trees, this one finds names such as Borwadi, Chaphyachiwadi, Jambulwadi,Vadachiwadi. A Thakur hamlets called is never a conglomeration of different castes and creeds. The community is self contained and lives in exclusive settlements on high attitudes thus keeping themselves aloof from the other castes as mush as possible. Therefore the Thakurs live by themselves.

Economic Life

The economic position of the Thakur is determined by the amount of grain he holds, number of ploughs, numbers of livestock and size of the house are other criteria for economic status. Agriculture is the main source of income and he mainly cultivates rice, nagli and vari. Stock-breeding is also an important activity. Fishery is mainly for house consumption. Thakurs work as laborers either in the fields, forests , road constructions or on farms of rich people.

Selling fire-wood, black berries (Karavanda and Jamun), mangoes, palas leaves and baskets is yet another source of earning cash. They also exchange grains with local traders for different things which they require for daily use. The expenses of the Thakurs are few, these wants are restricted to bare necessities. Food requirements as such is meagre. Taking loans from the local money lenders for festivals, marriages, death rituals, etc. has been practice of the Thakurs since time immemorial. This has therefore given an opportunity to the Sahukars to exploit the tribals from different perspectives such as bonded labor, indebtedness, sale of girls, etc. This trend has been recently diminishing in the area.

Family Life

A family is usually formed of a man who is the head of the family, his wife and children. Married daughters must live with their husbands, since the family types of Thakur society are patriarchal, patrilineal and patrilocal. Married son either continues to live with the father, or gets separated and makes a new home. Married brothers do not live together. In a Thakur family every member does some work or the other. The women folk rear children and are in charge of the kitchens. Old women look after the younger children. In a Thakur village nearly all the families are related. Mutual help is seen and co-operation is more evident among the members of the same Clan. The fact that each member plays a part in running the household has resulted in a friendly family atmosphere.

Marriage

Marriage is one of the most important events in the life of a Thakur. Preparation for it starts with the selection of a bride. There are certain kuli (clans) or families which cannot inter-marry.

The padirs cannot marry the padirs, but they can marry the pardhis. Age at marriage for the boys is usually 16-17 and the girls it is 14-16. A Brahman is usually consulted to fix an auspicious occasion for the wedding.

Having approved of the bride in preliminary talks, the settlement is ratified by the ceremony of betrothal which is called supari phodane. This action is symbolic of finalizing marital relationship to proceed with further ceremonies marriage usually takes place at the bride's house. The Thakur marriages are usually celebrated late in the evenings in the month of Margashirsha and Magh. i.e in the winter after the harvest. Tuesday is strictly avoided.

There are three types of functionaries for the marriage ceremony. Two of them are couples. They are called umbarya and umbari and pitarya pitari respectively. The female partners of these two couples must be married according to "lagna" rites.

The pitarya pitari as the term signifies, represents the ancestors. The umbarya and umbari are entrusted with the construction of booth. The third functionaire are vahulies, and generally are unmarried young girls who are to do all the menial work. The dej or bride price is given both in cash and kind. The amount varies from Rs. 150.00 Rs. 300.00 and in kind 2-3 bags of rice. This depends on the economic status of the families involved in marital relationships.

Kinship

The Thakur relationship system is in no way a classifying system today. The father and father's brother are addressed as baba, mother and father's wife -ai. The step father -Kaka, a step mother is mothi or dhakti - ai depending in whether she is elder or younger. The elder brother's wife may also is vadhai meaning elder mother. The husband of the mother's elder sister- Baba. The mother's sister is moushi. A man is addressed as Javai not only by his wife's father but also by his father's brothers and cousins. Father-in-law is addressed as mama and father's sister phui.

Brother -in-law as Bhauji and younger brother as a bapu. Wife's sister as sadin.

Younger people are addressed by names, while older people by formal names. Por is a term used affectionately for children. Some kinship terms of ka Thakur are different from Ma. Father is addressed as aba. Wife's elder sister is known as Sasu. Younger sister-in-law Sali, great grandfather Ajya, Mother's sister is addressed as dhakti. Son's wife's parents and daughter's husbands parents as vyahi. Husband's elder brother as dir. Younger brother's wife and also sons wife as uhus/vahare.

Religion

The Thakurs supernatural beliefs are mainly expressed in ritual and magical practices. His attitude towards his deities (deva) is one of fear and dread. Each of them is a potential from doing him harm than with an expectation of some positive good. His pantheon consists of a number of deities. Among them are the village gods whose names are as follows: chedhoba, vaghoba, khambya Bhairi, etc. The Hirva represents peacock from the animal world. Munja, Khais and Vetal come from the spirit world, the virdev and supali represents the ancestors. The majority of are of stones smeared with red lead. Kanir dev is yet another god of ear who is appeared when a patient suffers from severe ear ache.

Sun is the most powerful of all gods and the mother earth is his wife. Moon is his brother and water again has brotherly relationship with sun and moon. The lightning, and Holi (festival of fire and goddess of fertility) are sisters of the sun, moon and water. These five cosmic elements play an important role in the Thakur cultural system. The village god is a brother of the sun and lives with the people. He goes to see the sun on sundays and tuesdays.

The Satvai is a goddess of fortune and fertility. She writes the life span of an individual on his forehead for lord Brahma. Brahma forms an individual's foetus in the mother' womb. A person's atma (soul) is present just below the sternum. The soul leaves a person's body through the mouth, eyes or nose, because one of these are open when the soul leaves. It is believed that the Satvai sends yamraj to take the person's soul.

The Thakur deities are regularly worshipped and their divine rites are performed as and when the situation demands. Failure to perform certain divine ceremonies and rituals may result into health hazards and terrifying calamities. The deities need constant attention of the Thakur devotees.

The Thakur's belief in spirits and ghosts are not very different from those of the plain farmers. According to the Thakurs they are performed as and when the situation demands. Failure to perform certain divine ceremonies and rituals may result into health hazards and terrifying calamities. The deities need constant attention of the Thakur devotees.

The Thakur's belief in spirits and ghosts are not very different from those of the plain farmers. According to the Thakurs there are four species of ghosts namely the Khais, munja and the Vetal. These evil spirits are responsible for bringing about troubles and sickness.

Death and Funerals

The Thakurs have elaborate rituals which are carried out after death.

A dead person is placed on the floor with the head pointing south. Few ornaments of little value are buried in the grave. The waste chord is cut before the grave is closed (Among the ma, the obsequies are performed at the earliest on the seventh and latest on the tenth day after death. When a woman dies in childbirth a ring of the dhanvel creeper which represents her child and some thorns of the asana plant believed to prevent the deceased woman from becoming a ghost,are placed by her side in the grave. When a pregnant woman dies, the Ka cut open her abdomen, remove the foetus and bury it separately.

Tuesday and Saturday are considered inauspicious and the obsequies in such cases are performed a day earlier. On the annual obsequial day, which falls on the new moon day of Bhadrapad, food offered to the deceased is placed on the roof. Once during the first year rice and the dhal and vegetable must be offered on the grave.

On the tenth day in case of married males, ninth day in case of married females seventh day in case of bachelor's spinsters the ritual of soul migration is performed to send his/her soul to heaven. The ceremony is presided over by a Brahmin Priest.

Villagers gather at the house of the host at noon without a formal invitation. A drum which can be heard through out the neighbourhood serves as an announcement. The host provides his guests with food. With this the ceremony gets over. In body symbolism chapter, death rites are explained in detail.

Maternal and Child Health Care Beliefs and Practices of the Thakurs.

Ever since independence, the principal national aim has been to secure improvement in the quality of life for the Indian people. Adequate health and family welfare services is one of the most important components of improved quality of life. Towards this end, the government of India has been making all efforts and has committed to provide "Health for all by 2000 A.D." by signing the WHO sponsored Alma Ata declaration of 1978 (N. Bhaskar Rao, 1988 : vii).

The scene today is disheartening in spite of the intensive efforts on the part of the government and voluntary organization, the level of acceptance of family planning and acceptance of utilization of health and MCH services is low.

Research studies in MCH and family welfare have pointed out that the services provided by the government agencies namely PHC's and sub-centres were inaccessible. The grass-root level workers and the higher authorities show lack of initiative, enthusiasm and concern for the various activities of the PHC's and the sub-centres. Lack of adequate training among the health workers leading to a low level of confidence among them and their inaccessibility surfaced as the main reasons for low level of utilization of government health facilities. There is a high rate of infant mortality mainly due to the following reasons.

i. incorrect perceptions of the beneficiaries towards the PHC's and the sub-centres.
ii. lack of appropriate motivation and educational efforts.
iii. the under - utilization of maternal (pre and post delivery) and child (immunization, nutrition) health care services.

To improve the quality of life among the rural and the tribal masses, health education and motivation are the main media which can impart sound and correct knowledge to them. The common notion of the programmes dealing with Health Education and Motivation is that the target population is foolish and needs to be educated. It is observed that health education programmes many a times show lack of knowledge of the cultural beliefs, practices, traditions about health and diseases and their system of health care. Due to this glaring loophole the heath education and motivation are often weakly planned and implemented with minimum or no follow-up programmes. All the same, many a time health education is mistaken for health publicity and health education aids. No thought is spared to understand peoples perceptions, customs. beliefs, practices and their traditions regarding health and disease.

Communication a major tool in health education helps to further the process of equipping the people with facts, ideas and attitudes which will help them make a better choice toward improving the quality of their life. But this tool has not been appropriately implemented in health education programmes.

The application of appropriate and effective health communication is no doubt, culture-specific. In every society there exists the people's very own communication media, their network processes which are functional and have been existent even before the advent of modern science and technology. People in tribal and rural areas have a definite and a systematic pattern of communicating information to relatives and friends and other community members. These people are able to successfully convey information regarding funerals, auspicious ceremonies weddings, meetings etc. Thus it is observed that a definite and culture specific pattern of communication operates. Hence it becomes necessary to document the people's system of communication and then base the health education programmes on what is available traditionally.

Traditionally women as mothers, wives and sisters were providers of health care within the home (Shiva and others 1992 : 38). This was at the family level. At the societal level there are medical practitioners. Had vaidus are known as bonesetters. Herbalist (vaidu), shamans (Bhagats) and the midwives (dais) to provide health service to the sick in their community.

The people's (emic) concepts of preventive, promotive, curative and destructive medicine is symbolically and meaningfully interwoven inn their culture. Thus all actions, chants, gestures, utterances, songs, holy objects, words, rituals and ceremonies associated with maternal and child health care are meaningful within their cultural frame of reference. This chapter highlights the various symbolic and meaningful elements associated with maternal and child health care beliefs and normative practice of the Thakurs.

Food Habits of the Thakurs

A. General Diet of The Community :

The data collected through interviews and observations revealed that the Thakurs consume the following food.

CEREALS :	Rice is their staple food.
MILLETS :	Nagli (Eleucine Coracana), Vari (Panicum Meliacea)
VEGETABLES :	Brinjals, Potatoes, Tomatoes, Amaranthus, bhaji, French Beans, cabbage, cauliflower etc.
PULSES :	Toor dal, Udid, Hulga, Peas.
FRUITS :	Fruits such as bananas, chikku, oranges are rarely consumed by the Thakurs. Their diet includes seasonal fruits such as Zizyphus jujuba, Mangifera indica, Carissa carandis, Ugenia jambolina, Emblica officinalis etc. These are gathered from the forest.
OILS :	Besides groundnut oil the Thakurs manufacture oil from Mahua seeds (Bacia latifolia).
CORM :	Dioscorea bulbifera is used by the Thakurs very often. They go in search and the same in the woods especially during famine. Dioscorea is believed to be highly beneficial for women after

	delivery as it increases production of breast milk. Its local vernacular name is "dudh kand", "dudh" refers to milk and "kand" is corn.
NON-: VEGETARIAN	Fish, meat, pork are consumed occasionally. Dry fish is regularly consumed.
MILK & : MILK PRODUCTS	Consumption of milk and curds is rare among the Thakur adults and children.

B. Hot and Cold Concepts of Diet :

Ethnologists in many parts of Latin America have pointed out that important ideals concerning health and sickness are based on hot and cold qualities in nature. Certain illnesses are believed to having been caused due to intake of "hot diet or substances" and treated with cold remedies, while sickness believed to occur because of intake of cold diet or substances are treated with hot remedies (Schutlur Mary, 1979 : 160).

A favourable and parallel consideration is given to hot and cold diet as well as to the ideals concerning health and sickness believed to be caused by the hot and cold qualities in nature and in diet. The Thakurs classify all the food items and even medicine into three categories viz. 1. hot 2. cold 3. lukewarm.

Some of the foods classified as hot by the Thakurs are wheat, vari, bitter gourd, brinjals, potatoes, coriander, gram, peas, toor dal, papaya, banana, fish, eggs, meat, chicken, jaggery, monitor's meat and pork. The local liquor prepared from Mahua flowers (Bacia latifolia) is also included in this category.

The foods classified as cold are Nagli (Eleucine coracana), Cabbage, Cucurbita, Onion, Cauliflower, Tomatoes, Ambadi bhaji, Mango, Orange, Karvanda, Jamun, Watermelon, Emblica officinalis, Lime, Milk, Curds, latex of Ficus hispida and Coconut water. Rice is classified as "lukewarm" i.e. the combination of hot and cold category. In cold reason hot foods are prepared and preferred and vice versa.

Medicines taken by them are also classified into hot and cold. Thus to treat cold and cough a medicinal herb (Allium sativum) believed to be hot is administered. The Thakurs believe that excessive consumption of hot and cold foods cause illness. Consumption of too hot and cold foods are considered a taboo for pregnant woman as it is believed to affect both mother and child.

Who Eats First : A Tragic Reality :

Almost all Thakurs eat twice a day except during the cultivation season during which the adults eat thrice a day. The Thakurs have black tea in the morning and breakfast-cum-lunch at 11'O clock and their dinner is at 7 p.m.

The women who spend major part of their time cooking, fetching water, collecting firewood, doing household work, child rearing amd doing their bit where agricultural work is concerned are a neglected lot. This negligence extends into the sphere of diet. The adults male and children eat first. The left overs are later consumed by the women folk.

Women who are regarded as the second sex, the lesser sex, the weaker sex do not enjoy an equal health status as compared to the men. They are deprived of the right of eating along with other family members. This pattern of men and children eating first is also common among the Nawapur tehsil, Dhule district (Tribhuwan Robin & others, 1992 : 9).

Quantity of Food Consumed :

The diet of the adult females is slightly less as compared to the adult males. The children and the older folk consume more or less the same quantity of food.

The table given below depicts the quantity of food consumed by the Thakurs.

C. Diet of Pregnant Women

Pregnancy is considered a natural event in a woman's life and hence no special care or diet is recommended for a pregnant woman. She follows the normal diet as during other times. Raw papaya, banana and dioscorea bulbifera are taboo for the pregnant woman as it is believed that the excess heat in the above may lead to an abortion.

Pregnant women refuse to consume the iron tablets given by the P.H.C. It is believed that the heat in the tablets leads to an abortion, or the foetus enlarges and delivery of such a child as believed by some Thakurs is difficult for the woman. Drinking excess black tea (without milk) is also believed to lead to an abortion.

D. Diet after Delivery

A special diet of rice porridge (kanji) is given to the new mother for a period of 15 days. Kanji is prepared in the following manner. Rice is ground and then boiled in large quantity of water. The kanji is believed to increase the production of breast milk. As stated earlier, rice is considered to be lukewarm and hence it is believed to produce lukewarm blood in the mother's body which in turn is converted into lukewarm breast milk which is easily digested by the newborn.

Too hot and cold foods are a taboo for the new mother, it is believed that too hot or cold food if consumed affect the temperature of the mother's blood and hence the breast milk may in turn be affected and cause illness to the child. Yet another food item (Dioscorea bulbifera - dudh kand) is believed to increase production of breast milk.

E. Foods Avoided After Delivery

Solid foods are avoided by a new mother for they are not digestible. It is believed by the Thakurs that after delivery the stomach and the intestines need rest. Solid foods are also avoided as they are believed to cause thickening of the breast milk which is difficult for the child to digest and is believed to cause digestive disorders in the child.

Hot foods such as potatoes, brinjals, black tea, spices, jaggery, chillies, papaya, gram etc are avoided as they are believed to create heat which results in the breast milk becoming hot and leads to diarrhoea in the case of the child.

Among the Mavchis - a tribe residing in the north-west of Maharashtra, fish and meat are avoided as they are believed to cause vaginal infections in the mother. Sour foods are also avoided as they obstruct the flow of the impure blood discharge. The Mavchis believe that the greater the flow of the impure blood discharge the better it is (Tribhuwan Robin, Khatri Maya, Ganguly Meeta, 1992 : 7). Similarly a Thakur midwife (suine) also sees to it that all the impure blood is removed out as it is believed to be harmful for both the mother and the newborn if retained in the body of the mother.

F. Diets of Infants and Children

The Thakur mothers do not breast feed the newborn for five days after delivery. The cholostrom milk is squeezed out on a cloth and washed with water. The Thakurs believe that the food and water consumed by the woman leads to the formation of blood which is further converted into breast milk. During the pregnancy period menstrual blood does not flow out and is retained in the body. It is believed to be evil. The child survives on this blood. The Thakurs believe that some of the menstrual blood is retained in the body and this blood due to the spermatic (sticky) effect makes the breast milk thick and sticky.

Thus this sticky and thick nature of the breast milk is believed to be indigestible and causes diarrhoea and dysentery in the new born. This milk sticks to the internal lining of the child's intestines due to which it is unable to defecate which results in bulging of the stomach.

In some cases upto the fifth day (after birth) the child is given honey, cow's milk and water. Mothers breast feed their infants till their stomach is full. Infants are breast fed for a period of ten to twelve months. Weaning foods are introduced after the sixth month and the solid foods include dal, boiled potatoes, rice, kanji etc. Cow's and goat's milk are used as supplementary food. Among the Mavchis buffalo milk is avoided till the fifth month as it is believed to be heavy and indigestible by the infants (Tribhuwan Robin and others 1992 : 8).

G. Diseases Prevalent among Mothers and Children

The staff of Kashale PHC including the Medical Officer of the staff and Medical Officer of Ayurvedic Dispensary runby the Academy of Development Science and a practising homoeopath were kind enough to give valuable information on the common ailments prevalent among the mothers and children of the Thakur tribe.

Common Ailments Among Mothers :

1. Anemia, 2. Malnutrition, 3. Worm infection, 4. Sexually transmitted diseases, 5. Spontaneous abortion, 6. Fungal infections, 7. Dental caries, 8. Malaria, 9. Tuberculosis, 10. Eczema, 11. Boils, 12. Scabies, 13. Abscesses, 14. Diarrhoea, 15. jaundice.

Common Ailments Among Children :

Some of the common health problems identified among children are:

1. Scabies, 2. Cold & cough, 3. Sore-eyes, 4. Fungal infections, 5. Worm infestations, 6. Boils, 7. Measles, 8. Dental carries, 9. Fever, 10. Abscesses, 11. Diarrhoea.

The disease causational concepts of the Thakurs are separately highlighted in chapter IV.

H. Personal Hygiene

The term personal hygiene includes all those personal factors which influence the health and well being of an individual. In a brood sense it comprises of a range of day to day activities such as body care, bathing washing, care of clothes, hair, teeth, skin and nails, cultivating good habits regarding diet, sleep, exercise etc and on the whole a systematically organized way of healthy life. Any disruption of these activities may impair health. It's a matter of individual health responsibility (Park, 1986: 19).

It was observed, that the Thakurs tie their cattle inside their huts/houses as they believe the cattle to be family members thereby inviting dirt and diseases into the house. Women do not wear any footwear as they cannot afford them. Washing clothes is not regular though bathing is which is done without soap. The women tie a cloth around their waist while bathing which is left to dry on the body itself. After the bath the sari is tied tightly over the cloth. Such a practice ensures that the skin does not come in contact with the air which leads to more often than not various fungal infections.

I. Rituals and Ceremonies

The term ritual according to Edmund Leach (1968 : 524) should be applied to all. "Culturally defined sets of behaviour, that is to the symbolic dimensions of human behaviour as such regardless of its explicit religious socials or other contact". Every ritual and ceremony is performed to achieve some thing. Thus ritual is a purposeful act performed with intentions. Given below are some of the important rituals and ceremonies which are associated with the Thakur maternal and child health system.

Menstruation and Rituals of Purification :

Menstruation is considered to be a socially recognized state of pollution. A girl who is menstruating for the first time is not allowed to wash clothes in flowing water, which according to the Thakurs is the Ganges. Doing such an act defiles the Ganges and leads to an incessant flow of blood like the flow of river. A menstruating woman keeps herself aloof for four to five days. She does not cook nor does any household activities. The Thakurs believe that food prepared by a menstruating woman may cause illness. Thus a menstruating woman is socially dislocated from the society because it is believed that social interaction with her may bring trouble to the community.

After the menstrual period i.e. on the fourth or fifth day the woman takes a bath and washes her clothes. She then lights an incense stick after which she is eligible to interact with the society and perform her duties. This cleansing of her body symbolizes her purification from the evil menstrual blood. The purification rite thus symbolically places her back into the social system.

Concepts and Normative Behaviour During Pregnancy :

The Thakurs believe that first the soul (atma) and later on the bodily parts of the foetus develop. It takes two and a half months for a girl child and four months for a boy child to develop completely.

A pregnant woman does not interact with a barren woman during her term of pregnancy as she is believed to have an evil influence over the would be mother and her child. During the solar eclipse, pregnant women do not cutvegetables nor cook. They are not allowed to look at the eclipse for it is believed that the child may be born with cleft lips. Pregnant woman who cut vegetables during the solar eclipse are believed to deliver congenitally deformed children.

Several beliefs are attached with a pregnant women. One of them, if milk begins to ooze from the breast of a pregnant woman and her bodice gets wet with it, the child is believed to be still born. If the nipples grow black, the Thakurs think the child will be a boy, if they turn grey, it will be a girl. The period of pregnancy is longer if there is a boy in the womb and shorter if a girl. With a boy her face grows pale, her cheeks sunken and her neck is lean and drawn.

Childbirth :

When a woman feels her time is near, she goes home, changes her sari, wraps a piece of cloth round her loins and lies down supine on a rough blanket in the inner chamber resting her head on a folded cloth. She is assisted and attended to by the suine (midwife) and potdhari (suine's helpmate). If there is much delay or the delivery is difficult, charmed ash is brought from a Bhagat and applied to the forehead of the parturient woman. Another measure is to wet a part of her husband's loin cloth in a little water and to give the water to the ailing woman to drink. Placing herbs such as plantain (Musa paradisica) roots and/or the root of Rui-milkweed (Calotropis gigantia) are placed at the nape of the neck and are supposed to be efficacious. The delivery posture is east-west, with the mother's head points towards the east while her vaginal opening (ninth opening/darvaza) points/faces the west, where Satvai (Goddess of fortune and life span - Mother Earth) dwells. This position ensures that the newborn should be first seen by the Mother Earth who bestows fortune and life on every newborn.

Treatment of Umbilical Chord :

The suine uses a sickle (koyati) to cut the umbilical chord (nal). Of late due to the influence of the PHC's some of the suines use a razor blade which is rarely sterilized before use. The umbilical chord is buried outside the western wall of the house. This is done to prevent it from becoming an object or device of witchcraft in order to harm the newborn. The symbolic aspects of the burial of the umbilical chordare highlighted in detail in the chapter on body symbolism. For five days the mother takes bath with the child and the water is allowed to flow over the umbilical chord so as to quicken its decay. On the fifth day the child is offered to goddess Satvai (Mother Earth). The new mother does not back the west till the fifth day till the ritual of offering of the child and her (Mother Earth) completing the task of writing the life span of the child is over. If the mother backs the west she shows her displeasure about the birth of her child and invites the wrath of Satvai who kills the newborn. This belief is supported by ample evidence where the newborn and the mother have become victims of the wrath of Goddess Satvai (Mother Earth) as a result of breach of this taboo.

Preventive Rituals :

It is commonly believed that most of the prolonged illnesses seen in children is because of the effect of evil eye. To ward off the effect the Thakurs tie a string containing black and yellow beads on the wrist of the child. This is known as Dithmani. The black and yellow colour is believed to absorb/neutralize/ward off the effect of the evil eye. Similarly among the Mavchis a black thread (mangadhya) is tied around the neck of the child. It serves the same purpose. (Robin Tribhuwan and others; 1992).

For five days after childbirth the mother has to keep indoors, this is a preventive measure, she may become the victim of some evil spirit.

Cultural Norms Imposed on a Barren Woman :

A barren woman is not given the same treatment as a normal/fertile woman receives. Her biological incapability is her major handicap and this decides the type of treatment she received in her daily life and on auspicious occasions. She bears a social stigma.

Following are some restrictions laid on her as far as social interaction is concerned.

a. A barren woman is not allowed to enter the room where a woman is delivering a child. It is believed that the barren woman may cast an evil eye which carries with it jealousy and hatred. The child may fall ill or even die.

b. She is prohibited from attending auspicious occasions like birth ceremonies, naming ceremonies, marriage etc.

c. The shadow of a barren woman is not allowed to fall on a fertile woman as this may bring barrenness in the fertile woman.

d. Her presence in any promotive, productive and curative ritual as far as health is concerned is prohibited as she is considered unproductive. Thus she is an outsider at such times leading to a clear demarcation between sterility and fertility.

e. A barren woman is not allowed to wear kunku (red powder) in the parting of her hair. This kunku is symbolic of menstrual flow. Her not wearing kunku is symbolic of her not having menstrual flow. A widow puts a black dot on her forehead, this symbolically means she cannot have sex with anyone for she is the property of her dead husband.

Thus a barren woman does not enjoy good social and mental health in the field of social interactions. But when a barren woman dies, she is given a different burial treatment. The rites performed are dominant with fertility symbols and rituals so as to ensure her fertility in heaven.

Rites Performed on the Death of a Barren Woman :

A barren woman's dead body is royally treated and ritually blessed to ensure her fertility in heaven or in the life to come. Her body is first bathed and then wrapped in a green blouse and sari. A part of her sari is filled with dry fruits. This ritual is termed as 'oti bharne'. Her body is bathed with turmeric and dry copra. She is offered green bangles and kunku (red powder) is put in the parting of her hair.

Significance and Meanings Attached :

a. The wrapping of the green blouse, sari, offering of the green bangles and application of the turmeric symbolize the wish of the Thakurs that her soul should be a fertile bride in heaven.
b. The application of copra on her body also symbolizes her fertility in heaven. The Thakurs apply copra to a girls body when she attains puberty. This indicates that she has become fertile. A sterile/barren woman is also treated similarly as the ritual symbolize that she (her soul) is already menstruating and she is now fertile.
c. The putting of kunku in her hair is symbolic of the menstrual flow she is expected to have in heaven during her next birth.
d. The filling a part of her sari with dry fruits, the custom of 'oti bharne' is symbolic of blessing her womb so that she is fruitful.

The Thakurs believe that men are never sterile or incapable of procreation. This disorder occurs only in the women, and hence, women are socially blamed.

CHAPTER - IV

ILLNESS IDEOLOGY

Every culture, irrespective of its simplicity and complexity has its own beliefs and practices regarding health and disease, it does not work in a meaningless fashion. Every system of culture tries to treat diseases in its own way. The treatment of the disease varies from one group to another. (Choudhari B. 1986 : 289).

Interpretations of the cause of a given disease depends much on the native's perceptions of the pathogenic agent or force responsible for the cause, the cultural situation or context in which the condition of ill-health has occurred, and the degree of disruption of a patients relationship with the pathogenic agents.

Interpretations of the origin and cause of illness starts the family level, with initial diagnosis to search for meanings. Suggestions and suspections regarding the possible origin and cause of illness is contributed by family elders, relatives, friends and village elders. Their suspections are confirmed by the Medical practitioners, who use culturally recognized methods of diagnosis to track the origin and cause of illness.

Disease Causation Concepts

Disease etiology is an important indigenous medical phenomena, of any community and precisely stems out from the meaning system (culture). It becomes a guiding principle for attributing an origin and cause of a disease to the intervention of a given pathogenic agent and there by in making decision to choose ethnomedical therapy.

The causes for different ailments or diseases as attributed by Thakurs from their point of view are as follows :

1. Possession of evil spirit.
2. Sexual intercourse with spirits.
3. Sexual intercourse with menstruating women.
4. Evil eye.
5. Witchcraft and Sorcery.
6. Disruption of human relationship with ancestral spirits.
7. Disruption of human relationship with cosmic entities and forces.
8. Disruption of the relationship of Thakurs with other tribes and caste groups.

9. Failure to perform divine duty.
10. Deviance from cultural set norms and order of house construction/ design.
11. Loss of basic bodily equilibrium due to entry of excessive heat or cold in the body.
12. Breach of social pollution taboos.
13. Disruption of man's relationship with the flora and fauna.
14. Wrong combination of diet.
15. Disruption of man's relationship with his deities.

1. Possession of Evil Spirits

Every human society believes in the existence of good and evil spirits who are directly or indirectly responsible for causing illness. Evil spirits taking control of body, mind and soul is a very common phenomena observed in ethnomedical accounts. This section of the data chapter highlights the Thakur concept of human body as a spiritual symbol.

The Thakur's believe that if a bachelor or a spinster dies, his or her soul does not go to heaven but moves on the earth troubling and causing illness to human beings. On enquiring with many Thakur's as to why these spirits are left on the Earth to trouble people, they said both spinsters and bachelors do not go through the process of marriage, their sexual desires are not fulfilled, they do not get inner joy of rearing children and establishing home.

The souls of such cases become evil spirits and move on the earth to trouble living beings. It is also believed that if a woman who dies during her delivery, does not go to heaven but, stays on the earth because of her attachment and love for her child.

Evil Spirit that attack the human body

The Thakurs classify three types of evil spirits namely, Munja, Khais and Hadeli.

The spirits of the bachelors, spinsters and mothers who die during delivery are believed to take the form of these evil spirits which do not go to heaven but remain on the earth to trouble human beings.

Chaphekar L.N. (1960:91) has also reported about the nature of these spirits.

a. Munja

A Munja is a white skinned male evil spirit with a long staff. His staff has a bell (ghungru) at the anterior end. Munja always keeps a blanket (ghongdi) on his shoulder. He wears a white loin cloth round his waist and a shirt (bundi). He moves in the jungle.

b. Khais

A Khais is a tall and a blue-black coloured male evil spirit. He does not wear a shirt. He puts a loin cloth round his waist. He is a strong wrestler. He mostly troubles women and strong men. His feet are of reversed type i.e. the heels are in the front and the toes behind. He loves tobacco, liquor, non-vegetarian food and of course blood.

c. Hadeli

A Hadeli is a female evil spirit, dark skinned with long hair (kept open) and has hair all over her body. The open hair and the presence of lot of hair on the body are symbolic to the Hadeli's urge to have sex or of being a loose character woman. She wears a green sari which symbolizes her desire to be a bride while she was a human being.

These three spirits namely, Munja, Khais and Hadeli live and move in the jungle during the nights. They are also believed to be very active during the new moon (Amosha) and full moon (Poornima) nights. The Peepal tree (Ficus religiosa) and banyan tree (Ficus Benjamina) are the abodes of these spirits.

Types of Illness caused

The evil spirits are believed to cause two types if illness namely,

1. Temporary illness by which a person is able to survive.
2. Permanent type of which a person is killed and discarded from the world of human beings.

Temporary Possession

The Thakur's believe that temporary illness causes neurotic tension to the patient. He or she behaves abnormally. The symptoms of a person possessed with evil spirits are headache, fever, shivering and abnormal behaviour.

In the case of temporary illness the evil spirits demand things like coconut, meat or blood. The Bhagat (Shaman) is consulted if one is suspected of having possessed by evil spirits.

He then talks ritually to the spirits and enquires why he got hold of the patient. On finding out his demands he is given the required things so that he leaves the person. Temporary possession does not cause a patient much harm as does the permanent possession.

Permanent Possession

The second type of possession is a category which reveals the analysis of Thakur concepts of spirit possession. Diseases such as albinism and congenital deformities which are scientifically considered as genetic disorders are socio-culturally interpreted by the Thakurs as a result of sexual contact of an evil spirit with a woman who gives birth to an albino or a congenitally deformed baby.

2. Sexual Intercourse with Evil Spirits

The concept of albinism

The Thakurs believe that an albino child is born as a result of sexual intercourse of a woman who gives birth to it with a male evil spirit named Munja. A Munja is a white skinned evil spirit, whose soul does not migrate to heaven for his desire to go through and enjoy family life, sex, desire to rear children is not fulfilled. Hence he troubles women mostly.

It is believed that a Munja picks up a woman who is sleeping next to her husband, has sex and as a result a albino child which is white skinned (abnormal like a Munja) is born. Sometimes he may attack a woman in the jungle and do the needful. Illness episodes have revealed that Munja at times takes the form of the woman's husband and has sex with her. Thus the body of an albino shows dominant genetical trait of a Munja.

A Thakur believes that the soul, body and the mind of an albino totally belongs and resembles to a Munja. It is different from the human bodily order and is classified into evil bodily order.

Since the albinos are considered as offsprings of Munja, he can be harmful both to the woman and the Thakur society, after all he falls into the evil category.

To get rid of this evil one, the Suine (midwife) with the permission of the family head, kills the child by putting a basket smeared with cowdung on the albino child, pointing his or her head towards the evil south and leaving him to die of suffocation.

When it gets dark, the Suine along with one or two male members of the family bury's the child. Out of the 20 midwives which were interviewed informally for 3-4 sessions, nineteen have reported that they have killed at least five to six albino children. On enquiring as to why the children are killed the midwives gave the following explanation -

1. On the fifth day at 12 in the afternoon when the Sun God is right above our head, Goddess Satvai who resides in the West and who is the Goddess of Fortune and fertility is worshipped.

The very same night at 12'o clock, she comes to visit the child and writes his fortune on the forehead. This action symbolizes the starting point of the child's life as a member of the Thakur society.

Since this Goddess is the most supreme power who writes fortune of the people and also has the right to take their life (atma), she is also responsible for the formation of foetus in the mother's womb. On the fifth day when she comes to visit them, the house is cleaned and smeared with cowdung. Menstruating women, if any, are sent out of the house. There is no sign of uncleanliness. The way is thus made to welcome theholy one.

Now, the albino is an offspring of the evil spirit. The holy and the most supreme Goddess Satvai and the evil cannot come together. They are two separate entities, one is holy (Satvai) associated with life and the other is evil (munja) associated with death. To avoid the meeting points of evil and good which are binary oppositions the albino child is killed.

2. Since these albinos are considered to be the children of Munja (the evil one) they can be harmful to both, the mother and the Thakur society as such. The rationalisation here is that living Thakurs can only interact with other living Thakurs and the ancestral spirits can interact only with good ancestors. The living ones cannot therefore have any social interactions with the evil dead (Munja) which is an intermediary phase between life on earth and life in heaven.

Here, the question arises as to why a basket is used to kill albino children. The interpretation given by the midwives goes as follows - for five days a child born is kept in a basket which is not smeared with cowdung. The Satvai has control over it for five days. On the fifth day the Satvai is worshipped in order that she writes the fortune of the child and gives the charge of the child to the respective family. In the situation, the dorsal posture of the basket is exposed to light with the child's head pointing towards all other directions except the evil south, symbolizes the continuity of its life whereas the upside down posture of the basket with cowdung smeared on it, covering the child creates darkness, pointing the child's head to the evil south symbolizes death.

The act of turning the basket upside down demarcates a clear cut line between life and death, between good (Holy Satvai) and the evil (Munja).

Congenital Deformities

In cases or instances where the child is born with severe deformity, such children are considered to be the offsprings of Khais as they are deformed and are black in colour. In this case also the Khais has sexual intercourse with a women similar to that of Munja, and hence the similar practice is followed to kill the khais' child too.

Chaphekar (1960) also reports the killing of such children but does not answer what meanings are associated with these practices. The midwives have certain criteria to recognize that the child is an offspring of the evil spirits which are as follows :

1. While the child is being delivered the place smells of meat.
2. The child has teeth/tooth which he uses to bite.
3. The child is deformed.
4. Thr frontal bone is hard.
5. The woman finds it difficult to deliver because sometimes the child's head is too big.
6. The child's colour is white (albino) or black like the khais with severe deformity.

The umbilical cord if such children is not buried near the house for the act of burying the umbilical chordis symbolic of the child's attachment to the family, house and the village in which he is born.

The placental waste, umbilical chord is buried along with the dead body of the child, thereby symbolizing the detachment of the evil with the living good.

Symbolic Aspects of Albinism & Congenital Deformities:

The entire set of normative actions and ritualistic behaviour that the Thakurs associate with excommunicating/getting rid of albino and congenitally deformed children, are seen very much as meaningful and rational by the Thakurs. Their conceptions about albinism and congenital deformity cross cuts into other domains of their social life. Given below are some examples of domains which are cross cut by concepts albinism and congenital deformity.

1. *Marriage* :

It is common belief among the Thakurs that the soul of a married person goes to heaven. However, bachelor's and spinster's souls are not admitted heaven for they are believed to be thirsty souls of the worldly pleasures. They believe that the soul of a bachelor and/or spinster does not migrate to heaven but it dwells on earth for it has not enjoyed the married life.

2. *Sex* :

Marriage is a prerequisite of having sex and therefore the Thakurs get their children married at avery early age. A person who dies without getting married his soul does not go to heaven, it stays on the earth and becomes evil for it has not had an opportunity to enjoy sexual life which was possible only through marriage. Since their desires are not fulfilled they attack women to have sex and hence albinos and congenitally deformed offsprings are born.

3. *Evil Spirits* :

The concepts of albinism and congenital deformity also expresses the Thakur concepts of different types of spirits, who have sexual intercourse with women and thereby produces deformed children. Munja and khais are the two male evil spirits, while Hadeli is a female evil spirit.

4. *Body Deformity* :

Albinism and congenital deformity is associated with deformity and abnormality of the human body. The Thakurs compare human body with universe which is pure and holy. The bodies of albino and congenitally and deformed children haveno form and hence it is evil and associated with darkness and hell.

5. *Concept of Soul* :

This behaviour also reflects the Thakur concepts of souls. The good souls that go to heaven and the bad souls which take the form of evil spirits and remain on the earth to trouble people.

6. *Concepts of Jati* :

Illness episodes have projected the Thakur ideology of Jati or caste conceptions. In many cases the Thakurs attribute the male evil spirits to a Jati group (kathkari, Mahar, Mang or Muslim). It would be narrated in the episode that a Muslim Munja (male evil spirit) picked up a Thakur woman, made her unconscious and had sex with her and hence a Munja (albino) was born.

7. *Death* :

What is considered to be evil or a product of evil (Albinism and Congenitally deformed offspring) should be sent to the evil world and cannot grow with good (human beings). Thakurs therefore kill their children either by choking their throats or by using suffocation method by putting a basket smeared with cowdung and leaving the child to die of suffocation.

8. *Rituals of Fortune* :

The Thakurs perform rituals of fortune on the fifth day after the delivery. This ritual is performed in order to offer the child to mother Earth (Satvai) who writes the fortune of the child in the night. In case of Albinos and congenital deformed children this becomes impossible.

9. *Killing of Albinos and Congenitally Deformed Children:*

The action of killing the albino and congenitally deformed children although is legally not permitted according to the law, the Thakurs still kill these infants and bury them during the nights to save their skin from the cops. They feel that taking the risk of killing the infant is more important and meaningful than to let it grow and invite trouble for the mother, her husband and the society at large. They take this risk because they see a meaningful logic in performing these actions.

10. *Body Purification* :

A woman who delivers an albino or a congenital deformed child is considered to be physically polluted by the male evil spirit. Hence rituals are performed to remove the entire evil effect that is in her. Her abdomen is pressed to remove the blood (symbol of evil). Her breast milk is squeezed out. She is given bath everyday for 12 days and before she has the first sexual contact she takes bath, applies charmed ash from the hearth on her forehead and lights an incense stick. This way her body getspurified. Water, ash again symbolize agents of purification in this context.

11. *Conflict with Other Social Groups* :

In real social life the Thakurs categorize the Kathkaris (a neighbouring tribe) the Mahars, Mangs and Chamars (the untouchables castes) and the Muslims, lower than the Thakur in social hierarchy. This is because of their dietary habits. Kathkaris eat rats, goose, monkeys, owl, dead cattle etc, while the "cow and bull" (considered holy by the Thakurs) also find a place in their diet.

This conflict of purity and pollution that exists at social level is expressed by the Thakurs at spiritual level in their belief that the evil spirits of Mahars, Mangs, Chamars, Kathkaris and Muslims have sexual intercourse with Thakurs women as a results of which congenitally deformed children and albinos are born. The concept of albinos and congenital deformity of the Thakurs express their hatred, conflict with the above said social groups.

3. Sexual Intercourse with Menstruating Woman

Tribal concepts of menstrual blood and associated behaviour have been differently interpreted by various anthropologists. Mead (1938, 1940) in her account of the Mountain Arapesh of New Guinea and Ian Hogbin's first account (1935-5) of the Neighbouring Wageo point out that menstrual blood is dangerous and menstruation strengthens the woman because it is a means of discharging from the female body the dangerous fluids received from the opposite sex during intercourse.

Douglas (1970, 1975) highlights behavioural concepts which the tribal folk associate with menstruation and also their concepts of purity, pollution, male superiority over females, the social differences between males and females, rites of purification and so on. Thus it is clearly visible that meanings which the tribal associate with menstrual behaviour cross cut structures of other social domains and thus this behaviour becomes meaningful to the natives from an emic perspective.

Menstrual blood according to the Thakurs is dark, evil, hot and corrosive (with reference to the penis) and is thus impure and considered a pollutant. Due to the above qualities attributed to the menstrual blood, it is believed (by the Thakurs) man having sex with a menstruating woman comes in contact with the pollutant (menstrual blood) which spoils his blood and his body starts degenerating and becomes deformed. Similarly food cooked by a menstruating woman if consumed by a man or woman leads to their being inflicted with leprosy. Sexual intercourse with women of other types castes and even prostitutes causes leprosy and sexually transmitted diseases according to the Thakurs.

Thus Thakurs adopt certain preventive measures. The menstruating woman is a social outcast for the menstruating period. She does not perform any household nor occupational activities. She does not interact with either the family or tribal community. She is given food in separate dishes. After the menstrual period is over she goes to the river takes a bath, bows in the eastern direction, comes home, lights an incense stick and is then free to interact with the family and the community. For more details refer episode no. 29.

4. Evil Eye (Drishti Lagne) :

The "evil eye" belief - primarily means that someone can cause harm by just looking at a another's property or at any other person. This is found in many parts of the world, though not all of it. (Maloney C. 1972:V). Some people might think of this belief as simple a superstition or classify it among the occults, but what is one person's superstition of occults, is another person's belief or religion. Anthropologically we try to understand what is meant by an evil eye belief, who casts the evil, who/what can it strike, under what circumstances and why how such apparently strange superstition arise and how does it fit into the social and cultural systems and why does it persist in so many different parts of the world today.

The features which are common to the belief of the evil eye in most ethnomedical accounts seem to be limited to the following points -

i. power emanates from the eye/mouth and strikes some object or person.
ii. the struck object is of value and its destruction or injury is sudden.

iii. the person who has cast the evil eye may be oblivious that he has caused the destruction.
iv. the affected may not be able to identify the source of the power (evil).
v. the effect of the evil eye can be detected or its effect modified/ mollified or complete cure is possible by particular rituals, devices or symbols.
vi. the belief helps to explain or rationalize sudden sickness, misfortune, loss of possession such as animals or crops. (Adams & Rubel 1967; Barth 1956; Elworthy 1895; Foster 1972 & 1965; Gifford 1958; Hastings 1908; Maclagan 1902; Meerloo 1971; Schock 1966; Seligman 1910 & 1922; Simon 1973; Spooner 1970 and Vuorela 1967).

Whether or not it may be accounted universally,the evil eye is a wide spread phenomenon. It is an element of symbolic and religious system. (Spooner 1972 : 279). The Thakurs explain -

i. the actors responsible for casting the evil eye.
ii. the target / victim.
iii. the source/power which casts the evil eye.
iv. the reason why it is cast.
v. beliefs concerned with evil eye highlights relationship of the tribe with other neighbouring tribes and caste groups.
vi. also highlights the manner in which this belief operates in their cultural situation / context.
vii. the rituals/precautions taken to ward off the effect of the evil eye.

Persons/Actors Responsible for Casting the Evil Eye :

In depth interviews conducted with the heads of house holds (above 45 years) revealed that the following persons could be normally responsible for casting the evil eye.

1. Vanjuti (barren woman) :

A barren woman is believed to cast an evil eye on the fertile women and their children due to her biological inability to bear children. Thus a vanjuti is given a lower status in the society hence the cause for jealousy.

Her unfulfilled desire to bear children forces her to perform actions which bring harm to the health of fertile women and children. The Thakurs believe that her barreness itself is converted into an evil power which is used to harm the newly born, newly wedded girls and new mothers. Thus barren women become socially stigmatized and are not allowed to participate in many social rituals, functions etc. Thus her frustration often becomes the cause for her jealousy and she casts evil eye and/or becomes bhutali (witch).

2. Bhutali (Witch) :

The witch or the bhutali is endowed with a special evil power to cast an evil eye and cause harm to anybody. She is believed to perform two roles.

i. cast evil eye.

ii. perform black magic or rituals of destruction.

According to the Thakurs most of the witches (Bhutali) are widows who do not enjoy a married life like other women. Some of them may be Bhagatins (female shamans) who give up practicing good, (white) medicine and take up black magic. Thus 'white medicine' implies in this context the giving up of preventive, promotive and curative measures of medicine and taking up or adopting black magic which brings about destruction.

Bhutala (Sorcerer) :

A sorcerer or Bhutala is a person specialized in performing black magic or rituals of destruction to harm people's health. He has special power which he emits from his eye and casts evil eye to bring harm.

Members of Lower Tribes and Castes :

According to Thakur's social hierarchy neighbouring tribes like Kathkaris and caste groups such as Mangs, Mahars, Chamars and Muslims are lower to them. The Thakurs interact with them in the market places, fields, rivers etc. The Thakurs believe that members of these groups are also at times responsible for the evil eye which causes harm to the health of the Thakurs. Thus the Thakur concept of evil eye also throws lights on their social hierarchy and interaction with other groups.

Enemies :

Where there are friends, there are enemies - says the Thakur. Conflicts, fights, heated arguments are part of social interaction and interpersonal communication. When sickness, fever or ill-health among children is observed following a conflict/fight etc, the cause is immediately attributed to the casting of an evil eye by the opponents/rival.

General Category :

Under this category any person who is jealous of the Thakur's property, health, good hunt, talent, personality, food etc casts an evil eye. Here the main motive is hatred, envy or jealousy.

The Source of Power from Where the Evil Eye is Cast :

Every society believes in the existence of malevolent and benevolent spirits. The benevolent spirits are responsible for luck, happiness, peace and the good happenings whereas the former are responsible for unhappiness, troubles, misfortune illness. Thus they have evil power with them.

The Thakurs believe that the person/actor responsible for the evil eye gets the power from the following sources.

i. Dith Bhut : The evil spirit of "Drishti" (evil eye).
ii. Evil Spirits : Munja, Khais, Pisha, Hadeli are some of evil spirits from whom power is drawn to cast an evil eye.
iii. Rakshas (giants) of the south : The Thakurs believe that there are giants residing in the south which give evil power to cast an evil eye.
iv. The magicator the evil look : Chaphekar (1960) points out that new born on whose eyes blood falls while the umbilical chord is being cut grow up with the power to cast evil eye. Such people are believed to be empowered right from birth.

The Reasons for Who And Why Does He/She Become Victims Of Evil Eye :

The analysis of the Thakurs concepts of evil eye points out that any person who has material possession like clothes, television, radio, watch, food etc or who is healthy, doing well in his occupation, has a good crop or a person who is healthy, talented or a woman who is fertile generally become victims of evil eye.

Thus putting in a nutshell the whole concept of evil eye rests on the presence of two groups i. the haves ii. the have-nots.

As is evident the haves become the targets of the have-nots. The operation of evil eye and its effect is however interpreted simultaneously depending on the contribution rendered from family, elders, village elders, relatives, friends and the medical specialists dealing with the effect.

The Bond Between Social Relationships And Evil Eye :

The belief regarding the evil eye and its execution within a social context reveals the Thakurs concepts of social hierarchy, social interaction, relationships and the conflicts within and with other social groups. Thus the Thakurs firmly believe that the Kathkari (neighbouring tribe) and other lower caste groups like the Mangs, Mahars, Chamars and Muslims etc are experts in casting the evil eye and are believed to frequently cast evil eye on the Thakurs. This does not mean that the Thakurs spare their own brethren. Even within the tribe there are people (as discussed above) who cast evil eye.

The upper caste groups such as Brahmans, Marathas, Agris, Gujrathis, Kunbis, Mahadeo Kolis, Dhangars, Sutars, Lohars, Kannadis are classified as Dev Jatis (God like jatis/groups) and often attribute the casting of evil eye and the practice of witchcraft and sorcery to the members of the Davanjati (Rakshas/giant like groups) like the Mahar, Mang, Chamar, Wadari, Muslim caste, Thakurs & Kathkari tribe.

The existence of the social hierarchy gives rise to social difference in the greater interactional system (i.e. there is interaction between the members of the Dev Jati and Davan Jati) and highlights the social conflict which often expresses through the evil eye and which is remedied at a spiritual level. The various rituals performed to ward off the evil eye effect or nullify the evil eye effect are highlighted in the chapter 'Ritual Healing'.

5. Witchcraft and Sorcery :

Witchcraft is the term used in general discussion to cover all forms of supernatural influence bringing illness, misfortune or death to its victims (Wintrob R.M. 1973:320). The essential belief is that any individual jealous of another's achievements, advantages or abilities whether in love, business or politics can arrange an evil spell to be cast on the adversary. To do this the perpetuator must consult an intermediary, knowledgeable about supernatural phenomena through whose skill and for a suitable fee the spell will be effectively placed.

These intermediaries are called witch doctors, sorcerers, medicine men, shamans, Ju-Ju men, native healers, houhgans, root workers, bush doctors etc.. Such people are considered equally effective in removal of spells and treatment of victims of witchcraft and sorcery and in casting of spells (Wintrob R.M. 1973:320)

To cast the spell, items belonging to or representative of the victim are brought to the intermediary. An article of clothing, hair or nail, excreta, umbilical chord, earth over which he has recently walked or a carved image, a doll, or a lime symbolizing the victim (Wintrob 1973:320, Middleton and Winter 1963, Evans Pritchard 1937, Marwick Max 1952, Reynolds Barrie 1963, Turner 1967, Douglas 1963).

When Evans Pritchard first made the distinction between witchcraft and sorcery, he clearly intended to define the same in Zande culture (1937, 21). Azande believe that a witch performs no rite, utters no spell and possess no medicines. An act of witchcraft is a psychic act. But the sorcerers do it by performing magic rites with bad medicine. Witchcraft in short, may be unconscious and involuntary though it is often intentional, inherited and inherent. Sorcery, on the other hand is always conscious and voluntary, is taught and often bought. Witchcraft operates directly and sorcery indirectly through spells, rites and medicines. This dichotomy verbalized and explicit among the Zande is not made in many societies. The concept of witchcraft and sorcery differs from one community to another.

The Thakurs believe that both, witches (Bhutali) and the sorcery (Bhutala) intentionally or consciously cast black magic spells to harm or kill an individual.

1. Both Bhutala and Bhutali use charmed objects such as nagli grains (Elevane coracana), Vari grains (Panicum mallicea), bones of dogs, goats and human beings which are by magic placed in the body of the victim in order to harm/kill him/her (refer episode nos. 2, 3, & 4).
2. Besides placing charmed objects, rituals of destruction are performed by chanting evil mantras to bring about misfortune, trouble, illness or even death to the victims by Thakurs witches and saucers.
3. Also,it is believed by the Thakurs that a tasteless powder or decoction ritually prepared may be sipped into the food/drink of the intended victim so that he succumbs to the spell - often the victim develops pain, vomiting, diarrhea, intense tumors and at times agitated destructive behaviour. The effect of the spell is that he may suffer a sudden bad crop, rejected by the spouse/lover, unexpected political downfall and aat times the spell may be fatal.
4. In order to cast a magic spell items belonging or representative of the intended victim are brought to the Bhutala to Bhutali. Articles, clothing, hair locks, nails, stained clothes of a menstruating woman, umbilical chord, blouse stained with breast milk, blood urine, excreta or a carved image of the victim are used.

   Thus the Bhutala or the Bhutali perform rituals of destruction to harm the victim. All articles brought are symbolic of the victim.
5. The most effective form of black magic prevalent in the Thakur belief system is known as "Muth Marne". Here the Bhutala uses a charmed lemon as a missile to harm or kill the victim. (Chaphekar 1960 : 90). After careful scrutiny, it was discovered that the Bhutalas are the one who perform this ritual.

A Bhagat (shaman) was asked why a lemon is chosen as a missile, he answered the lemon symbolizes the atma (soul) of the victim.

The Bhutala gathers thorns of any tree growing in the south direction (Rakshas disha - evil direction) and recites chants of the destruction and pierces the lemon with the thorns. The act of facing the south direction symbolizes the appeal Bhutala makes to resident evil spirits to give him the power to kill. The insertion or piercing of thorns in the lemon symbolizes the killing of the soul of the victim as the lemon is symbolic of the soul.

The Bhagat was asked what would be his role if a patient who had a victim of the "Muth Marne" ritual came to him. The Bhagat replied if the patient seeks help before the ritual or while the ritual is going on he (Bhagat) has the power to turn the same missile to destroy the sorcerer and thus save the patient (victim). He also added that sorcerer performs such rituals in the night in secret places.

Chaphekar points out that witchcraft is generally practiced by old women. If the villagers are convinced that an evil act is the doing of an old witch, they take measures, decided by the Panchayat (Village Committee) to put an end to her wicked activities. Her tongue is pierced and she is forced to drink water of a tannery (Chaphekar 1960 : 138,139).

An interesting episode goes as follows. Padu Dore of Thakurwadi had four buffaloes and to his dismay he discovered that his buffaloes were giving less milk lately. He doubted that someone had cast a spell on his buffaloes. To confirm his doubt one night he stayed awake and watched his buffaloes. To his surprise at about 1 p.m. a calf suddenly appeared and suckled the buffaloes. The next day he consulted the Bhagatin (female shaman) of his own village. She instructed him accordingly. The next night also Mr. P. D. stayed awake and kept a vigilant watch. At about 1 p.m. a calf appeared and began to suckle. Mr. P.D. hit hard with a hard staff (musal) on the back of the calf which ran in the direction of the Kathkari hamlet making noise/screaming like a woman.

The following day Mr. P.D. consulted theBhagatin who ritually found out that the buffaloes' milk was being suckled by a Kathkari Bhutali (witch). It was soon discovered that the Kathkari Bhutali was suffering from a severe backache (as a result of Mr. P.D.'s hard blow on the back on the previous night). Mr. P.D. along with his sons had a fight with the Kathkari Bhutali and her son. She confessed and assured him that she would stop this practice.

Chaphekar (1960:176) reports a case where a village was infected by an epidemic of guinea worms. A Thakur village had employed a Muslim to caste an evil spell on the village. Thus the Thakurs believe that Kathkaris, Mangs, Mahars, Chamars and Muslims who are lower in social hierarchy cast evil spell on the Thakurs to hurt or to kill them. The reigning motive behind these evil spells are hatred, jealousy, envy etc.

The Thakur concept of witchcraft and sorcery projects the social status and roles of witches, sorcerers and also reflects the Thakurs ideology of social relationship, hierarchical gradation, interaction and social conflicts within and outside the tribe with members of other caste groups residing in Karjat region.

6. Disruption of Human Relationships with Ancestral Spirits :

Ancestor worship amongst the Thakurs deserves to be noted (Chaphekar, 1960:89). The male ancestor spirit is known as "Supali". The Thakurs believe that all their ancestors (vad-vadil) are in heaven (swarg) which is in the east. During "Pitra Amosha" (new moon night) in Bhadrapad (August-September) the Thakurs stay awake and perform the Dhambdi Dance all through the night. The Dhambdi dance is performed by the older folk to invoke the ancestral spirits. It is believed that the ancestral spirits come down to visit and dine with the Thakurs. The next day the spirits move about in the Thakur hamlets.

The next day the Thakurs prepare food and some of it is thrown in the eastern direction. Some of the food is placed on the eastern part of the roof. Throwing the food in the eastern direction symbolizes offering the food to the ancestral spirits which reside in the eastern direction. The food placed on the roof if eaten by crows signifies that the spirits have visited the house and are happy with all the members. Thus the Thakurs share a close relationship with the ancestral spirits and there is harmony between the two.

Failure to satisfactorily perform any ritual concerned with the worship of ancestral spirits such as failure in offering food, liquor, tobacco, bidis, etc means inviting warth and troubles of the ancestral spirits. Ancestral spirits are believed to cause illness due to disturbance of the family member's relationship with them (refer episode no. 23).

Illness in some cultural situations or contexts as interpreted by the Thakurs as an expression of the disruption of the relationship which exists between them and the ancestral spirits. Thus through the health behaviour of the Thakurs the inter-relationship between the Thakurs and their ancestral spirits is easily and clearly understood.

7. Disruption of Human Relationship with Cosmic Entities and Forces :

Whatever the natural aspects of space, it is like every other part of the nature, given meaningful configuration in the culture of any people and different people construct space differently to a greater or lesser degree. The cultural patterns of different societies offer different means by which special perceptions are developed, refined and ordered. The spatial concepts of different societies also vary with respect to the degree of abstraction attained. (Hallowell, 1955).

Human beings live in a meaningful universe, not a world of bare physical objects. (Hallowell, 1942). Interpretation of the cosmic entities and the forces differs from one society to another. For instance, the belief that sun, moon and earth are creators and/or supreme powers is prevalent among many Indian tribes (Vidyarthi and Rai, 1985:242).

Hallowell (1955) describes vividly and clearly the way in which the saulteaux, a North American Indian Tribe, conceive of space, the way in which they order it and the way in which that ordering in turn becomes a part of their experience of it. Within the cosmos certain spiritual entities both (good and evil) are given specific location highlighting nature's concept of direction symbolism (Parson Elsie, 1939 : I, 98-99); (Alexander 1916 : 286-287); (Hallowell 1955 : 184-202).

In order to understand the Thakur conception regarding their disruption with cosmic entities and cosmological forces, it is very necessary to probe into their belief system and interpretation of how they perceive the space, the entities and forces in it and their relationship.

a. Human Body and Universe :

Thakurs believe that the human body is nothing but an image of the cosmos. They correlate the ten openings of the body namely eyes, nostrils, ears, mouth, atma (soul), wrist pulse, Naval, urethral/vaginal opening, pulse of the feet and the anal opening to the ten planets. These planets are referred to as 'Baya' (sisters of mother earth). The earth is positioned at the fifth position in the hierarchical gradation of the planets. The Thakurs believe that if they misbehave or deviate from the divine norms, these planetary spirits visit their body and cause skin diseases such as smallpox, chicken pox, measles, boils etc. These diseases are interpreted sometimes as the visitation of the "Baya" to mother Earth. Since the soul (atma) is also positioned at the fifth position it is a symbol of Mother Earth, who is visited by all these planetary spirits.

In another ritual that is the ritual of soul migration which is performed on the 9th day in case of a married female and 10th day in the case of a married male, 7th day in the case of bachelors and spinsters after their death. Ten rice flour balls are released ritually in the river water by a close relative of the dead person. These ten rice balls are symbols of the ten planetary spirits including Earth, which merge into the universe after the death of a person. This ritual is discussed in detail in the body symbolism chapter.

Even the entire body physiology and anatomy according to the Thakurs is governed and controlled by cosmic elements namely, 1. Light - Tej, 2. Fire - Agni, 3. Wind - Vara, 4. Water - Pani, and 5. Earth - Dantari

They believe that life giving fluids such as blood, milk, semen are the products of the water and food juices. Food is pushed in the stomach with the help of wind (vara). Blood circulates in the body because of the wind. A person is able to excrete due to pressure created by the wind in the intestine. Food is digested and converted into juices which are further converted into blood, urine and sweat due to Agni (fire) and water which help to boil the solid food to liquid form (juices) which are assimilated in the body in the form of blood and waster juices into urine and sweat. Water which is taken into the body keeps the body organs alive. The light which is present in the eyes helps the Thakurs to see things. A blind person does not have light (Tej) in his eyes.

Blood circulates in the body in an anticlockwise (right) way. Anticlockwise movement is considered to be an auspicious movement, because the sun moves in an anticlockwise manner from east to west, so does the moon and the clouds and wind. The whole cosmos according to the Thakurs moves in an anticlockwise fashion. Most rituals therefore reflect or express the anticlock movement.

Besides the role of cosmic elements in governing and controlling the body physiology and anatomy. The worship of cosmos and the objects in it is a very common phenomena among the Thakurs. The Sun, moon and water are considered to be brothers while lightening and Holi (Goddess of Fire) are sisters. Mother Earth (Dantari) has nine sisters (Baya) planetary spirits. All these are supreme most powers. The sun is the most powerful of the above said entities. If these powers are not worshipped or given due recognition, they cause illness.

Thakurs are supposed to maintain good relationship with the cosmological entities and forces in order to maintain good health. The moment there is disharmony orimbalance in their relationship with these forces or entities, it is likely that misfortune or illness is invited. Besides good cosmic entities and forces there are evil forces also in the cosmos that dwell in the south (Rakshas (Giant) disha). These evil spirits and forces cause illness and death.

Good cosmic forces are more powerful than the evil cosmic forces and spirits. Thakurs therefore maintain a good relationship with the good forces. During the marriage rite twigs of Ficus glomerata and Tectona grandis are tied to a pole. The Ficus glomerata symbolizes the moon while Tectona symbolizes the sun. These objects are symbolically brought into the marriage ritual to ward off evil forces that my cause harm or bring about trouble during auspicious occasions. In many instances good cosmic spirits are given due respect and play a curative, preventive or a promotive role as far as the health of the Thakurs is concerned. The moment human beings become dishonest and unfaithful to these entities and forces, they bring about trouble and misfortune. Refer illness episodes 5, 13, 19, 26, 28 for more details and body symbolism chapter. Thakurs hence have set ideas about the order of cosmos which means good health and disorder expresses their ideology of illness and misfortune due to the disruptions of their relationship with the cosmos.

Directional Symbolism and Spatial Orientation :

East is considered to be the direction of life because the sun rises from there. North is believed to be holy as it is the abode of Gods, West is auspicious as the earth dwells towards the west opposite the sun. Most rituals (Auspicious) are performed facing the east, north or west. These rituals may include rituals of marriage, child birth, fertility, hunting, healing and so on. The south is an inauspicious and evil direction for the Thakurs as it is inhabited with evil forces and giants. The Thakurs do not point their heads towards south and sleep for it is believed south is meant only to point the head of a dead person while burying him.

Elsie Clews Parsons reported that the Pueblo Indians usually avoid sleeping with the head in the orientation given the dead in burial (1939; I, 98-99).

A similar belief Hallowell (1955) pointed out concepts of sauteaux the directional flow of wind from the north in a myth by stating the evil action brought forth by winds flowing from the north. On the contrary, the Thakurs believe that wind flowing from south bring about misfortune and sickness. The directional ordering of the Thakur spatial universe, therefore, is one that penetrates into other spheres of social life.

8. Disruption of Thakur Relationship with Other Tribes and Caste Groups :

Illness episodes and the in depth interviews have shown that sickness in certain cultural contexts occurs as a result of disruption of the Thakur relationship with other tribes and castes. As any folk society tends to interact with other social groups inhabiting around it so also the Thakurs interact with other tribes and caste groups inhabiting around their settlements.

Infact, a Thakur defines his social world around him into two categories of social groups (jatis) namely Dev (God like) jatis and Davan (evil/giant) jatis. The Dev jatis includes following caste groups. The Brahmin, Gujrathis, Maratha, Kunbis, Agris, Dhangars, Malis, Lohars, Sutars, Mahadeo Kolis, Kannadas and the Nhavis while the Davan jatis include Thakurs, Mahars, Chamars, Mangs, Muslims and Kathkaris. There is a general belief that the members of Davan jatis practice witchcraft and sorcery, cast evil eye and harm or kill people using destructive rituals. The members of Davan jati are also believed to cause social pollution and bring about illness. For instance a member of Davan jati is not allowed to participate or even cast his shadow in a healing rite of the Marathas and Brahmins.

The Thakurs believe that the social groups which are lower to them in hierarchy cause illness and bring about misfortunes to them. Illness episodes have shown that how evil spirits of the Kathkari tribe trouble the Thakurs and likewise the evil spirits of Muslims (ref. episode nos. 14, 15 & 46). They also believe that lunar and solar eclipses are caused because their Gods, the Sun and Moon are blocked by the spirits of Mang and Mahar caste group. These spirits try to swallow the God (Moon and Sun) of the Thakurs (ref. episode no. 8).

The very word "Dev" which means God is given to the "Devjati" who are very much superior to the Thakurs in all aspects. The Thakurs depend on the Brahmins for important rites such as wedding rite, death etc. for ration, clothing, loans, employments etc on other "Devjatis". The "Devjatis" are like Gods for the Thakurs since they depend on the "Devjatis" for many reasons.

Thakurs owe a lot to the "Devjatis" at the social level. These gratitudes to the "Devjatis" are expressed to them in the healing rite normally "Jagran" in which the planetary spirits "Baya" are believed to take the form of "Devjatis" and visit the body of a Thakur. The names of these "Baya" reflect the caste name and they are Brahmani Baya, Gujrathi Baya, Marathi Baya, Kolani Baya, Agarni Baya, Kannadi Baya, Mahar Baya and so on. These caste groups are worshipped at the spirit level and symbolically express the gratitude which the Thakurs show them for the benefits they get from the "Devjatis" at the social level. Probably Thakurs might have historically designed this cultural practice of worshipping their superior caste groups.

Illness is thus caused by both Devjatis which include skin diseases such as chicken pox, measles, boils, body sores etc. and possession of evil spirits, fever, severe stomach ache, death etc. caused by the member of the "Devjatis". Disruption in the social relationships at the intersocial group level is believed to bring about illness. The Thakurs not only live in their own social system as one unit but are a part of the greater social system namely the Devjatis and the Devjatis residing in Karjat area. The chapter on body symbolism discusses this issue in detail.

9. Failure to Perform Divine Duty or Rite :

A Thakur's attitude towards his deities (diva) is one of fear and dread. Each of them is a potential source of danger. He offers prayers to them more to dissuade them from doing him harm than with the expectation of some positive good (Chaphekar, 1960 : 87).

The Thakurs classify the divine beings based on their power and supremacy over other Gods. This hierarchial gradation is as follows.

I. Sun : Most supreme power in the universe.

II. Mother Earth (Satvai) : Goddess of fortune and fertility.

III. Moon (Brother of Sun), Water (Brother of Sun), Baya or planetary spirits (Sisters of Mother Earth), Lightening (Mother Earth's sister), Holi (Goddess of Fire).

IV. Village Gods : Waghyadev, Chedoba Bhairi, Khambyadev, Hirwa, Secret Goddess spirits of Devjati.

V. Other deities : Khandoba, Kanhoba, Bhavani, Hanuman, Mariai.

VI. Clan Gods : Kanhirdev etc.

VII. Ancestral Spirits : Virdev and Supali.

It was observed that besides these major deities there are a number of other objects and forces, animals which are worshipped by them. Every God or Goddess has imposed certain normative obligations on the human beings such as offering the first grain, a sacrifice or a coconut. Besides these there could be other restrictions. For instance, during the solar and lunar eclipses, pregnant women must not cut vegetables for it is believed that the child would be born deformed. She must prevent herself from eating food because they believe that an evil force covers the sun therefore it is dark. This evil darkness (which symbolizes death) falls on the food which if consumed may harm the foetus.

Secondly, if a village God is not offered a goat by the villagers every year, he may bring an epidemic or troubles. A tiger is worshipped so that he does not eat their cows. During the Pitra Amosha the ancestral spirits are invoked so that they come down on the earth. They are given food. Any failure to perform any divine ritual or duty is believedto invite trouble or illness. The Thakurs also believe that sometimes illness is a divine sanction. A person has to pay for his deeds on the earth therefore he falls sick. Illness is not only punishment for wrong doings or deviance but, in some cases it is also taken as a divine honour. For instance, skin diseases such as measles, chicken pox, boils, sores etc. are believed to be caused due to visitation of Goddesses (Baya). Refer Illness episode no. for more details.

10. Deviance from Culturally Set Norms and Order of House Construction / Design :

The Thakurs believe in a typically culturally designed pattern of building a house which according to them resembles the cosmos. There are rituals of finding a suitable place/location, its cleansing, the anticlock placement of the poles, the directional symbolism and other symbolic forms in constructing a house is very meaningful to the Thakurs. Reflection of the cosmos in constructing a house is an auspicious thing. Hence a house which does not depict an image of the cosmos (holy) is evil and invites sickness, misfortune and troubles. Episode No. 5 gives a detailed account of how a person falls ill on deviating from the culturally set norms and order of house construction / design. The Thakurs believe that living in a house as prescribed by their traditions is like living within the cosmos (divine beings) while shifting from their traditional houses or adopting new types is like inviting evil spirits and forces to live with them.

11. Loss of Basic Bodily Equilibrium Because of the Entry of Excessive Heat or Cold in the Body :

In many areas of the world, including Latin America, South East Asia and South America one finds prevalent notions derived from Hippocratic humoral therapy or comparable ideas of Indian Medicine, that health depends in part on a proper balance between "hot" or "cold" (Foster, 1953; 1967; Jelliffe, 1956; Polgar, 1962; Nash, 1965; Hart, 1969) (For interpretation relating this actiology in Mexican communities to the social outlook of peasants, see Foster 1967 and Ingham 1970).

Associated with this therapy is the prescription of detailed precaution to maintain to prevent chilling in a Gautemalan Mayan community : keeping oneself covered, avoiding cold water and foods which are classified as "cool" and not getting caught in the rain (Adams, 1953)

The Thakurs classify factors viz. hot and cold as being responsible for ill-health.

A. Consumption of too hot or too cold diet.

B. Exposure of human body to cold or hot environment

i. working or walking in hot sun.

ii. exposing oneself to too cold environment.

iii. entry of cold breeze in the body through the nostrils.

iv. getting caught in the rain.

The Thakurs differentiate between temperature hot and chilly hot foods. Chilly hot refers to the pungent taste while temperature hot refers to the hot or cold intrinsic qualities of food excess of chilly hot foods causes diarrhoea or dysentery. Consumption of temperature hot foods is harmful for the stomach. Too cold foods if consumed cause cold, cough, pneumonia, etc according to them.

If a person is working in extreme sunny, hot climate a Thakur believes that his blood gets burnt up and most of the times such persons are believed to get sore eyes. (refer episode no. 39). Exposing oneself to too cold air is harmful and causes cold, cough and pneumonia. Similarly if one gets caught in the rain he is likely to fall ill.

There are number of restrictions imposed by the Thakur culture on a new mother. She is not to eat too cold foods because it is believed that if she consumes too cold foods, her blood would become cold and in turn her breast milk which is a product of her blood will also have that cold effect which will get into the child's stomach and he will suffer from cold and cough. In a like manner hot food may convert her blood hot and subsequently her breast milk hot and this hot milk will have an adverse effect on the child's digestive system and hence it will suffer from diarrhoea and dysentery (refer episode no. 37). The section on Maternal and child health care beliefs and practices gives a list of foods classified into hot and cold by the Thakurs.

What is caused due to a hot diet, air or water is treated with cold diet. Cold water/juice or herbal medicines have cold intrinsic qualities. In a like manner what is caused by a cold diet, air, water is treated with hot diet, hot medicine, hot water not inhalation and fumigation.

Besides entry of hot and cold elements in the body, Thakurs also believe that certain foods and fluids if consumed change the colour of body fluids such as blood, breast milk, urine, semen, muscles, sputum, stools etc. Colour hence becomes a criterion or symptom to locate or trace the type of illness in certain cases. For instance, eating excess of Badisauf (Foenicum vulgare) is believed to change the colour of blood to yellow and hence skin, eyes, nails of a patient turn yellow. These symptoms are indicative that a person is suffering from jaundice. If a person spits blood, they believe that he is suffering from TB. Severity of diarrhoea and dysentery is judged on the basis of the colour of stool when a patient has severe cold his mucus is watery and green in colour. The blood of a leprosy patient is greenish yellow. Black blood is a symptom of old age while orange is a sign of adulthood. Change in the colour of blood from red-orange-black is symbolic of aging. This change of bodily fluid colours becomes a criterion for tracing a category of illness (Refer episode no. 25 for more details).

12. Breach of Social Pollution Taboos :

The word pollution in the scientific sense literally means to make foul or impure. There are scientific explanation about water, air, noise pollution etc. The data on Thakur ethnomedicine has pointed out their belief regarding "social pollution" - which I would like to define as the symbolic actions, objects, substances, wards, gestures, utterances etc within a given sociocultural context are believed to create social distances, cause illness, bring about misfortune, invite warth of Gods and Goddesses and facilitate severe illness. "Menstrual blood" (vital) for instance is believed to be "evil", "pollutant", "black" and "hot" in nature. It causes diseases such as leprosy on account of sexual intercourse with a menstruating woman or consuming food cooked by her. A menstruating woman does not attend a healing rite for her presence is believed to aggravate the patient's suffering. She is not to interact with her family members nor other tribesmen. She is socially dislocated from her society for a short period for five days and taken back after the cleansing rite. Thus "menstrual blood" as a substance is socially interpreted as pollutant by the Thakurs . It creates social distance, it is believed to bring about misfortune and illness (refer episode no.: 11 & 29). A barren woman is prohibited from attending or entering a house where delivery takes place. Her very presence is believed to harm the mother or child. She is believed to have come there with evil intentions and to make use of her evil power to harm the new mother or the child, out of jealousy and envy cause she is not fertile.

Similarly the Thakurs believe that food prepared by a Kathkari (lower tribe) if consumed, causes stomach upset. Kathkaris are lower in status than the Thakurs and eat unclean food and therefore they are socially termed as unclean. Thus what is prepared by an unclean person is likely to pollute a person's health or biological system as it were.

During the healing rite (Jagran) the Thakurs do not allow menstruating women in that house to participate in the ritual. They believe that "Baya" - planetary spirits or the sisters of the Mother Earth are sterile and hate anyone who menstruates. If a menstruating woman deviates from this taboo and pollutes the environment. She aggravates the warth of "Baya" and ultimately the patient suffers their warth. Similarly drunkards are not allowed to attend the "Jagran ritual" for alcohol is believed to be a "pollutant" in this context and cannot be coupled with a divine situation. Members of other caste and even Thakur tribe are purified by sprinkling cow's urine on them so that their minds may be purified before they attend the ritual. This is done to avoid the "Baya" getting annoyed and causing more trouble to the patient.

13. Disruption of Man's Relationship with Certain Flora and Fauna :

Plants and animals have been profoundly interpreted as cultural symbols in different human societies. Some plants and animals hold sacred values while others are either evil, abode of evil spirits or source of black magic. A plant may be a religious symbol in one society may not hold true for the other society. People have reverence for sacred plants and animals. The Thakurs believe that Tiger (Vaghya), Snake (Chedha), Peacock (Hiriva) etc are Gods. They believe that if a Tiger God if not offered a sacrifice, they fear that it will eat their cattle. He is therefore worshipped diligently every week and a sacrifice is offered to him every year. A Thakur does not kill a cobra for he believes that its female partner will take revenge and kill him or one of his family members. Cobra is their God (Chedoba) Mr 'S' of Lobhyachi wadi was bitten by a cobra in the summer 1990. He interpreted that he had unknowingly urinated on the anthill where the cobra lives. That very same evening Mr 'S' was bitten by a cobra. Thus the cause of cobra biting him was linked up with disruption of his relationship with the cobra through the act of urinating on the anthill. He was later given herbal medicine by Palu Lobhie - Herbalist of Lobhychi wadi.

Irrespective of the cobra being so dangerous, it is interpreted as a symbol of deity. In the like manner Tigers are considered to be Gods and pleased at the spirit level so that they do not kill their cows and even themselves. Tulsi (Ocimum sanctum) is considered to be holy and also Rui (Calotropies gigantia) which is a symbol of Mother Earth. These plants if stepped upon in a ritual context are believed to cause disease and more specifically sterility as they are symbols of fertility. They are worshipped and appeased by barren women for want of children. Shid (Bauhinia racimosa) symbolizes 'Sun' on Dasera (festival) day. It causes disease if it is not worshipped.

Besides sacred plants and animals, the Thakurs also believe that there are plants and animals which have evil power or which can be used as magical means or abode of evil spirits. For instance Ficus religiosa (Pipal), Ficus benyamina (Vad) are abode of Munja, Khais and Hadeli (evil spirits). If these trees are cut the evil spirits will disturb human beings and bring forth a state of illness.

So is the case with Owl (Ghubad). If it sits on the house where a child is born, it is believed that the child dies. If a fox is shot or killed its spirit trouble the Thakurs. Thus disruption of relationship with certain flora and fauna brings about illness (refer episode 49) for more details.

14. Wrong Combination of Foods :

The art of combining foods is essentially cultural. Every society has got its own style of preparing food and a set pattern of combining foods. Some societies eg. The Indian society prefers spicy or chilly hot foods, while chillies are enemies of the Africans. Besides having beliefs about how foods should be combined and consumed there also exist beliefs regarding what food is not be combined with another. This concept could be turned as wrong combination of diet.

Ayurveda has pointed out the do's and dont's of wrong combinations of diets. Salim Shah (1993) is his unpublished thesis on the study of Leucoderma pointed out that Leucoderma is caused due to wrong combination of foods. Many of his respondents have stated that eating fish with milk causes Leucoderma (kode).

The Thakurs believe that a person get Leucoderma if he combines fish with curd in his diet. At the same time tea and curd taken together cause stomach upset or even if curd is taken just five minutes after a person has taken tea he or she starts vomiting. One must always eat Bhakar (coarse bread) after eating banana and then drink water. The rationale here is that banana is cold in nature and if water is taken after eating it, a person may get cold. Bhakar (hot) therefore neutralizes the effect. Banana and tea cannot be consumed together as they are believed to create heat in the body.

15. Disruption of Man's Relationship with His Deities :

The Thakurs have been always aloof from other castes and tribes. Even if there are 15-20 houses they would make a hamlet. They are used to staying in a closed society. Thakurs have faced economic and political security, as they are below the Davan jati (evil social group). The upper castes and tribes have always exploited the Thakurs.

The only source of security for them was their deities - the village Gods and Goddesses, clan Gods, and so on. Any deviance as far as the relationship of Thakurs with their deities means ill-health or misfortune. Episodes have highlighted Thakur concept of illness due to warth of Gods and Goddesses. Given below are 50 illness episodes which depict tribal illness ideology, body symbolism, vitual healing & health seeking behaviour is an ethnomedical system of a tribe.

EPISODE NO. : 1

Aim

To gain an insight about the Thakurs concepts of congenital deformities from an emic perspective.

Background

Gangu Khandi, 18 years, married female. Her maiden hamlet was Khondyachi wadi. After her marriage she resides in Chaphyachi wadi. She narrates her experience of having a congenitally deformed child when she came for her first delivery to khondyachi wadi.

Course of Events

A married girl goes to her parents house for her first delivery. This is a custom followed by the Thakurs. Gangu was sent by her in laws residing in Chaphyachi wadi to her parents house in Khondyachi wadi for her delivery. As her time was nearing Gangu complained and cried in pain.

She kept saying that something is biting/cutting her womb. During delivery she had a hard time and the room was filled with an unusual foul smell.

She gave birth to a boy who was deformed. He was dark, hands and legs were very small. One of the arms was shorter, head was abnormal, the tongue was on the dorsal side of the child.

The attending midwife (suine) of Khondyachi wadi Bhagi Nama Dhole immediately consulted Gangu's father. It was decided the child should not be allowed to live. She put a basket smeared with cowdung on the child whose head was pointing south and left it to die of suffocation.

In the meantime one of Gangu's relative was sent to Chaphyachi wadi to convey the bad news to her in-laws and to summon her husband. That the very night the child was buried with his dorsal side pointing upwards.

Gangu was asked "why was child born deformed ? How did this happen?" Initially she laughed and hesitated to tell. By this time her mother joined in and both were of the same opinion. They said that the child belonged to Khais (black skinned male evil spirit) because the child had a dark complexion, hair on his body and abnormal features. 'When and how did Gangu come in contact with the Khais?' Gangu was silent. Her mother replied 'Once Gangu went to the forest to collect firewood, as she was tired, she sat under a tree to rest and fell asleep. It was during the time that she was asleep that the Khais had sex with her ('Khais Gangila Zombala') and hence the child was born deformed.'

'Why did you not let the child grow?' Promptly Gangus mother answered, "The child would have killed my daughter, her husband and many other people in Chaphyachi wadi. It is an evil spirit and how can we allow it to grow ? It impossible for such a thing to happen".

Analysis

Male evil spirits having sex with the Thakur women is a very common belief among them. There are two types of evil spirits Khais (black skinned) and Munja (White skinned) who bring trouble to a Thakur woman. In the case of Gangu, Khais had sex with her and she delivered a deformed child.

On enquiring with Gangu's mother why do evil spirits trouble a woman sexually. She replied that when bachelors die, their soul (atma) does not go to heaven, it lingers on in this world seeking the desires of family life. Their sexual desire is unsatisfied. Hence they have sex with a woman.

"Why is the child buried with the dorsal side up ?". Gangu's mother replied by doing so the evil spirit is prevented from returning again to trouble the woman and her people. Such infants are killed by the Thakurs as they are evil (offspring of either Khais or Munja) and are permanently done away with. They cannot live in the good Thakur society. When

Gangu's husband was asked if certain rituals were performed to cleanse her (his wife Gangu) as she had contact with Khais, he answered "yes, she has to remove all the impure blood after the delivery thus cleanse her body. She takes bath for five days. She is massaged with groundnut oil especially the vagina and the abdominal parts. This is done by the suine (midwife). It takes nearly a month or two for the woman to become pure before she can be accepted by her husband. After this, the first time she has sex with her husband she has to first have a bath and offer a coconut to the village God.

EPISODE NO. : 2

Aim

To highlight the origin and course of prolonged wounds and the suffering caused by it, as attributed by the Thakurs in their medical system.

Background

Jaithu Pardhi, Sarpanch (village headman) of Kautewadi hamlet, Kashale village, 55 years, married, a member of the Thakur tribe.

Course of Events

Jaithu's right hand little finger had become crooked and had lost neural sensation. He was bitten severely by a 'crab' about ten years of ago. This incident occurred during the monsoon when he had gone to hunt crabs in the river on a rainy day.

Jaithu washed the wound applied a paste of the leaves Tridax procubens and tied the wound with a piece of dirty cloth. The next day he found the hand had swollen and the wound was so painful that he literally cried in pain. He continued home treatment for about two weeks but in vain.

Jaithu's friend Ganpat, an elderly man advised him to consult aa Bhagatin (female shaman) to find out the origin and cause of the suffering. The bhagatin's consultation day was Tuesday (devacha var). So Jaithu consulted her on Tuesday, she heard him patiently. She slipped into a trance. Hair let loose, her body moved in an anticlock direction. She was trying to find the cause of the suffering.

After 15-20 minutes she come out of her trance and told Jaithu that he had become a victim of witchcraft. She applied some herbal medicine on Jaithu's little finger. Jaithu continued his treatment, she applied the medicine for the next 4-5 days. Each day Jaithu paid her one Rupee and twenty five paise for her services.

The bhagatin's treatment showed good results. One fine morning when he opened the cloth bandaged around the little finger and pressed the wound for the 'pus' to come out, to his surprise out fell four-five grains of vari-a millet (panicum species).

Jaithu narrated his experience to Ganpat and to thebhagatin. She told him that it was definite that he had become a victim of witchcraft. She told him that some woman had used witchcraft and had filled vari in his (Jaithu's) little finger, the biting of the crab was only an excuse. (khekada chavalyache nimit hote).

Jaithu pondered over this thought and realized that a woman from the Kathkari tribe had asked him for some vari, which he had refused to give. He was then convinced that the same woman by using witchcraft had filled vari in his little finger of the right hand so as to cause him severe pain and suffering.

Analysis

The Thakurs attribute to the kathkaris a lower status in their social hierarchy because the diet of the kathkaris include rats, bandicoots, monkeys, foxes, beef, crows etc. Such a diet is considered by the Thakurs as unclean and polluted and such dietary behaviour is associated (according to the Thakurs) with evil beings like Rakshas - giants. Thus the Kathkaris are considered an evil tribe doing evil deeds like black magic, witchcraft, sorcery etc.

When an illness occurs after some kind of deal or interaction with the kathkaris, the Thakurs believe that the cause of such illness is due to witchcraft and sorceric spells performed by the evil kathkaris. The Thakurs believe that the kathkaris take revenge out of jealousy and hatred so as to cause prolonged illness. An example of this belief is Jaithu's suffering when he refused to give vari grains to a kathkari woman.

Usually the family elders are the first ones to find out or trace out the origin and cause of illness. At times relatives, village elders and friends also give advice. Lastly it is the Bhagat (male shaman) or a Bhagatin (female shaman) who confirms the doubts and notions of these people by performing diagnostic rites.

EPISODE NO. : 3

Aim

To highlight the Thakur concepts of witchcraft as expressed in their illness experience due to disruption in their social ties.

Background

Dhakti Ganu Ughda, married, resident of Borwadi, Pathraj village, cut her finger while harvesting paddy. Dhakti's age is 35 years.

Course of Events

It was the harvesting season, Dhakti was helping her husband Ganu to harvest paddy. Sometime later Dhakti cut her left hand index finger severely. The cut was bleeding profusely. Seeing this Ganu immediately tied a piece of sari around the cut without applying any medicine.

Dhakti opened the bandage after three days. The cut had become a wound which gave her great pain. She consulted a herbalist who gave her herbal medicine to apply. Dhakti does not know what medicine it was. The wound was deep. She continued treatment for two weeks but her wound did not become any better. Her appetite also was greatly reduced due to the pain.

Her husband Ganu suspected that Dhakti had become a victim of black magic. He then took her to Malu Lachka, the Bhagat of Borwadi. Malu cleansed himself by washing, took a metal pot (tambya) with some water and put in it holy ash from the hearth and spun the pot clockwise so as to diagnose the cause of Dhakti's illness and pain. While doing this he chanted mantras. He interpreted that a "Bhutali" (a Thakur witch) had filled dog's meat in Dhakti's index finger and the cut was only an excuse to cause her pain and suffering. Malu gave her a herbal oil to apply on her finger. He also performed some rituals so as to ward off the evil effect. When Dhakti's wound was healed she says a piece of dog's meat fell out of it. Dhakti put the piece of meat into the fire to destroy its power.

Analysis

The practice of witchcraft and sorcery is very common among the Thakurs. According to them such practices exist because of jealousy and/ or hatred among the family, clan, inter-tribal or between tribe and caste groups. In the case of Dhakti a "Bhutali" (witch) from the village caused trouble because of jealousy.

It is believed that animal flesh, bones, grains against such as nagli, vari are used as magical objects to harm the enemies by performing black magic rites. Acts of black magic and sorcery thus depict conflicts taking place between family members, clan members, interclan, inter-tribe or between a tribe and caste group.

EPISODE NO. : 4

Aim

To investigate the 'cause' attributed by the Thakurs to prolonged wounds according to their medical system.

Background

Rakhmi Phasal, a married woman, 32 years old, resident of Kautewadi hamlet - Kashale village, had a wound which caused her inexplicable pain and suffering for 20 days.

Course of Events

In the year 1989, in the month of February, one fine morning Rakhmi was scrubbing the household utensils. She cut her finger while scrubbing an old frying pan (tava).

She quickly washed her hand, applied groundnut oil and bandaged her finger with a piece of sari. She opened her bandage only on the fifth day and saw that the wound was filled with pus. She again applied oil and tied the wound. She had suffered a lot in the past five days.

Rakhmi's husband and father-in-law decided that she should be taken to the Bhagat (male shaman). The Bhagat diagnosed her problem using the metal-pot (tambya) technique i.e. he let a metal-pot filled with water move in clockwise direction for 5-10 minutes. In the pot is put a pinch of ash from the hearth.

After having diagnosed Rakhmi's problem Janu Bhagat interpreted that Rakhmi had become a victim of witchcraft and she must see a Bhagat from Mattewadi (a hamlet 5 km. from Kautewadi).

The next day Rakhmi was taken to the Bhagat in Mattewadi. Using the same diagnosis technique, he too interpreted that Rakhmi had become a victim of witchcraft practiced by a Kathkari woman. He gave Rakhmi some herbal medicine for a week. Rakhmi offered a coconut and a bottle of local liquor to the Bhagat when her wound was healed.

When Rakhmi recollected, she remembered an incident which occurred in the Karjat market. Rakhmi had bargained with a kathkari woman about the chillies she was selling. In the end she had refused to buy the chillies from the woman.

Analysis

According to Rakhmi the prolonged pain and suffering she had endured was not because of a natural cause i.e. the cut in her finger, but was a deliberate attempt to harm her. This view was later confirmed by the two Bhagats who also believed that Rakhmi was a victim of witchcraft.

Whenever the cause of witchcraft and sorcery was to be found it was always attributed to the doings of kathkaris, Chamars, Mahars, Mangs, Muslims and Wadaris. These are the caste and tribal groups, placed lower in the hierarchy of social status by the Thakurs and are believed to practice witchcraft and sorcery.

EPISODE NO. : 5

Aim

1. To highlight how illness experience crosscuts meanings of human body as a social, religious and cosmological symbol.
2. The various conceptions of a Thakur involved in house building.
3. To study the material culture.
4. The explore the concept of evil spirits.
5. The explore the symbolic aspects related to childbirth.

Background

Mrs. Dharma Pardhi, 28 years, married female. Both she and her husband Mr. Pardhi were working for a voluntary organization viz. Academy of Development Science (A.D.S.) Their native settlement Borwadi is 1 km. away from A.D.S. Mr. Pardhi worked in a dairy and Mrs. Pardhi worked in the cafeteria. Their working hours required both of them to be most of the time at the A.D.S. Hence they were given a house near the dairy on the campus itself.

The A.D.S. has built good concrete houses for its employees. This house (given to Mr & Mrs Pardhi) did not meet the Thakurs concept of house building. The Pardhi family stayed on the A.D.S. campus for seven years. During this period they changed their home twice for a number of reasons. Some of the major reasons are highlighted in this episode.

Course of Events

During this period of seven years Mrs. Pardhi faced a lot of trouble and was sick on several occasions.

Illness and Trouble in the New House

During the first year, in the new house on the A.D.S. campus, Mr & Mrs Pardhi often fell sick. Either or both of them would fall sick every month. The following year two of their pet cats died and their son suffered from chicken pox in the third year.

Request for a new House

After suffering from a spate of calamities spread over a period of three years, the Pardhis decided to request the authorities for a change of house. They believed that this house was unlucky for them.

Setting of the New House

The second house allotted to them was also near the dairy. It had many cultural drawbacks according to the Thakurs. To enlist them, the door of the house faced south. The southern direction is believed to be evil, the hearth (chulah) was in the north-eastern direction, there was no 'Mothur-med' (the first pillar which symbolizes the Sun God), there was no 'Aada' (a horizontal jamun wooden pole fixed below the roof) This 'Aada' symbolizes the sky. There was no central place for grinding rice. Overlooking these cultural drawbacks Mr & Mrs Pardhi lived in the second house for a period of four years.

Disaster in the Second House

Mr & Mrs Pardhi found that after shifting to the second house their luck and fortune had taken a turn for the worse. Trouble, sickness, misery were their constant companions in the second house. The calamities which came upon them can be enumerated as follows -

1. Constant prevalence of sickness in the family for seven years.
2. Two cats died in the first house.
3. One calf died in the second house.
4. Both Mrs Pardhi and her son suffered from chicken pox.
5. The construction of the house did not meet the Thakur's cultural building style.
6. Mrs Pardhi lost her job as the cafe incharge in the A.D.S. cafeteria.
7. The 'Baya' - a band of Goddesses symbolizing the planets would visit Mrs Pardhi every Tuesday and Thursday and would go into a trance.
8. Their village God 'Bhairi' - considered to be the brother of the Sun God (life giver) appeared to Mrs Pardhi in her dreams and would tell her to change her house from A.D.S. campus to Borwadi (their native village).

On Consulting A Bhagatin (Female Shaman)

'Mrs Pardhi, did you discuss your problems with anyone?' Pat, came the reply 'Yes, of course I consulted a Bhagatin of Kotimba village.'

The Bhagatin was given Rs. 1.25 to diagnose the origin and cause of the troubles and illnesses which fell on the Pardhi family.

The Bhagatin lit an incense stick, offered a coconut to the 'Baya' - the planetary Goddesses. She then went into a trance during which she moved in a clockwise direction and started reciting the mantras. She interpreted that Mrs Pardhi's trouble and sickness was because of the warth of the 'Baya'. The 'Baya' were annoyed with the Pardhi's because they stayed in the A.D.S houses which were not built according to the culturally recognized norms of the Thakur society. Mrs Pardhi was asked to shift back to Borwadi and was given a necklace (Gala patta) made of aluminum, which symbolizes that Mrs Pardhi was a devotee of the 'Baya' She was also instructed to offer a coconut to the Baya after shifting to her native settlement in Borwadi.

From A.D.S. To Borwadi

When Mrs Pardhi heard the divine instructions from the Bhagatin and the call of the Baya, she discussed the matter with her husband and her in-laws. They also agreed and so Mr & Mrs Pardhi shifted out of the A.D.S. premises. They settled in a culturally designed house and are living here since the past two years. When asked about any troubles, they replied 'We are perfectly happy and free from all troubles.'

Analysis

Mr & Mrs Pardhi firmly believed that a Thakur house brought good luck and a house built by the A.D.S. brought ill-luck to them. They gave information about the cultural significance of building a house (in a particular way) which is nothing but a reflection of cosmos. The cosmos in turn is a reflection of the human body and therefore there is a very close relationship between the human body and the cosmic objects that exist in the universe.

Layout and Construction of a Thakur House

When a Thakur builds his house, he abides by the cultural rules and regulations regarding the building of a house. Thus, the various rituals and ceremonies, concerned with every step of house building are religiously followed. Some of the rituals are concerned with finding a suitable place for the house, digging the Earth and placing the first pillar (Mothur-med) which symbolizes the sun, worshipping the pillar, fixing in the anticlockwise direction the remaining three pillars and so on. These rituals are symbolic and meaningful to the Thakurs.

1. The Mothur Med (The support of the house)

A wooden pillar of teak is known as mothur med. The head of the house digs a hole five feet in depth and puts some gulal (red powder) and rice grains in the hole. Then, five men including the head of the family erect the pillar firmly into the hole.

The pillar is symbolic of the sun, head of the Universe and the hole symbolizes the mother Earth. The fixing of the mothur med into the hole is symbolic of the sexual relationship between the sun and the earth (male and female cosmic forces). A coconut is offered which symbolizes the spermatic flow of the sun, into the earth. The rice placed in the hole symbolizes the fertility of the family. The participation of males symbolizes their dominance and their sexual role. Thus fixing of the mothur med is meaningful and symbolic of establishing a family.

Thus the mothur med is very significant in building a house as it is symbolic of the Sun (the life giver and supporter if humanity). The next phase is that of worshipping the mothur med. The head of the family ties a black cloth tothe pole. In the cloth are various things viz, Biba (Semicarpus anacardium), Halad (Aurcuma Domestica), Supari (Areca catechu) and gulal (a red powder). These objects are ritualistically tied to prevent and ward off the external evil effect on the house. The mothur med is fixed towards the south-east.

The Fixing of Other Three Poles

After the mothur med is fixed the other three poles are fixed in an anticlockwise manner. This is done because the Thakurs believe that the sun moves in an anticlockwise direction from the east to the west round the earth. They also believe that the wind, clouds and other cosmic movement is also in the anticlock direction.

2. The Hearth (Chulah - Goddess of fire)

Towards the south-east next to the mothur med is the hearth. It faces the west. This is so done, so that the woman while cooking should face the east - the direction of life because the sun rises there. The fire of the chul symbolizes 'Holi' a goddess of 'Agni' (fire) who, the Thakurs believe is the sister of the Sun. The chul is thus holy and a symbol of purity, as it contains fire which helps to purify and cook raw food.

The ash (Surya Rakhad) in the chul is considered holy and symbolizes the body of the sun. All medical practitioners including Bhagats and Bhagatins (male and female Shaman), Vaidu (herbalist), had vaidu (Bone setter), Midwife (Suine), the Mantrik (Snake and Scorpion sting specialists) and the potdhari (help mate of the midwife) use the holy ash for performing healing rites.

The Purification of the Hearth

Although the hearth is believed to be the symbol of purity, it is cleansed and purified ritually on many occasions. One such occasion is on the solar eclipse. On this day the hearth or the chul is not used at all, which means that Thakurs do not cook on this day. It is believed that the Sun (Life giver) is covered with darkness (evil) and hence all the food items and water lose their power and strength and become evil. The evil effect of darkness pollutes the almighty Sun and makes it impure and blocks the light giving holy rays of the Sun. After the eclipse, all vegetables, grains and other food items are washed ritually with water (the purifier and brother of Sun).

The Thakurs especially the pregnant women fast on solar eclipse. After the eclipse is over, the hearth is plastered with cowdung and water. This act symbolizes the purification and cleansing of the evil effect of darkness on the hearth. The ash from the hearth symbolizes the remains of the Sun and the hearth or chul is symbolic of the Goddess of Agni (Holi). These two, symbolize the company of the divine forces with the Thakurs. Some other occasions on which the hearth is purified are -

1. During the 'Pitra Amosha' (a festival of ancestral spirits). The Thakurs believe that their ancestral spirits come and visit them.
2. On the fifth day after the delivery to welcome the 'Satvai' - the mother earth. It is believed that she comes in the form of a bird or an animal to write the 'life span' of the new born by making a mark on the child's forehead.
3. The hearth is plastered when a menstruating woman completes her menses. Before she cooks she must bathe, wash her clothes and then purify the hearth by plastering it.

Cowdung thus symbolizes an object which holds the power to ward off evil effect, purify and also neutralize the evil effect. When a person is affected with or by the evil eye, cowdung is ritually used to absorb the evil effect.

Thus, presence of the hearth and its position in the south-east is very meaningful to the Thakurs.

3. The Kitchen, Dining Cum Delivery Room

The kitchen where the hearth is placed is used for cooking and dining, It also doubles up as a place for delivery. The pregnant woman lies down facing the west about five feet away from the hearth. The delivery posture is never North-South as south is the direction of death, while north, east and west are directions of life.

4. Sleeping Place

The central place in the house is used for sleeping by the Thakurs. It is in this area that the rice is ground and pounded. In the center of the room there is a hole known as 'Ukhali'. 'Ukhali' is made of stone and is used for pounding rice and to separate the husk. Pounding is always done by the woman.

5. Cattle Shed

Cattle are looked upon with great affection and considered to be children by the Thakurs. Hence they are tied in the house itself. This is so because the livelihood of the Thakurs depend on the cattle.

6. The Rakshas Disha (The evil south)

The south (direction) is believed to be the dwelling place of evil spirits, giants and bad forces. It is therefore termed as "Rakshas Disha". Even the air and wind which blow from the south are believed to bring illness, trouble and death. As the south, symbolizes the direction of death, the Thakurs bury their dead with the head pointing to the south.

Even while sleeping or resting, the Thakur never sleeps with the head pointing south. He rests, pointing either North, East or West. It is believed that magicians, witches, sorcers get their evil powers from the south. All evil acts are performed facing south.

7. The East "Ungvat Baju"

Of all the directions, the east is believed to be the most important of all. The main significance attached to the east is that the Sun (life-giver) comes up (rises) from here and hence all good activities, rituals and ceremonies are performed facing the east. Some of the rituals are given below.

1. Diagnosis of illness (performing diagnostic rites).
2. Collection, preparation and administration of medicine is done facing the east.
3. All village GODS face the east.
4. Drummers performing Dhambdi (dance performed by elders) and Gauri dance (dance performed by youngsters) facing the east.
5. Rituals connected with offering food, sacrifice and coconut are performed facing the east.
6. All actions, rituals and ceremonies which aim to bring good fortune to the Thakur society are performed facing the east.
7. The air/wind which symbolizes life is believed to flow anticlockwise from east to west.

East is believed to have a good effect on Thakur life and thus is symbolic of "life" and "good omen" heaven (swarg) is believed to be situated in the east.

8. The Mavalat Disha (The West)

The west direction is the direction of "Goddess Satvai" (The Goddess of fortune, life span and fertility). Goddess satvai is none other than Mother Earth. She faces the sun in the west, while it is in the east. The wind blowing from the west carries with it the spirits of "Baya" - the nine planets (Sisters of mother Earth). On the fifth day after the delivery the Satvai comes from the west to visit the child and to write its life span on the forehead.

9. The Dev Disha (The Holy North)

The Thakurs believe that the Northern side of the earth is slightly tilted. There are nine lakh steps in this direction which take a person to residence of the Gods.

10. The Entrance

The Thakur is guided by the cultural norms and he is allowed to let the entrance of his house face either in the North, East or West direction but never in the Southern direction.

If the entrance faces the south it is an open invitation to sickness, sorrow, trouble and even death. To the door post are tied five chillies and a lime. The lime is believed to absorb the evil effect while chillies which symbolize hotness (fire) are believed to ward off the effect of the evil eye.

11. The Burial Place of the Umbilical Chord

The umbilical chord is buried outside the wall which is in the west. On the inside of the wall is the bathing place of the mother and the new born. The bath water flows out on the umbilical chord buried outside and decays it, thus the chord disappears and is prevented from becoming an object of sorcery and witchcraft.

The ritual of burying the umbilical chord is interesting as it reflects the symbolic and meaningful elements associated with the Thakur's conceptions of sex, fertility, delivery, womanhood, black magic etc. The suine (midwife) takes a palas leaf (Butea monosperma) on which she places the umbilical chord (Nal), the placental waste (Var), rice (chaul), coin (paisa). This leaf is placed in such a way that the apex of the leaf points towards the east and the leaf base towards the west.

Diagram IV : 1. showing Umbilical Chord Burial Ritual

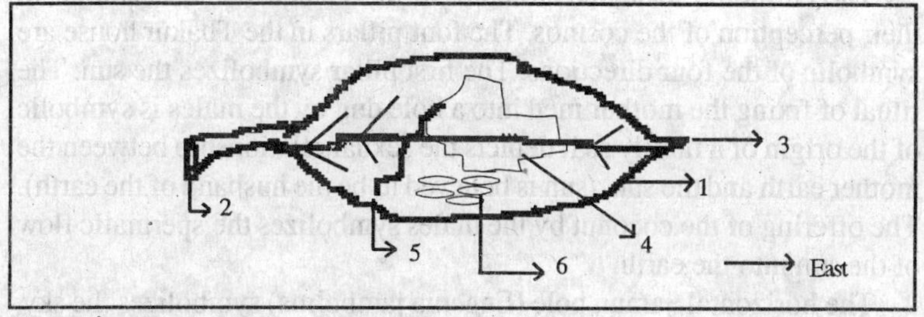

Meanings

1. The leaf is symbolic of a fertile woman.
2. The apex symbolizes her head.
3. The base of the petiole symbolizes her vaginal opening.
4. The var symbolizes the womb.
5. The nal symbolizes the child.
6. The rice on the leaf is symbolic of continued fertility.
7. The east west position of the leaf symbolizes the sexual and delivery posture of a woman.
8. The dorsal surface of the leaf is symbolic of the woman's desire for children and sex. Chaphekar (1961) reports that if the midwife turns the leaf over onto the ventral side, it (the act of overturning) symbolizes the woman's desire of not having or conceiving any more children.

12. The Anticlock Movement

The fixing of the main pillars of the house starts with the fixing of the mother med. The remaining pillars are fixed into the ground in an anticlock direction. This practice is observed because the Thakurs believe that the sun and the whole cosmos move in an anticlockwise direction. Most rites which are performed to bring good fortune to the Thakurs are performed in an anticlock movement. The rotation in such movements is also anticlock in direction. For instance, the moving of "tambya" in the diagnostic ritual, the dance movements, moving of the bride and the groom around the sacred fire also is done in the anticlock direction.

After fixing the four pillars in the four directions, a small wooden plank of the jamun tree (Eugenia Jambolina) is fixed in the center of the roof. It symbolizes the sky. A coconut is tied to this pole. The water in the coconut symbolizes the rain and the coconut the clouds. The Thakurs worship the jamun pole (sky) during construction in the belief that doing so will prevent the house from leaking.

The Thakur House as a Symbol of Universe

The culturally designed structure of the Thakur house is similar to their perception of the cosmos. The four pillars in the Thakur house are symbolic of the four directions. The first pillar symbolizes the sun. The ritual of fixing the mothur med into a hole dug by the males is symbolic of the origin of a family as it depicts the sexual relationship between the mother earth and the sun. (sun is believed to be the husband of the earth). The offering of the coconut by the males symbolizes the spermatic flow of the sun into the earth.

The horizontal jamun pole (Engenia jambolina) symbolizes the sky. The coconut hung on the "Aada" - the jamun plank symbolizes the clouds and the water in it symbolizes the rain. The offering of a coconut by the Thakur is an appeal to the sky not to let the roof leak.

The three directions, north, west and east are believed to bring the life giving air, while the south is believed to be evil and brings trouble, illness and death to the Thakurs. The anticlock direction followed during building a house by fixing the poles in symbolic of the anticlock movement of the Thakur Gods 'Sun' and his brother 'Moon'. Even other cosmic forces such as wind, clouds, seasons are believed to move in an anticlock direction. The Thakur house thus is a symbol of the cosmic outlook of the Thakurs.

The Human Body and the Cosmos

The Thakurs categorize the human body into a universal whole. According to them the human body comprises of ten openings viz, the eyes, the nose, the mouth, the atma (the region below the sternum), pulse of the wrist, the naval, the vaginal opening, the pulse of the feet and the anal opening. These ten openings symbolize the ten planets in the cosmos. The planets are similarly ordered like the openings in the body. The Thakurs believe that just as the universe exists because of the sun. The Thakurs believe that man is able to see because the sun supplies light to the eyes during the day and the moon supplies light at night.

The blood circulation is also anticlockwise in direction just like the movement of the cosmic objects and forces in the universe. The body survives because of

1. Light : The source is the sun and the moon.
2. Water : believed to be the brother of the sun & the source is clouds and earth.
3. Wind : Comes/blows from north, east and west directions.
4. Food : Made up of earth, sun and water.

The Thakur defines life within this framework and therefore the body is closely related to the universe. Due to this close association the "Baya" (cosmic Goddesses) visited Mrs. Dharma Pardhi and asked her to leave the A.D.S. the construction of which did not fit into the cultural framework of the Thakurs.

Reason for Mrs. Pardhi's Illness and Troubles

Mrs. Dharma Pardhi thus attributed all her illness and troubles to the fact that they i.e. she, her husband and their children, did not live in a culturally designed house of the Thakurs which resembles the human body and is a symbol of the universe. The order of the body and universe must be similar or should resemble in order to have perfect harmony.

This harmony was clearly absent in the A.D.S. house in which Mrs. Dharma Pardhi lived with her family.

Thus this illness episode cross-cuts meanings of many institutions such as material culture, cosmic perceptions, the notion of evil spirits, the concept of human body as a cosmic symbol etc.

EPISODE NO. : 6

Aim

To investigate the manner in which the Thakurs co-relate the cause of illness and failure to participate and perform a ritual related to ancestral festival.

Background

Mr. A.J., married male, aged 60 years, resident of Khondewadi narrates his illness experience and attributes the cause of his ill-health to failure to perform and participate in ancestral rites.

Course of Events

Mr. A.J. took ill following a festival known as "Pitra Amosha" (a festival of ancestral spirits) celebrated by the Thakurs during the rainy season. Mr. A.J. had high fever, he did not consult any physician but kept on drinking cold water. His son Mr. K. was worried and called the bhagat home. The bhagat observed Mr. A.J. carefully and then performed the diagnosis rite and interpreted as the course as wrath of ancestral spirits (wad-vadil) Mr. A.J. had indeed failed to participate in the "Dhambdi Dance" - which is performed all night long on the no moon night (of Pitra Amosha) to welcome their ancestral spirits from heaven and invite them to stay with the respective family for a day. The next day, some food is placed on the palas (Butea frondosa) leaf and placed on the roof. When the crows come and eat this food it is considered that the ancestors have accepted the food and are happy with the Thakurs. Prior to placing the food on the roof a little of the food is thrown towards the east. This action symbolizes the offering of food to the forefathers. Mr. A.J. had failed to perform the above ritual of offering food and had also not participated in the Dhambdi Dance. Thus the ancestral spirits were angry and he had fever. The bhagat applied some charmed ash on Mr. A.J.'s forehead and asked him to offer a coconut to ancestral spirits which he faithfully did. Mr. A.J. was completely cured within the next three to four days.

Analysis

The Thakurs share a very close relationship with their ancestral spirits. Every year on "Pitra Amosha Night" all the old folk of the village perform the Dhambdi dance all through the night to invoke the ancestral spirits to stay with them for a day. This practice has been going on since time immemorial. The next food is prepared and placed on the eastern side of the roof. This action is symbolic of their (Thakur's) respect to their forefather. The Thakur society has been isolated from the main stream and if at all there is any interaction then it is one of the exploitation. Hence to release their tensions and to look for help, the Thakurs turn to their forefathers who are believed to come down from heaven and stay with them. Thus this festival is of great significance for the Thakurs.

Mr. A.J. had high fever following this great festival in which he did not participate nor did he perform the ritual of offering the food though he was the head of the family. Thus his illness was interpreted as the wrath of ancestral spirits. Thus the episode highlights the relationship the Thakurs share with their forefathers (ancestral spirits), the rituals performed to involve the spirits and offering a food to satisfy them.

EPISODE NO. : 7

Aim

To understand the Thakur's concept of causation of boils and the treatment as perceived by them from an emic perspective.

Background

Mr. A.T., married male, aged 40 years, bhagat by profession, resident of Khondewadi, explains the Thakurs concept of origin and cause of boils and the treatment given thereby.

Course of Events

Mr. A.T.'s son, Mr. S. was suffering from boils in the summer of 1991. He had a big boil under his armpit. Mr. S. was 13 years old then. Mr. A.T. said that, many people suffered from boils in that summer. Mr. A.T. describes this event as visitation of "Mamadev" (the moon-brother of the planetary spirits.

On enquiring from Mr. A.T. who is mamadev and what was the purpose behind his visitation, Mr. A.T. being a bhagat was well versed with the beliefs and practices of the people replied almost without delay that the moon is mamadev and he visits people to check their deviant behaviors.

"Mr. A.T. does the moon cause boils ?". "yes, he does". "Is the moon evil ?". "No, he is God, the brother of the almighty sun". "Then why does he cause boils ?". Pat came Mr. A.T.'s reply "people are becoming very selfish and have forgotten God to check their deviant behaviour the moon causes boils".

"Mr. A.T., how does the moon get into the body ?". Mr. A.T. replied "The moon comes in the form of hot air along with the other female spirits - the "Baya" who always have with them a "Gavli" - caretaker (the moon)".

"Mr. A.T., how do you know that the moon has visited a person ?". Mr. A.T. replied "The person/patient gets fever, starts shivering, then scratching and then the boil is visible. "What treatment did you give your son, Mr. S. ?". "Mr. A.T. replied that a ghat (representation of the moon) is set and worshipped from five to fourteen days till the boil is healed. The ghat is set up using a metal pot on the mouth of which a coconut is placed. The flowers of 'chapha' (plumeria rubra) are spread below.

Until the patient does not get well songs of praise are sung to the sun, moon and Baya in order to please them so that they may peacefully leave the body of the patient. The patient is given cold diet and precaution is taken to see that menstruating woman does not enter a house where a 'ghat' is established. On either the fifth or fourteenth day the patient is given a bath known as 'pani ghalni'. The ghat is then put into a basket and left outside the village boundary.

Analysis

Boils are believed to be caused due to the visitation of 'mamadev' (moon) and the Baya. These cosmic objects enter the human body through the medium of hot air which makes the body fluids. viz. blood, water mucous etc. hot and erupts out through the skin pores and in visible as boils. A boil being bigger in size that those caused during chicken pox and measles is believed to be a symbol of the moon (Mamadev).

The Baya always move with mamadev (moon). In the case of boils it is only the moon which erupts out through the skin and not the Baya. Thus the boil is a symbol of the moon which checks the deviating behaviour of man. Thus by the visitation the moon (second divine force) is believed to create social order at a symbolic level using a physical medium (human body). Thus the human body gets a divine status in such a cultural context due to the entry of the cosmic spirits.

EPISODE No. : 8

Aim

To highlight the Thakur's perception, regarding how cosmic disorder (solar eclipse - grihan) influences their health.

Background

Mrs. A.N. married female, aged 43 years, a resident of Naldewadi, narrates how she suffered from ill-health because she broke a cosmic taboo on a solar eclipse day.

Course of Events

It was solar eclipse and every adult in Naldewadi was fasting. Mrs. A.N. could not control her hunger, she made herself a bhakar (bread) and chatani (chilly paste) and had it for lunch. In the evening when her husband returned from his work she again broke her fast with the husband. He was not aware that she had eaten during the day.

The next day Mrs. A.N. suffered from dysentery and vomiting. She immediately recollected the previous day's mistake. She told her husband who scolded her and then took her to the bhagat of Saraiwadi. He was told of Mrs. A.N.'s mistake. He diagnosed the cause of her illness and interpreted that her food was polluted because the darkness (evil force) had blocked the light of the sun's life giving rays.

"Mrs. A.N. why did the food get spoilt ?". She explained, "the sun God was covered with darkness (evil force) due to this the life giving rays were blocked. As a result of this the water that is used for cooking gets polluted by the evil effect of darkness and pollutes the food. So I suffered from dysentery and vomiting".

"Mrs. A.N., can you tell something about the darkness or the evil force that covers the sun". Mrs. A.N. explained,"the darkness is the spirits of the Mangs and Mahars (lower caste groups)". She then asked "Have you ever seen a cobra or any snake catching/swallowing a frog ?". "yes" said the researcher. She then continued, "in the very same way the spirits of Mangs and Mahars try to engulf our sun God. But these spirits leave our God in the evening".

Mrs. A.N. further added that if a pregnant woman eats food on a solar eclipse day, she may have an abortion because the evil effect falls on the food she consumes and her blood becomes polluted. Since the foetus survives on the blood it is aborted this happens if she is four or less than four months pregnant". "Mrs. A.N., what if the woman is more than four months pregnant ?" She replied "then the child is still born, my sister when she was pregnant, cut vegetables on the solar eclipse (grihan) day, when her child was born, it had a cleft lip (cut in lip)", Mrs. A.N. "How is cutting of vegetables related to deft lips ?". She answered,"We Thakurs believe that plants have life, during the solar eclipse they do not get the life giving rays of the sun and struggle for life. If a pregnant woman hurts life (plants/vegetables) she is punished by the sun God who cuts any part of her child's body.

"Mrs. A.N., What happens if a Mahar or a Mang caste member enters your village during the solar eclipse ?". She replied, "We do not communicate or touch the person neither do we go to their village. But if by mistake one touches a Mang or a Mahar the person has a bath immediately and purifies himself". "How do you break your fast on the polluted day of the solar eclipse ?". She explained, "We go and fetch fresh water from the well (Navin pani) and then cook our food and eat it".

Analysis

It is surprising to know that when there is change in cosmic order there is drastic change in health behaviour of the Thakurs at a social level. All medical practitioners compulsorily fast. Pregnant women abstain from consuming food or cutting vegetables as this may lead to abortion or still birth. This highlights the relationship Thakurs have with their Sun God as a very important and meaningful one. They believe he is the creator and sustainer of life and during a solar eclipse (when he is in trouble) the entire life in the universe is troubled.

This episode also expresses their ideology of the cosmic order, and if it is disturbed it influences human health because the human body is nothing but aan image of the cosmos. It also expresses their perception about the lower caste people i.e. the Mangs and Mahars whose spirits are believed to block the life giving rays of the Sun.

EPISODE NO. : 9

Aim

To investigate the origin and cause of a severe ear aches, as perceived by the Thakurs in a given cultural situation.

Background

Chahu Rama Thorad, married male, aged 50 years, resident of Khondewadi narrates his experience of severe ear ache.

Course of Events

It was somewhere during the year 1970, about 22 years ago (according to Chahu) his son Gotiram got married. A week later after the marriage Chahu suffered from a severe ear ache. His father Rama advised him to put the cooled oil of Mahua seed (Bacia latifolia) in his ear. Chahu continued this treatment for five days but he got no relief.

He was then instructed to see Ambo Thorad, the bhagat. Ambo use the culturally designed and accepted method of diagnosis i.e the metal pot technique. He recited the "Nadiche mantra". Ambo interpreted the cause of earache as failure to perform a divine duty. Chahu had indeed failed to offer a marriage reception food to his clan God "Kanir dev" - ear God. This failure resulted in him being punished by the God.

Ambo instructed Chahu to offer a coconut to the clan God (kul dev - kanir dev). He also gave a powdered preparation to be mixed with Mahua see oil and to be put in the ear. He applied charmed ash on Chahu's forehead. Chahu offered a coconut and continued Ambo's treatment for two weeks. He was cured.

Analysis

What is introduced through the spiritual world, has to be healed spiritually and hence a spiritual curer is consulted. Although Chahu's problem was attributed to failure in performing divine duty. Ambo combined herbal treatment with magico-ritualistic therapy so as to give Chahu physical and psychological treatment.

The fact that Chahu went to a Bhagat and did as he was instructed emphasizes that there is great meaning attached to his form of health behaviour. Thus the earache in this context was due to the intervention of the Clan God. The Clans re believed to be the offshoots of their clan Gods who hold right over the clan.

EPISODE NO. : 10

Aim

To highlight the provision made by the Thakur culture to fulfill the desire of material objects while the patient is in a stage of ill-health.

Background

Mrs. Z, married female, 28 years, resident of Nagyachi wadi narrates her experience of chicken pox.

Course of Events

In the summer of 1992, Mrs. Z suffered from chicken pox which started with symptoms such as shivering, fever, itching. Her father-in-law consulted Walku Thorad - the bhagat of the hamlet. He diagnosed it as a visitation of the Baya - planetary spirits. He instructed Mrs. Z's father-in-law to establish a "ghat" - a symbol of Baya. For two days there was "jagran ceremony" held in the house of Mrs. Z. Her neighbours and family members sang praises to the Baya.

On the fifth day, while the drums (Dholki) were being played and people were singing the bhagat got into a trance and questioned Mrs. Z (who was possessed by the Baya) what did she want. Mrs. Z answered on behalf of the planetary spirits that she wears a necklace, green bangles and green coloured blouse piece. The Bhagat said that what was asked for will be given. The next day Mrs. Z's father-in-law bought the articles and the next evening the Bhagat offered these along with a coconut to Mrs. Z who was no longer possessed by the Baya.

The researcher asked Mrs. Z aa strange question. He asked her, "how many blouses do you have ?". Mrs. Z hesitated and then answered "two". "Do you like to wear ornaments, Mrs. Z ?". She asked, "How do you know ?", and further added that the Baya were able to assess the needs of the body when they visit.

"Mrs. Z, did the Baya know that you did not have a blouse ?". She replied, "If they do not know, then who will know", she also added, " if we deserve something from our soul we get it and when the Baya visit they understand our needs and we are accordingly rewarded. In my case I di not have more than two blouses so they provided me with one".

Analysis

The Thakur community is very backward in economy. Though the women are fond of ornaments, clothes etc, they cannot have them at the social level hence they desire and get it at a spiritual level. Mrs. Z also said that some women get saris, towels, anklets, necklaces and other ornaments during the visitation of Baya.

Thus analyzing a step further, it is observed that the Thakur culture has designed ways and means to meet the economic needs of individuals. The offering of blouse, sari, Rs. 10-25 to the midwives and a towel, bottle of liquor, loin cloth or a feast to the male practitioners is nothing but an exchange of goods and services to meet their needs.

The Thakurs are too poor to eat chicken regularly so when a sickness occurs in the family, a chicken is sacrificed to the pathogenic agent during the healing rite. The blood is offered to the pathogenic agent and the flesh is consumed by the family and the Bhagat.

Also every year a goat is sacrificed to the village God so that he protects the village from ill-health and misfortune. Thus the blood is offered to the God and the meat is consumed by the village. This ritual also symbolizes the need for social get together.

EPISODE NO. : 11

Aim

To highlight the co-relation of leprosy etiology with that of breach of a dietary taboo during menstruation as attributed by the Thakurs.

Background

Tuli Hindola, a leprosy patient, married, female of 32 years, a member of Thakur community, resident of Bhalewadi, now resides on the outskirt of Bhalewadi. She attributes the cause of her disease to failure to abide by a dietary norm during menstruation.

Course of Events

Tuli is married to a primary school teacher who deserted her when she was affected by leprosy. She was 29 years then. Tuli has been ex-communicated by the people of Bhalewadi and now resides on the outskirts of the village in a small hut.

Origin and Cause of Leprosy

According to Tuli, she is affected by leprosy because she cooked and ate food during her menstrual period. When asked whether her husband and children had also eaten the food. She replied, "No, I have no children and that afternoon my husband had gone to the tehsil headquarters at Karjat for some school work".

Development of Deformity

Two months after she ate the food cooked by her during the menstrual periods, Tuli developed a big patch on her left thigh. Within some months similar patches were seen on the body. When it came to a point that her nose started showing signs of deformity her husband then suspected that she was suffering from leprosy. He prohibited her from going out of the house, due to fear of social stigma. She would go out only for defecation either in the early morning hours or late in the evening.

When Tuli's deformity was quite noticeable, her husband reported the matter to the "khot" (village headman) who suggested that Tuli be ex-communicated and that her husband should re-marry as Tuli was sterile. Thus Tuli was sent out from the family circle and presently resides outside Balewadi.

Analysis

The Thakurs believe that food cooked by menstruating woman causes leprosy is certainly meaningful within their cultural frame of reference. Menstrual blood is impure, black, evil, hot and corrosive in nature. Anything which comes in contact with it is contaminated or polluted. Food is converted into blood in the body. Food cooked by a menstruating woman is converted into blood which is polluted black, evil, hot and corrosive in nature.

The serious offense of cooking food during menstruation means to incur the wrath of "chul" (the Goddess of fire or Agni). The chul or hearth is believed to be sacred as she represents the Sun God who according to the Thakurs is the giver of life. It is because of the chul that Thakur cooks food and survives. Cause of leprosy is at times associated with the wrath of "Chul" as she cannot stand impurity that is a menstruating sitting in front of her and cooking food.

This hot, corrosive and impure blood spoils the pure blood in the body and starts destroying the body tissues which results in the deformity of the body. The Thakurs believe that what is pure must remain pure and any contact with impurity makes it impure. Thus what is socially recognized as impure is discarded out of the social system and hence leprosy patients are ex-communicated and do not interact with other members of their society.

EPISODE NO. : 12

Aim

1. To study the socio-cultural and behavioural aspects associated with leprosy within the Thakur culture.
2. To explore their concepts of the origin and cause of leprosy.
3. To explore the interaction of a leprosy patient with other members of his society.
4. To study the Thakur's concept of body image and leprosy cure.

Background

Pandu Bhima Pardhi, male Thakur, 28 years, resident of Chinchwadi, is a leprosy patient and is ex-communicated by his fellowmen. He lives outside the village in a small hut.

Course of Events

Pandu is suffering from leprosy since the last two years. He narrated his illness experience by classifying it into various phases.

Disease

Leprosy is locally known as "Raktapiti" in the Thakur community. It has two other local names "Kushtarog" and "Zadi".

Origin and Cause of Leprosy

Pandu was affected by leprosy when he was 26 years. He narrated that it is believed by the Thakurs that if a man has sex relations with his wife during her menstrual period, he is affected by leprosy. Pandu disregarded this belief and had sex relations with his wife Pali, two years ago when she was menstruating. he believes that he is paying for his past act now. He was asked "why and how do women suffer from leprosy ?". To this he replied that there are several causative factors and went on to highlight them.

1. If a man has sex relations with a menstruating woman.
2. Consuming food prepared by a menstruating woman causes leprosy.
3. Body contact with a leprosy patient causes leprosy.
4. Leprosy is also caused if the soiled clothes of the menstruating woman are touched.
5. When a viper (zadya) bites its poison causes leprosy. Thus leprosy is also locally known as "zadi" because it is believed to have been caused by "zadya's poison".

Symptoms of Raktapiti

It began with small white patches. Pandu misunderstood them for leucoderma. Leucoderma according to the Thakurs does not have social stigma and is hereditary. When deformity set in, he was worried. As he stayed in a nuclear family he was able to conceal his deformity for sometime.

Immediate Reactions of the Family members

Pandu lived with his wife and their son in a separate hut in Chinchwadi. When his wife came to know of his deformity, she was worried that her husband would be ostracized by the community. After much contemplation she reported the matter to her father-in-law who spoke to the village headman (khot) and to some elders. They together discussed the issue and it was decided that Pandu would stay on the outskirts of the village where he would be served food by his wife. He was to refrain from interacting in any manner with the other members of his community. Pandu's wifc would place some food for him néar a tree outside the village and Pandu would later pick up his meal and eat in his hut. Pandu was restricted from entering the village.

Concept of cure

"Is there a cure for Raktipiti, Pandu ?". He replied, "No, because it is a curse of the Gods for his misdoings and failure to perform a divine rite or duty. No medicine man or practitioner can cure 'Raktapiti'".

Why is it then that some patients are cured when they take the P.H.C. (sarkari davakhana) medicine ? Pandu replied, "they are cured because they go to the P.H.C. in the initial stage of the disease". "Why didn't you go and try the PHC medicine ?". To this Pandu's reply was, "I was afraid that people would get to know of my disease and stigmatize me".

Leprosy and Body Image

"Pandu, what causes body deformity ?". He replied, "A leprosy patients blood is not pure red and normal, instead it is black or greenish blue in colour. This kind of blood degenerates the human body like the slow poison of 'zadya'" (viper) does".

"How do you know that the colour of the blood of a leprosy patient is black or greenish blue ?". Pandu explained, "We, Thakurs do not bury the dead bodies of leprosy patients but cremate them. If we bury them, the leprosy worms (kidas) may come up from the soil and cause leprosy. When we cremate the body greenish blue fumes and smoke are seen coming out of the patients dead body. Hence a leprosy patient's blood is black or greenish blue in colour. It is also believed as people grow old their blood turns black. Black blood is symbolic of the end of life or the last phase of life.

The various systems in the body of a leprosy patient do not function normally because the blood of such a patient is not pure red, neither does it have strength and does not circulate fast in the body. It brings about degeneration of the body which leads to deformity which is the opposite of form. Deformity is the last phase of life for a leper. It is believed that the leprosy patient's atma (soul) also becomes polluted as a result of the impure blood in the body.

Analysis

The Thakurs believe that menstrual blood is evil, black, hot and corrosive in nature. A man having sex relations during this period with a woman gets leprosy as this menstrual blood is believe to enter into the man through the male genital organ (penis). It is also believed that a man/ woman who consumes food prepared by a menstruating woman is affected by leprosy. It is believed that the evil touch of such a woman spoils the food. Food and water contribute towards the formation of blood. The evil touch makes the food evil which in turn produce evil blood. This blood circulates in the body bringing about degeneration and pollution of both atma and body. Deformity begins to set in. Deformity is an antithesis of the form which is considered to be divine.

That which is not "normal" and "divine" does not find place in the normal society and in normal situations, and hence the physically deformed individual is stigmatized and dislocated from the other members of the society who have a divinely prescribed and accepted "form" (body). The Thakurs believe that the human body reflects the characteristics of the cosmos and the universe. Universe is pure and holy while deformity is not. The pure and holy is God made while impurity and evil is "Rakshas like". Hence that which is Rakshas (giant, abnormal, deformed) is dislocated from that or from those who are divine or natural.

It is believed that women and children are affected by leprosy due to their interaction with leprosy patients. A leprosy patient's touch is evil. When he talks his atma liberates foul and evil breath and this evil breath causes leprosy in those who come in contact with him.

TheThakurs believe that leprosy can also be caused due to the bite of a viper (zadya). Such leprosy is termed as "Zadi". They associate the gradual process of body deformity with the slow effect of the vipers deadly poison. The gradual loss of neural sensation in fingers and toes is associated with the slow movement of the viper. The white spots which are early symptoms of leprosy are associated with the black and white stripes on the viper's body. The whole human body becomes deformed and inactive which symbolizes the vipers inactiveness and laziness.

However, on the tenth day after the leprosy patient's death the Thakurs perform purification rituals to purify the soul of the dead patient and therefore ensure its migration to heaven. Although a leper does not enjoy social significance on earth, he gets a chance to interact peacefully and happily in heaven provided the purification rite is performed on the 10th day after death.

The preventive aspect with regards to leprosy is to ex-communicate the leper out of their social system. Leprosy as a disease thus highlights the social interaction, the death concept, the body image, the Thakurs concept of environment etc.

EPISODE NO. : 13

Aim

To explore the directional symbolism the Thakur associate with sleeping posture, sexual posture and its relation to ill-health/death.

Background

Mr. A.S., married male, aged 58 years, a bhagat by profession, resident of Saraiwadi explains the Thakur's concept of sleeping and sexual posture and its relation to directional symbolism.

Course of Events

Mr. A.S. suffered from high fever when he unknowingly slept with his head pointing south. This was brought to his notice in a vision in which the sun God asked him to purify himself by drinking cow's urine and by offering a coconut to the village God - waghoba. Mr. A.S. did as he was instructed, he also drank a decoction of Leucas-aspera mixed in water.

On enquiring the significance of the south direction Mr. A.S. said that the south direction is evil, there are giants (Rakshas) residing there. The wind that blows from the south, causes ill-health. The Thakurs bury their death with the head pointing south. "Where do the Thakurs point their heads while they are engaged in sex ?". Mr. A.S. replied, "they may point either east (ugavat baju) or west (mavalat baju) or north (dev disha) but never south. Even when a woman delivers her head points east and the vagina points west because satvai resides there and she should be the first one to see the child. Also a woman cooks facing the east and the hearth is situated always towards the south-east. if a woman cooks facing any other direction it may cause ill health or even death.

Analysis

In this particular context the Bhagat emphasizes that directions play an important role in,health. The east is the direction of life as the Sun God dwells there, North is the direction where Gods reside and west is the direction where satvai dwells - she is the Goddess of fortune and fertility. The south is believed to be evil, as the "Rakshas" (evil giants) reside there. South symbolizes death. Even the wind that blows from south is believed to cause illness. No auspicious rituals are performed facing the south. It is because of this reason the Thakurs do not point their heads to the evil south while sleeping, nor during sexual intercourse and delivery which have got implications of creating and bring forth life. South symbolizes death, evilness and darkness. While east symbolizes life. North holiness and west direction fertility.

EPISODE NO. : 14

Aim

To highlight the Thakur concept of Albinism from an emic perspective.

Background

Mahadev Padir, 17 years, bachelor, student of Std. IX at the Donger Pada Ashram School, resident of Gadwadi Pathraj Grampanchayat narrated the following episode which occurred in his family.

Course of Events

Mahadev's paternal aunt delivered the second son. He was born an albino. The attending midwife helped deliver the child. After delivery, she consulted the father) Mahadev's uncle) and it was decided that she would kill the child. The midwife took a basket smeared it inside and the outside with cowdung and inverted it (the basket) on the child. After and hour the child dies of suffocation. The dead body was taken and during the night by the midwife and buried. She was assisted by the father and some elderly people. The body was buried with its dorsal side facing the sun. This is done as an act of preventing the evil spirit (in the dead body) from leaving the body. The midwife was paid Rs. 40/- for the services.

On enquiring with Mahadev why the child was killed. he answered he was the child of a white male evil spirit - Munja. Mahadev was asked what is the co-relation between a human child and the evil spirit. He replied Munja is white skinned male evil spirit. He is the spirit of a bachelor who died without having a family and sexual life. he craves for the sexual life and as a spirit takes revenge. "Mahadev, how did the munja come in contact with your aunt ?". Mahadev replied, "My aunt was picked up from my uncle's side as they slept. She was carried away by Munja who had sex with her and then returned her back to my uncle". "Mahadev why was the child killed ?". He answered, " The child was not normal, he was evil and whatever is evil is not eligible to grow with human beings. If such children are allowed to grow up they would bring doom on the village". "Mahadev, who kills the child and how ?". Mahadev answered, "This act is done by theattending midwife (suine) after consulting the father (of the child) or the head of the household. The midwife smears the basket with cowdung and inverts this over the child who dies of suffocation or at times she chokes the child by pressing the neck".

Mahadev has experienced another similar incident which occurred in the family of his paternal uncle's. This uncle's granddaughter was born an albino and was killed in the same way (refer genealogy). On enquiring with Mahadev from which direction did the Munja come from, Mahadev had another story to narrate. He narrated that about seven to eight years ago a Muslim albino bachelor was murdered in Tadwadi and it is his spirit which causes trouble to the people of the village. The spirit still lingers around the village and attacked his aunt and cousin sisters both then delivered albinos.

Analysis

The Thakurs have their own method of classifying normal and abnormal, good and evil.

Thus the albino child, who does not fit into the common framework is considered evil and whatever is evil is excommunicated totally. The Thakurs believe that good and evil cannot stay together and that what belongs to the evil world must be returned. Thus the albino children believed to be fathered by Munja are killed thereby sending them back. The burial position of the child is symbolic that the spirit would never trouble the family.

The Thakurs also believe the children born with congenital deformities are fathered by Khais (a black evil spirit). The khais has no form. These children are also killed and buried.

The normal acceptable form of the body is believed (by the Thakurs) to resemble the cosmos and therefore it is divine. What is good (the human body) is allowed to grow and be a part of the human society. Albinism and congenital deformities are exactly opposite to divine, and true form of the body and therefore belong to the evil cosmic forces and are therefore not a part of the human society.

Note - See Genealogy Below:

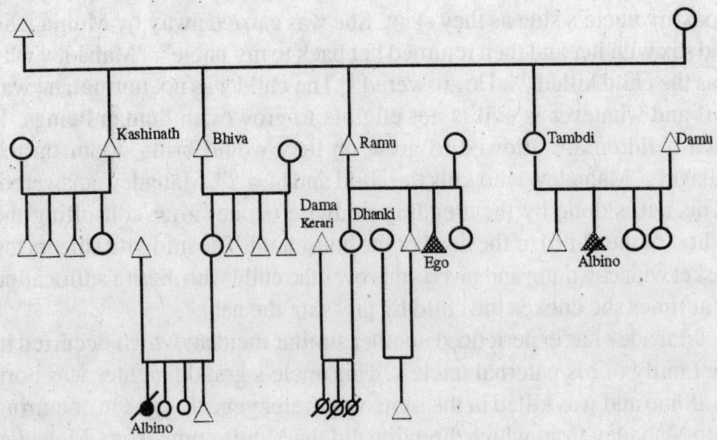

Aim

To investigate the Thakur beliefs and practices on possession of evil spirits.

Background

Budhya Katwara, married man, 26 years, resident of Thakurwadi - Kasahale village was possessed by an evil spirit sometime in the year 1980.

Course of Events

The first incident of this episode occurred in the year 1980 in the month of August (rainy season). Budhya accompanied by his friend Alo went fishing to the river Pej, which flows about 5 km. away from his house.

It was evening and the sun was about to set, Budhya had been fishing for nearly 3 hours and had caught nearly 1/2 kg of fish. He was set to go home when suddenly he spotted a big black crab and jumped back into the river to catch it. He did not get it. Alo had been watching Budhya and asked him why he had jumped into the river. Budhya told him about the black crab. Alo laughed and told Budhya that there was no such thing as a "black crab" and added that Budhya must have seen a ghost. Taking this incident in a light vein both walked back home as the sun had nearly set.

The next day at about 4 o'clock in the afternoon Budhya along with his friends again went fishing to the Shilar river about 2.5 km away from Thakurwadi. This time he had a larger catch, one kg of small fish and two black fishes (Mharal). Towards sunset the men started back home. On the way back Budhya's friend noticed that he (Budhya) suddenly started chewing raw black fish. A little while later Budhya got into a bush, full of cobwebs and continued chewing the raw black fish. His friends saw darkness in the bush. They were perplexed at Budhya's behaviour.

Three of Budhya's friend tried to pull him out of the bush but they felt that Budhya was stronger than them. They continued their tussle for about 15 minutes during which Budhya's head was hurt as he hit against a stone. Noticing the head injury one of the friends ran to call Kamli, Budhya's mother.

He was brought home with the help of the other men. The village elders advised Kamli, that she should consult the Bhagatin of Kotimba. They suspected that Budhya was possessed by an evil spirit. That night Budhya had fever, he did not eat and was unusually quite.

The next day when Budhya heard that he was to be taken to the Bhagatin, a Mahar by caste, he put up a lot of resistance. He behaved violently, shouting and breaking things in the house. It took three strong men to hold him and take him to the Bhagatin.

Diagnosis and Interpretation

The Bhagatin was informed about Budhya's unusual behaviour. She made Budhya sit, placed a burning incense stick and a lamp in front of him. Abir (black powder), gulal (red powder), a lamp and some rice called 'ghat' were placed in front of the Devi's (Goddesses) who help her diagnose the cause of illness.

Hair let loose, moving her head in a clockwise direction, the Bhagatin got into a trance making funny sounds. While in a trance, she took a whip and loudly said addressing the spirit, "I know you are a Khais (male evil spirit) and have attacked Budhya on Amosha (no moon) evening near river Pej. You tried to attack him in the form of black crab".

She then whipped Budhya and asked the spirit what he wanted. The spirit then demanded a sacrifice of a black cock and a coconut. Kamli agreed to do the needful. The Bhagatin then hit the evil spirit five times which then left Budhya making a loud funny sound. The Bhagatin then came out of her trance and said that the evil spirit was a 'khais' from the kathkari tribe. The following tuesday the cock was sacrificed and the village elders, Bhagatin along with Kamli's family feasted on the sacrificed cock. Budhya was cured and resumed his normal duties and behaved normally.

Analysis

The Thakur believe in three types of evil spirits which bring trouble and cause illness.

i. Khais - a strong male evil spirit, black coloured with inverted heels.

ii. Munja - a white coloured male evil spirit.

iii. Hadeli - a black coloured female evil spirit with hair let loose.

It is believed that when a bachelor or a spinster dies, their souldoes not go to heaven as they have not fulfilled their desire of marriage, sex and family life. These souls then become evil spirits.

The episode reflects Thakur's ideology regarding khais (Male evil spirit) being black in colour, consumption of raw fish, taking the guise of a black crab, attacking healthy and strong persons like Budhya, Budhya being possessed on Amosha (no moon evening), putting up resistance against three strong people, affinity towards darkness and craving for blood and hence the demand for a cock to be sacrificed.

The episode also highlights the Thakurs conceptions/notions of situations in which the spirits may attack. In the present episode the attack was on a Amosha eve (no moon night). Evil is symbolized by the colour black and the affinity towards such things as darkness. Black cock is sacrificed because the evil spirit is a male. Yet another very interesting fact highlighted in this episode is that of the evil spirit being a kathkari, inter group conflicts are a constant feature between the Thakurs and the Kathkaris because the kathkaris are placed lower than the Thakurs in the social hierarchy.

As they do not enjoy similar status at the social interactional level they both (Thakurs and Kathkaris) give vent to their hatred and jealousy for each other at a spiritual level. Social conflicts are interestingly solved at spiritual level through healing rites. The illness episode also depicts the social stigma attached to the Kathkaris as defined by the Thakurs. This stigma exists after death but at a spiritual level.

EPISODE NO. : 16

Aim

To investigate the Thakur beliefs and practices regarding the phenomenon of being possessed by evil spirits and to explore the symbolic elements that they (the Thakurs) associate with the illness caused by the evil spirits.

Background

Ganu Ughda, resident of Borwadi hamlet, Pathraj village, married,

48 years old, has a farm situated on the eastern side of his hamlet surrounded by forest.

Course of Events

One evening Ganu was returning to his home from his farm, carrying a head load of fodder for the cattle. All of a sudden a white dog charged at him for no rhyme or reason. To defend himself Ganu put down the fodder and picked a big stone and threw it at the dog. The dog ran away and disappeared.

Seven days later Ganu got fever. He used to feel sleepy, tired and shiver with cold. Interestingly this happened only at night. Ganu tried a decoction of Leucas aspera with water for 3-4 days but in vain. In the meanwhile people started suspecting that Ganu's illness was because of an evil spirit attack. Interestingly Ganu went to the P.H.C. (Primary Health Centre) but he felt no better.

Ganu's father went to consult a Bhagat from 'Dhotrewadi'. As usual the Bhagat using the metal pot (tambya) diagnosis rite diagnosed Ganu's illness. He interpreted the illness as being possessed by 'Munja' (a white male spirit). The Bhagat told them, that the white dog hit by Ganu on his way back home was none other than 'Munja'. The Bhagat gave the holy ash (Ibut - is the ash from the hearth (chula) which symbolizes body of the sun - the life giver) to put it on Ganu's forehead. he also instructed Ganu's father to sacrifice two male black cocks to the 'Munja'. This sacrifice should be offered near the place where the Ganu was attacked. After applying the Iboot on the forehead Ganu became allright. Two days later the cocks were sacrificed to Munja for freeing Ganu/leaving his body.

Analysis

Ganu's fever was caused because he was possessed by 'Munja'', a white male evil spirit which is culturally recognized by the Thakurs. This evil spirit took the form of a white dog and attacked Ganu apparently for no rhyme or reason. It is believed by the Thakurs that the evil spirits bring trouble and cause illness to humans.

It is also believed by the Thakurs that the spirits are very active on a dark night. Ganu was attacked on the beginning of Amosha (new moon night).

The symptoms of being possessed, as reflected in the episode, are high fever, shivering, quietness etc. Since the cause of Ganu's illness was attributed to spiritual intervention the person (socio-ritual curer) consulted was a Bhagat who gave 'Ibut'. Ibut is the holy ash from the hearth which in this context symbolizes the body of Sun (almighty life giver) integrating with the human body. It is believed to neutralize the evil effect which takes charge of the human atma (soul).

The sacrifice of black cocks is symbolic of the nature of evil spirits. Black symbolizes evil and consumption of blood symbolizes the Rakshas (giant) like nature of the deformed spirits.

EPISODE NO. : 17

Aim

To highlight from an emic perspective the Thakur's concept of sterility in woman as a state of the ill-health.

Background

Mrs. P, married female, ages 30 years, resident of Saraiwadi explains the socio-cultural aspects of sterility of a Thakur woman.

Course of Events

Mrs. P was married to Mr. D when she was 15 years old. Even 15 years later she did not bear a child. Five years after her wedding, her in-laws took her to the Bhagat to know the reason of her infertility. He interpreted that Mrs. P was sterile because her puberty rite was not performed properly. After this, the in-laws also consulted midwife who also declared Mrs. P was sterile.

The in-laws then told Mrs. P that they would get their son married for the second time (to a widow). The second wife bore two children.

This was beginning of a miserable life for Mrs. P. She ws constantly degraded and ill-treated by her in-laws. Even her parents did not show any sympathy. Her husband often beat her and she was not allowed to attend any auspicious ritual, touch a pregnant woman nor enter a house where a woman had delivered. Her status in the family and the society fell miserably. She did all the household work and often her husband quarreled with her. The second wife would at times attribute the cause of fever of her children to the evil eye of Mrs. P.

Even at societal level the above restrictions were observed and people stigmatized her as "Bhutali" - witch. The village Bhagat too in a ritual healing warned her husband of her evil deeds although she was never physically tortured. She could not raise her head and move about freely in the society.

Analysis

Mrs. P's parents attribute the cause of her sterility to witchcraft. They are of the opinion that Mrs. P's mother-in-law is responsible for Mrs. P's sterility. Mrs. P expresses this information on the oath of secrecy. her in-laws look down upon her due to her physical inability.

Thus The Thakurs classify sterility as ill-health and view the interaction of a sterile/barren woman with other members as social pollution in cultural specific situation such as marriage, turmeric ritual, birth ritual, delivery etc. Thus the sterile woman does not enjoy a good status while she is living.

On the death of a sterile woman, she is buried in a ritualistic way. She is wrapped in a green sari and the rite known as "oti bharne" is performed. The green colour of the sari is symbolic of a married woman. The ritual "oti bharne" is symbolic of ritually making her soul fertile. "Oti" - represents womb and "Bharne" means to fill. Thus this rite is performed to ensure her fertility in heaven.

EPISODE NO. : 18

Aim

The Thakur culture recognizes the concept of evil eye, This study aims to explore the concept of evil eye (Drishti) and its effect on a child's health.

Background

Hema Padir, married male, 35 years, resident of Borwadi, Pathraj grampanchayat narrated the origin and cause of his son's illness which he attributed to the cause of evil eye.

Course of Events

In the summer of 1990, Hema's son one and a half years old suffered from diarrhoea and vomiting. Hema's wife tried home remedies for four to five days but in vain. Hema's mother was of the opinion that the cause of the child's ill-health was due to evil eye.

Hema's mother then resolved to cure her grandson. She asked her grandson to face the south. Then holding some salt, few pieces of the broom stick and five chillies in her hand and chanting mantras, she moved her hand over the child's body in a clockwise manner five times and then dropped the articles in her hand into the burning fire of the hearth.

A black bead locally called "Dithmani" was then tied around the child's neck. The child was later taken to the P.H.C. and treated, after which he recovered completely. The healing process thus consisted of two types of therapies namely magico-ritual to ward off the evil effect and allopathic therapy to heal any biological disorder.

Analysis

Origin and cause of an infant's ill-health is mostly attributed to the effect of the evil eye, witchcraft, sorcery or wrath of Satvai (Goddess of fertility and fortune) by the Thakurs. Infants are considered to be pure, innocent and ignorant and a gift of God to mankind. The Thakurs believe that whatever is pure, beautiful and holy becomes a target of the evil forces and they cause harm through evil eye, witchcraft and sorcery.

The Thakurs believe that the Bhutala (sorcerer) Bhutali (witch), Wanjuti (sterile woman) or any other woman who is jealous of the child casts an evil eye or sends an evil force on the child. So as to cause harm to the child. The Thakur culture has made provisions to ward off the evil effect by performing certain rituals. The articles used to ward off the evil effect have specific significance. Chillies are symbolic of heat/hotness, salt is believed to absorb the evil effect of the latter and destroys it (the evil effect) by making a crackling sound. Brooms are used to remove dirt from the house and hence broom stick pieces are used as they are believed to remove the effect of the evil eye from the patient's body. The action of throwing in all the articles into the fire in the hearth symbolizes the purification of the patient and the total destruction of the evil effect. Making the child face the south is done because it is believed that evil resides in the south and attacks in the form of magical objects, black magical chants and the evil wind which blows from the south and carries the evil effect.

EPISODE NO. : 19

Aim

To highlight the origin and cause of Arthritis (vat) and the concept of physiology associated with it as believed by the Thakurs.

Background

Paddu Dore, married male, 80 years, resident of Thakurwadi, Kashale village, suffers from arthritis and explains on the basis of his illness experience the culturally held conceptions regarding the origin and cause of arthritis and the psychological factor associated with it.

Course of Events

Paddu Dore is suffering from arthritis since the last five years. He narrated his illness experience by stating that he had become a victim of 'vat' five years ago. he said, "I was returning from the field during the summer season and was sweating profusely. Before having lunch I decided to have a cold water bath and that very day in the evening I developed severe pain in the joints and had fever".

Paddu was asked, "Is this the only cause of vat ?". He replied, "No, there are many", and gave the following causes.

1. A person may suffer from vat if he has a bath with cold water when he is sweating.

2. When the body is exposed to cold air, the cold air causes scales to appear on the skin or the heels get cracked or the body becomes stiff.

3. The third reason why a person suffers from 'vat' is because there is too much or too less air in the body.

"Padu, what do you think happens when the proportion of air reduces in the body ?". Ha, Ha .... laughed Padu and asked the researcher in return, "Have you seen a deflated bus tyre ?". "Yes, of course", replied the researcher. Padu continued, "when the air in the tyre reduces, the tyre looses its original shape so also the human body becomes crooked and deformed".

Thus polio and epilepsy are classified under the 'vat' category and as the body becomes deformed during these diseases. "Padu, what happens when the air proportion in the body increases ?". Padu replied, "The stomach bulges and the body swells. There is a woman residing in Khondewadi who has a bulging stomach and her naval is also big. She suffers from 'vat' as a result of imbalance of the proportion of air in the body".

4. A person may suffer from 'vat' because of the 'Baya'. They are spirits of the planets in the universe. They visit the human beings when they are annoyed with them (humans). The 'Baya' enter into the human body either in the form of very hot or cold wind and cause joint pains.

"Padu, why does the proportion of the air become more or less in the body ?". He replied, "This happens because our body may not be in harmony with nature and the 'Baya'. "Padu, so wind is a very important element in our body". "Yes ! it is. It helps blood to circulate in our body, helps human beings to create speech, sound, burps, hiccups etc". "Padu, which other elements help the human body to sustain itself ?". To this Padu replied, "Water, light, wind, food, agni and body structure (mud)". The human blood, semen and breast milk find their source in water and are associated with survival and creation of life. It is believed that flesh and bones are strong because of food (khat - manure) and water. Blood circulation, sounds in the body, digestion and excretion are controlled by the wind. Agni (fire) is present in the atma (soul) and in the stomach (pot). Fire (heat) in the stomach digests the food. The fire in the atma keeps it glowing (alive). Light (prakash) is present in the body especially in the eyes, because of which human beings can see. The sun and moon (Almighty Gods) are the source of light and fire. The body structure is made up of earth and when man dies he becomes mud.

"Padu, all these important elements which constitute the body are they present in the cosmos ?". Padu laughed heartily and replied; "you people go to schools and are yet ignorant of the fact that the human body is nothing but an image of the universe, and all that which is present in the universe is present in the human body".

Analysis

The Thakurs attribute the origin of 'vat' to the following bodily complaints - body stiffness, polio, epilepsy, chapped heels, dry and scaly skin, joint pains, fits.

The causes of 'vat' are mainly attributed to the following factors - 1. imbalance of the air/wind proportion in the body, 2. having a cold water bath while sweating, 3. exposure of the body to excessive cold wind, and 4. wrath of the 'Baya'.

Thus the physiology of the human body is controlled by Agni (fire), light (prakash). The sources of these are the sun and the moon. The universe is the source of the wind. The body structure is made of earth (mud). Important life fluids such as blood, semen and breast milk have their source in water. To the Thakurs, the sun, moon and water are the almighty Gods and are brothers of each other. The Thakurs perception on body image cross cuts into meaning and symbols of other social spheres in life. These spheres include religion, hot and cold concepts, cosmology, nature and medicine. these spheres in life are inter-related into a meaning system.

EPISODE NO. : 20

Aim

To assess the concept of hot and cold humour that the Thakurs link with body sores.

Background

Ganpat Padir, male, married, 27 years, farmer by profession, resident of Khondyachiwadi of Pathraj village panchayat.

Course of Events

The summer of 1990 was a bad time for Ganpat. He was suffering from sores (of all sizes) and was covered with them literally from head to toe. His mother applied karanj oil (Pongamia pinnata). He was also taken to a vaidu (herbalisT) from Jamul wadi. The vaidu treated Ganpat for a week with herbal remedies. He diagnosed the cause of Ganpats ill health to the accumulation of heat element in the body. He said that Ganpat must have had too much of hot foods which aggravated the fire element in his body and therefore he got sores. The vaidu prescribed a diet which included cold foods and the medicine administered was also cold in nature.

When Ganpat was completely healed the vaidu was given a feast which included rabbit meat and alcohol. Ganpat's father had also promised Goddess Holi (Goddess of holi) that if she would cure his son, he (the father) would offer her a chick. Ganpat's father kept his promise and during the Holi festival made the promised offering.

Analysis

There prevails a very strong belief among the Thakurs that certain hot and/or cold foods if consumed in excess cause disease or bodily imbalance. Here, the patient was believed to have consumed excessive amounts of hot foods and so his diet and medicines were cooling so as to counteract the hot effect.

Another strong aspect this episode points out to is the appearance of Goddess Holi. it is believed (by the Thakurs) the Sun and the Holi control the fire element in the human body. Hence along with the physical or medical aspect of treatment there also exists a religious aspect which involves the appeasement of Gods or Natural forces.

EPISODE NO. : 21

Aim

To explore the causational and therapeutic concepts associated with cataract as perceived by the Thakurs.

Background

Antu Dharma Padir, male, married, 60 years, carpenter by profession, a member of the Thakur tribe, resident of Lobhyachi wadi narrates his illness experience.

Course of Events

Antu suffered from cataract from 1987-89. He was unable to see. When asked he said he had lost his vision. "How did you develop cataract Antu ?". He replied, "I am a carpenter and while at work small splinters of wood keep getting into the eyes and block the light so I could not see". "What remedies did you try ?". Antu replied, "I put monitor (Ghorpad) oil in my eyes. I also tried putting chilly powder. I continued this treatment for two years but in vain. People advised me to visit the Bhagat but my condition remained the same. In the year 1991, I dared to go to the PHC and was told to get operated. There was a cataract operation camp at Karjat. I got operated. Now I am allright and wear spectacles". Antu now professes more faith in allopathy.

Analysis

Antu attributed the cause of cataract to the entering of the splinters while he was at work. He also tried out all the traditional methods in order to find cure. having failed in his attempt he approached the PHC as the last resort and was cured. This helped him to have more faith in allopathy and also demonstrated the positive aspect of modern medicine which under normal circumstances is shunned by the tribe.

EPISODE NO. : 22

Aim

To probe into the medical system of the Thakurs so as to uncover the origin and cause of the prolonged unhealing wounds.

Background

Kamli Pardhi, wife of a Bhagat, resident of Lobhyachi wadi, 70 years and childless.

Course of Events

In the summer of 1990, Kamli went into the jungle to gather firewood. On her way back a thorn pricked her left foot. She could not remove the thorn completely. After a few days her foot was swollen and pus had accumulated in it. Mahadu, her husband applied the leaves of Dolichos ablab and bandaged her foot for five days. When he opened the bandage on the sixth day the wound had festered and caused a lot of pain.

Irrespective of a member of herbal remedies the wound would not heal. She was in great pain and the wound gave out foul smell. Mahadu did not let her go to the PHC, fearing amputation. Mahadu is convinced that Kamli's sickness is a result of witchcraft and it is done by some person from the village itself.

Analysis

In Lobhyachi wadi, maximum number of families belong to the Lobhie clan. Hence the name, Other wadis similarly get their names. Such as Padir wadi, Kaute wadi, Bhagatachi wadi etc.

In Lobhe wadi, there are very few families belonging to the Pardhi. Due to this there is constant friction directly and indirectly between the dominant Lobhie clan members and the Pardhi clan members. Mahadu owns more land than the Lobhie. This makes him an object of jealousy and hatred.

Thus Mahadu is convinced that due to jealousy and hatred his wife now suffers from the wound. Thus here, this episode reveals the inter-clan conflicts and the way it finds expression through witchcraft and sorcery.

EPISODE NO. : 23

Aim

To explore the Thakur's perception of visitation or intervention of ancestral spirits and its effect on human health.

Background

Kashinath Nama Dhole, married, 40 years farmer cum shopkeeper by profession, a member of the Thakur tribe and resident of Khodyachi wadi.

Course of Events

When Kashinath was a child of 10 years, his grandfather passed away. Within years his paternal grandmother also passed away. Kashinath was much loved by both his grandparents. Two weeks after the passing away of his grandmother, Kashinath look ill. He had high fever. His father Nama, tried the local method of treatment. He gave Kashinath the decoction of Leucas aspera.

For 4-5 days, the same decoction was administered. Kashinath showed little improvement. A bhagat by the name of Heeru was summoned. He used the metal pot technique of diagnosis and interpreted that the fever was due to the visitation of Kashinath's grandparents (ancestral parents) as he was very dear to them. The Bhagat told Nama, to go to kalam village and make two coin size statues of

1. Supali - female ancestral spirit
2. Virdev - male ancestral spirit.

These statues were made of aluminum. A cock and a hen were sacrificed as an offering to the ancestral spirits. The Bhagat and the family members partook of the feast. The Bhagat also gave Kashinath some decoction of herbs. Kashinath was completely cured and till today the statues of Supali and virdev are preserved safely.

Analysis

There exists very strong belief among the Thakurs that ancestral spirits visit their family and cause or bring illness for two specific reasons :

1. when the spirits visit a dear one.
2. when the spirits are angry if certain rituals are not performed.

In this case the fever occurred two weeks after the death of Kashinath's grandmother. It was in this cultural context that Kashinath's fever was interpreted by the Bhagat. The aluminum statues are still in Kashinath's house and are symbolic of fulfilling the sacrificial ritual of appeasing the ancestral spirits. Although the procedure of treatment was lengthy Nama preferred to continue it as the treatment was culturally acceptable.

EPISODE NO. : 24

Aim

To explore the Thakurs perception about the cause of tuberculosis.

Background

Govind Padu Pardhi, married male, 53 years, resident of Lobhyachi wadi, a member of the Thakur tribe, narrates his illness experience as a patient who suffered from tuberculosis.

Course of Events

Govind, nearly recovered from T.B. about 10 years ago, after undergoing treatment at Ulhasnagar Hospital. Later in January 1991, Govind suffered from the same complaints. this time, due to lack of finance, he did not go to Ulhasnagar Hospital for treatment.

He was spitting out blood, had high fever and became very weak. On enquiring why his sickness had worsened, he replied that he had not completed the earlier medical course and presently due to paucity of money he could not go to the hospital.

Cause of the Disease

Govind and his family members attribute the cause of T.B. to excessive drinking of alcohol. About 10 years ago, during the course of his treatment he was advised to abstain from drinking. Govind did not heed as a result of which his health continued to fail.

Treatment

Govind is now undergoing treatment (tablets and injections) at the PHC in kashale village. He has already taken 12 injections till date. He is of the opinion that because of the injections his urine becomes greenish yellow and adds that his lungs have got holes. He is convinced that the allopathic treatment which he is taking is effective and he will be cured.

Analysis

Govind is convinced that drinking excess of alcohol is the reason why he suffers from tuberculosis. He believes that alcohol is corrosive in nature and it burnt his blood and because of this hot blood there are holes in his lungs and his body is hot with fever. He believed that the tablets and injections have purified the dirt in his blood and cooled the blood. He says this with conviction as he can see the change in the colour of his urine.

Presently, it would be right to state the awareness of allopathic treatment for T.B. is quite high among the Thakurs. They are convinced that the cure for T.B. is only through the PHC. The Thakurs have witnessed the treatment and complete recovery of many T.B. patients like Govind Pardhi and thus their faith in allopathy has increased.

EPISODE NO. : 25

Aim

To understand the concept of <a. co-relation between the colour of the human blood and the state of health <b. the colour of the human blood and the stage in life <c. the colour of the human blood during jaundice, leprosy and snake bite.

Background

Mahadu Padir, married male, aged 68 years, resident of Lobhyachi wadi narrates his son's illness experience who suffered from Jaundice.

Course of Events

Mahadu's son Janu suffered from Jaundice in the summer of 1990 and was given herbal treatment. He got cured. On enquiring with Mahadu what is the cause of Jaundice, he replied that consumption of impure water and food turns the blood yellow and the following symptoms are visible, a. skin becomes pale and yellow, b. eyes becomes yellow, c. Nails turn yellow, and d. the patient becomes weak.

Mahadu was asked "what happened when a person is bitten by a cobra?". He replied, "The blood becomes blue". "Mahadu, does the colour of the blood change if the individual is affected by any other disease ?". "Yes, when a person suffers from leprosy, his blood becomes grayish black". Mahadu was also asked what happens to the blood when a person gets fever and how would one differentiate whether a person is healthy or not based on the colour of his blood. Mahadu had a classification for the different diseases or conditions,

1. Blue colour of the blood is an indication of snake bite.
2. Yellow colour indicated jaundice.
3. Grayish black colour was an indication of leprosy.
4. Dark black colour indicated menstruation.

The above colours of the blood are considered abnormal and an indication of ill-health. Mahadu also added that children and the youth (stages in life) are active therefore their blood is red during childhood and orange during youth. the two colours red and orange are associated with activeness, strength and power. Old people their blood becomes blackish and hence they loose their power of sight, hearing, speech, smell and feeling (touch).

"What maintains the red and orange colour of our blood, Mahadu ?". He replied, "In our body there is sun-light, which enables us to see. Agni (fire) keeps us warm. Water is converted into blood. Wind helps in circulation of blood and digests the food with the help of Agni. These elements in our body decrease as we get old and hence we become weak and powerless and the colour of the blood changes. If agni (fire) becomes less in the body. The wind in our body becomes cold and one feels cold and suffers from arthritis. If the light (sun light) decreases, one suffers from night blindness or becomes blind".

Analysis

Thus the Thakurs conception between the colour symbolism and health is highlighted. This episode also highlights the colour of the blood during the various phases of life and the Thakur's concept of strength and power. Thus diseases like jaundice and leprosy do not remain only at the biological level but involve symbolic and meaningful components which pervade the social system.

EPISODE NO. : 26

Aim

To highlight the culturally held perceptions of the Thakurs which provide a link between their concept of human body and the universe.

Background

Matti Mahadu Padir, married female, 70 years, resident of Thakurwadi, Kashale village. Matti was a traditional professional midwife (suine) by profession. She narrates her illness experience which provides a link between the Thakur's concept of human body and the planets in the universe.

Course of Events

Matti had been practicing midwifery for the last fourty years until in the year 1984 her helpmate (potdhari) a kathkari woman passed away. Matti is now old and keeps falling ill off and on. Her complaints centre around fever, cough, cold and body ache. She had tried several herbal medicines and home remedies which included branding of the joints with a hot iron rod. Shr also tried the P.H.C. medicines but none of the treatments had any effect on her. Finally, three weeks later her neighbour Aavdi advised her to consult the Bhagatin of Kotimba.

An interesting fact is that this particular Bhagatin (female shaman) belongs to the Mahar caste (an untouchable caste). Most Thakurs as well as kathkaris consult her as she belongs to the Davan jati which according to their social classification is a group associated with evil (giant like of Rakshas).

The Bhagatin got into a trance and interpreted that Matti had become a victim of the wrath of the Baya (the goddesses of the planets in the universe) and hence was suffering from continuous illness and suffering. Matti was asked, "why did the Baya get angry with you ?". She replied, "I did not perform a ritual of completing my service (Matti was a professional and traditional midwife) as a midwife". "Matti, who are these Baya ?". She answered, "they are the sisters of mother earth and are hierachially ordered in the universe. Mother earth is the fifth". Matti was asked, "How many Baya are there ?". She replied, "there are ten of them including mother earth".

"Matti, are these Baya evil ?". "No, they are goddesses". "Then why do they bring illness ?". She replied, "If a human being does not perform his religious duties, then the Baya cause illness and trouble". "Matti, what is the relation of Baya with the human body ?". Matti replied, "The human body is nothing but a representation of a universe". She further added, "which means that the body is a reflection of the universe". "Matti, which bodily features resemble the universe ?".

Matti first laughed heartily and then replied that the ten planets in the universe including the earth are arranged vertically, similar to the ten openings of the body. (daha darvaze). "Matti, which are the ten openings of the body ?". Matti gave the following ten openings - 1. Eyes, 2. Nose, 3. Mouth, 4. Ears, 5. Atma (soul), 6. Wrist pulse, 7. Naval, 8. Vaginal opening, 9. Pulses of the feet and 10. Anal opening (gupta darwaza).

She then explained, "Oh, its is so simple ten openings and ten planets". "Matti, what else in the human body resembles the universe ?". Matti's answer was that the human body has both masculine and feminine elements. The feminine elements or parts are the naval, vagina, little finger, soul and other openings. The thumb, urethra, testes, toes etc denote the masculine nature.

In the universe too there are masculine and feminine elements present. Stars, planets (Baya), lightening, wind denote feminine nature while the sun, moon, water who are believed to brothers denote masculine nature.

Just as the sun, moon give light to the universe so also light is present in the human body. There are is light in the eyes and it is because of this light that we are able to see. Agni (fire) in the atma (soul) symbolizes the sun. Sind is present in the cosmos and is also present in our body. The universe is made of soil, rocks and stones so also the human body is nothing but dust without life. When the human corpse is buried it decays and disintegrates and mixes with the soil. The water in the sea and the clouds is also present in the body. All important fluids of the body such as blood, semen, breast milk etc. are the products of water.

The mother earth has a husband wife relationship with the sun. So also the human male body has a husband wife relationship with the female body. The clouds, water and the sun all move in an anticlock direction around the earth hence water and blood in the body also move in the similar manner. the body cannot unction without the following cosmic elements light, fire, earth, food, water and wind which together form life. Hence the Bays are closely related to the human body.

"Matti, how did the bhagatin cure your illness ?". "the Bhagatin gave me 'Ibut' - holy ash from the hearth, which symbolizes the body of the sun, she also instructed me to give up my profession as the Baya desired this and advised me to wear an aluminum band around my neck which symbolizes that I am a devotee of the Baya and do not practice my profession".

Today, Matti is an ardent devotee of the Baya, does not practice her profession. She offered a coconut to the Baya for having cured her and also gave the Bhagatin Rs. 1.25 paise for diagnosing the cause of her illness.

Analysis

Thus the Thakur perceives the human body as a symbol of the cosmos and therefore the morphology and physiology of the human body bears resemblance to the universe. Therefore if social relationship with the cosmological objects is disturbed, then the human beings become susceptible to ill-health.

The body morphology consists of the earth (mud) and other planets. Agni (fire), hava (wind), Tej (light), Pani (water) are the four elements along with food which govern the physiology of the body.

The illness episode therefore attempted to cross-cut into the meanings associated with the Thakur concepts of body symbolism and cosmology and also attempted to demonstrate the manner in which the universe is ordered (as perceived by the Thakurs).

EPISODE NO. : 27

Aim

To uncover the Thakur concept of body symbolism and ethnophysiology that they associate with the origin and cause of scabies.

Background

Palu Kamlu Lobhie, aged 55, married male, a resident of Lobhiewadi, Pathraj Grampanchayat, a vaidu (herbalist) by profession narrates the culturally held beliefs of body symbolism and ethnophysiology associated with origin and cause of scabies.

Course of Events

Palu's son Sonu was suffering from scabies during the summer of 1992. Palu being a vaidu treated the disease by using herbal remedies. He made his son drink fresh juice of neem (Azadrachfa indica) leaves and applied externally the oil of pongamia pinnata seeds.

On enquiring with Palu about the cause of Sonu's scabies, he said that there may have been some problem with Sonu's blood.

When asked as to what was the problem he said that Sonu consumed a lot of jaggery before he had scabies.

When asked about the effects of jaggery on the body, he said that jaggery is sweet and if consumed in excess makes the blood sweet and invites 'kidas' (small worms) in the body.

When asked as to what happens next he said that the 'kidas' start living on the blood and are mostly present under the skin. These go on drinking water.

In the process of moving into the blood it causes itching. The movement of these 'kidas' and the effect of the sweets in the blood makes the blood hot and as much there are sores on the skin. The heat comes out through the skin pores and causes sores.

When asked as to why it was treated with neem leaves and Pongamia pinnata only, Palu replied that neem is bitter and cold in nature.

Its bitterness kills the 'kidas' in the blood and neutralizes the blood sweetness caused due to intake of excess sweets. It is cold in nature and hence neutralizes the heat caused due to intake of sweets in the body.

Pivli Rui (Pongamia pinnata oil) is applied externally because it also functions in the same way as neem except that it is applied externally, while neem is taken orally.

When asked as to what the PHC doctors applied for scabies, Palu laughed as said that they told them to wash the body with lifebuoy soap.

When asked whether they were right he said, what is the use of applying soap from outside when the origination of the cause (kidas- worms) is in the body ? The doctors should think about giving something internally to get rid of the kidas.

When asked about the different types of 'kidas' present in the body he said there were many of them Jantu (germ), Naru (guinea worm), Jant (Thread and round worms). When asked as to why they stay in the body,

Palu said that they like to live on human blood.

He said that our body is like a tree. The bones in the body are like the branches and skin of the tree. The flesh is like the bark (sal). The tree has hair on its body so also does the human body.

The tree bears fruits and the human beings bear children. There are germs and worms in the tree and so is the case with human body.

Both have atma (soul). Thus a human body very much resembles with a tree. Just as there are worms in the tree so is, the case with human beings. In Sonu's case the 'kidas' were 'Jantu' which lived on this blood and caused itching effect.

Analysis

The Thakur's concept about scabies is not merely interpreted as a physical health problem. It also considers/involves areas such as causational concepts, body physiological analogy which is a comparison between a tree and a human body and their interpretation of germs (Jantu) which arc harmful to both trees and human body.

This analogy itself is a proof how nature and culture are inter-related and how just a disease like scabies links itself conceptually with meaning and symbols of other spheres of life such as ethnophysiology, nature, healing causational concepts, classification of bitter and sweet substances and their effects on the human body.

EPISODE NO. : 28

Aim

To explore the Thakur's concepts about the cosmic forces which are instrumental in causing illness.

Background

Auvdi Padu Dore, married female, 64 years, resident of Thakurwadi of Kashale grampanchayat narrates the illness experience of her son Narayan who took ill because he was a target of the cosmic planetary spirits (Baya). This incident occurred when Narayan was six years old.

Course of Events

About fourty years ago in summer on the eve of the new moon night Auvdi was returning with the six year old Narayan from their farm. She heard a loud buzzing sound approaching above them and instructed

Narayan not to look up. Narayan being a playful child did not heed and looked up as the buzzing sound passed over them.

The next day Narayan had fever. Auvdi suspected the cause of the fever and informed her husband Padu about the previous day's happenings. Padu was afraid and decided to consult Bhagatin of Kolimba. Auvdi wrapped Narayan in a saree and took him to the Bhagatin (female shaman). The parents explained their problem to her. They offered her one rupee and twenty five paise to diagnose the origin and cause of their son's illness.

The Bhagatin lit an incense stick and displayed articles such as gulal (red powder), halad (turmeric), naral (coconut). These articles are used during worship. The Bhagatin's son started playing a small drum (dholki). The Bhagatin sat facing the east, hair let loose. She got into a trance and moved her head in an anticlock direction asking ritually the originator the cause of the fever what was the cure for the fever.

While the Bhagatin was in a trance, Padu and Auvdi requested the originator to cure their son and appealed that they were ready to do anything to get their son cured. The Bhagatin (now speaking on behalf the originator) replied that Narayan had come in the path of the moving planetary female spirits (Phirastya Baya) and therefore he was their victim. The Baya (goddesses) replied further (through the Bhagatin) that Padu and Auvdi must set up a 'ghat' (a symbol of cosmic forces - the Baya) and worship it for a fortnight and observe all the practices associated with this illness.

After sometime the Bhagatin came out of the trance. She then put 'Ibut' (the incense stick ash) on Narayan's forehead and instructed the parents to set up a 'ghat'. (An arrangement of a coconut in a metal pot with Plumeria flowers around). For fourteen nights the villagers could come to Padu's house and sing songs of praises to the Baya in order to please them. This singing ceremony is popularly known as the 'Jagran Ceremony'.

Taboos of the Jagran Ceremony

Auvdi Dore pointed out that there are number of taboos to be observed during the visitation of Baya for fourteen days.

1. No menstruating woman is allowed to enter the house where a 'ghat' is set up. Menstrual blood is a symbol of pollution and a evil pathogen. It pollutes the divine atmosphere. The Baya are therefore against it.
2. Narayan (patient) and his family members were not to eat meat or fish for those fourteen days. The Thakurs believe that if meat and/or fish is given to the patient, the Baya may cause him more trouble. The hot effects of meat and fish may add extra heat in the patient's

body, as there already a greater degree of heat in his body due to the visitation of Baya.

3. Drinking alcohol is also not permitted in the house where a ghat is set up. It is believed alcohol pollutes the divine situation.
4. A sorcerer and/or a witch is not allowed to enter the house, because where good (Baya) exists there evil (sorcerer - Bhutala and witch - Bhutali) cannot exist.

Treatment

On enquiring from Auvdi what exactly happens to the body when Baya visit a human being ?. She replied faintly, the Baya enter a human body through the medium of 'wind' (vara). This wind is hot in nature and therefore increases the body temperature high and therefore hot foods such as meat, fish, eggs etc. are avoided. Instead the patient is given the ritually collected sap of 'umber' (Ficus glomerata) root. The sap administered to the patient is believed to calm the patient (Baya).

On the fourteenth day Auvdi and Padu performed the ritual of 'pani ghalne' - pouring water. The patient was given a ritual bath by his mother. Auvdi said she offered a coconut for the Baya. The ghat was kept in a basket in the month 'paush' (Nov-Dec) outside the village. Narayan felt better after he went through all these formalities. The Baya then left him.

Analysis

Mother Earth (Dantari) according to the Thakurs has planetary sisters known as 'Baya'. These Baya live in the cosmos. The Thakurs believe that the Baya take different forms to visit the mother earth and the life existing on mother earth. They classify the Baya under two categories namely,

1. **Phirastya Baya :** or the moving planetary spirits. The phirastya Baya take the form of wild honey bees (the bigger species). Some times they take the form of hot wind and move about on the earth.

2. **Fodya Baya :** The second category is Fodya (meaning blisters & sores) Baya. They cause sores and blister on the body. The Fodya Baya take the form of various caste or social groups (Devjatis) and visit the patient.

Visitation of any of the above category means that the patient's body actually becomes a symbol of the Baya (cosmic/planetary spirits). The body automatically gets a higher (divine) status and therefore is worshipped. A 'Ghat' (a symbol of cosmos) is set up to ensure the presence of the Baya. The coconut symbolizes the sky and the coconut water (rain), the metal pot symbolizes the mother earth which is over arched by the sky (coconut). The water in the metal pot symbolizes the natural water which exists in mother earth. The flower on the apex of the coconut symbolizes the sun. The mango leaves symbolize the winds of all the directions. The plumeria rubra flowers symbolize the 'Baya' - sisters of mother earth.

This belief that the 'Baya' actually enter the human body is symbolic of man's intimate relationship with the cosmos. The Thakurs say that the 'pind' (human body) is nothing but the khand (cosmos). The ghat is set. The visitation of Baya is a form of social control which checks the deviant behaviour of the Thakurs such as eating excess non-veg, drinking alcohol, having sex with a menstruating woman etc.

Yet another interesting factor which plays a crucial role in the treatment - i.e. the sap of the Ficus glomerata tree symbolizes 'moon' and its sap the semen of the moon which given to the patient (Baya - females) satisfy their heat (sexual urge). The ritual of 'pani ghalne' again means the same thing. Water used to bathe the patient and the sap (umbarache pani) which is administered ritually is nothing but a symbolic indication of sexual satisfaction of the 'Baya'.

Physical experience of ill health is thus ritual perceived as an inter-play of the cosmological disruption of sex which is ritually patched up at the social level through a patient's body which according to the Thakurs is nothing but a symbol of cosmos.

EPISODE NO. : 29

Aim

To explore the Thakur's relationship between the concept of ill-health and the menstrual period.

Background

Pali Narayanan Dore, female, married, 30 years resident of Thakurwadi, narrates the Thakur's concept of the relation between the menstruation period and the state of ill-health.

Course of Events

Every month during 'vital' (menstrual periods) the Thakur women are supposed to sit in a corner of their dwelling place. She is not allowed to do any household chores. Her food is served from a distance to her.

She stays in the same place for five days, her movements and social interaction is restricted.

On the fifth day, after the periods are over she goes to the river, washes her clothes, has a bath, lights an incense stick to the Sun God, bows down facing east and the goes home. She is now free to interact with her family and other members of the community.

When Pali was asked about this temporary excommunication she was very shy and reluctant to answer. Gradually she came out of her shell and said that the menstrual blood 'vital' is evil and impure and therefore pollutes the atmosphere. While a woman is menstruating she is not allowed to cook as she is forbidden to sit in front of the chul (hearth) as the hearth is a symbol of Goddess Holi - the goddess of fire. If a menstruating woman touches or cooks the food the person/s consuming it will be affected with leprosy.

Analysis

Menstruation and the behavioural aspects associated with it reflect the following concepts of the Thakur society.

1. **Menstruation is a state of ill-health :** This stage is considered to be ill-health and the woman is socially and physically ex-communicated by her family and the other members of the tribe, as she is believed to be impure.

2. **Status :** During this period the status of the woman is further lowered and she does not participate in any ritual nor have any social interaction even with her own family members.

3. **Purification :** Since menstruation is associated with impurity and pollution, the Thakur woman performs the purification rite by having a bath in the river (Ganga - holy river). Water in this context is a symbol of purification as it cleanses the evil from the woman's body.

4. **Disease Causation :** Any interaction especially physical leads to being afflicted by disease. if a man has sex with a menstruating woman, it is believed that he will be afflicted by leprosy. Also if a woman/man consume food prepared by a menstruating woman she/he will also be a victim of leprosy.

5. **Hot/cold Concept :** The Thakurs believe that the menstrual blood is hot and corrosive in nature. If a man has sex with a menstruating woman, the hot effect of the blood is believed to circulate in the body

of man and degenerates the cells causing deformities as those observed in leprosy patients.

6. **Rest Concept :** A Thakur woman is a busy bee. All day long she is doing household chores, besides fetching firewood, water and also attends to agricultural activities. Thus to give her rest, the Thakur culture has designed this special period where she gets time off from her duties and can rest.

7. **Purity and Pollution :** The behaviour of menstrual woman expresses both pollution while she menstruating and purity when she purifies herself using water as stated earlier is a symbol of purity.

8. **Colour Concept :** The Thakurs attribute the colour black to the menstr..al blood and this colour in this situation symbolizes evil.

EPISODE NO. : 30

Aim

To investigate the Thakur's concept of the causation of common cold.

Background

Baban Padu Dore, married, male, 45 years old, resident of Thakurwadi (hamlet), Kashale village, narrates the Thakur's concept of causation of common cold.

Course of Events

During the monsoon season of 1990, Baban had a severe attack of common cold accompanied by a running nose. Baban was asked how did he get the cold. He said that he was working on the farm during the rains and walked back home with the head wet and exposed to cold air and water and therefore he had a running nose. Baban was asked why was mucous flowing out of the nose. He replied there are two worms present in the forehead between the two eyebrows and when they are exposed to very cold air and water they excrete mucous which is watery and comes out of the nose through the nostrils. When these kidas are exposed to normal temperature or slight cold they excrete less mucous and during such times the Thakurs take medicine or diet which is hot in nature.

Analysis

Thus even a minor ailment such as common cold cross cuts into the Thakur's concept of the physiology of the 'worms' (kidas) are believed to be present just above the frontonosal suture. This episode also reflects their concept of hot and cold. When a disease is believed to be caused by imbalance of the cold element or exposure of the body to cold air, diet or water, the water is then treated with medicines or diet which are hot in nature and vice versa.

EPISODE NO. : 31

Aim

To highlight the Thakur's interpretation of the causation of cataract and blindness and the manner in which these are linked to the wrath of the supernatural in a given cultural situation.

Background

Ganpat Pardhi, male, married, 65 years, resident of kautewadi (hamlet) lost his eyesight because of two accident on his farm. Today he needs the help of his grandson to move about.

Course of Events

When Ganpat was 40 years old, he met with an accident while working on the farm. He was threshing paddy with a stick, when the stick slipped from his hand and hit against the pole (mother) placed in the centre of threshing place and bounced back and struck Ganpat in his left eye. He immediately returned home and tied the leaves of vites negunds on the injure eye. This eye was allright and upto five moths after the accident he still had vision in his left eye.

Tragedy struck again the following year, while fixinga pole in the threshing place a pointed splinter went into his right eye. He consulted a vaidu but alas ! had lost his right eye.

His friend Jaithu advised him to consult a Bhagat. Ganpat consulted a Bhagat from Kautewadi. The Bhagat used the metal pot diagnosis technique and told Ganpat he had lost vision in both the eyes because he had failed to offer a sacrifice to the Guptadevi (secret Goddesses) who resided in his field. It was a custom that a cock should be sacrificed before threshing. And sure enough Ganpat had failed to offer the sacrifice for both the years.

Ganpat was asked who the Guptadevis were. He replied that they were planetary spirits (Baya) - sister of mother earth who visit the earth in any form to check human behaviour and further added that these Goddesses were present/residing in his field since the last generation. On enquiring whether the Bhagat had given Ganpat any medicine. Ganpat replied in the negative and added now it was not possible for anyone to do anything for him as the Baya had taken away the light (tej) from his eyes. (The sun is source of the light).

As a sign of repentance Ganpat had to offer the blood of a cock to the Goddesses. "why was blood offered, Ganpat ?". He replied, "there are two types of Baya. The Ratya baya (non-vegetarian) and the Chokhya Baya (vegetarian). In my field the Ratya baya reside and so to appease them a cock is sacrificed so that no harm is done to my family and the future generations.

Analysis

The Bhagat (Shaman) interpreted the cause of Ganpat's accidents as the failure to perform the religious duty towards the Guptadevi (Baya). The Bhagat's interpretation is based on cultural logic and from the cultural situation stems the reason for the accident.

The belief that Gupta devi resides in the fields is very common and perhaps is designed to impose social control through the religious medium. It is believed that if a person steals the crops of another then these devis bring misfortune to the thief. Blood was offered because these Devis are categorized as being non-vegetarian (Ratya) and vegetarian (Chokhya).

The Devis are classified on the basis of the dietary habits of the caste group. There are vegetarian and non-vegetarian caste groups residing in the same vicinity with the Thakurs. The Thakurs believe that the Baya take the form of the higher castes and hence the Baya accordingly are given names,

1. Brahmani Baya - Brahman caste (vegetarian)
2. Gujrathi Baya - Gujratis (vegetarian)
3. Marathi Baya - Marathas (warriors - non vegetarian)
4. Malani Baya - Mali (gardener - non vegetarian)
5. Kolani Baya - Mahadev Koli (tribe - non vegetarian)
6. Agarni Baya - Agri caste (non vegetarian)
7. Kannadi Baya - Stone workers (non-vegetarian)

The action associated with Ganpat's accidents brought to the foreground the Thakur concept of religion caste system, intervention of supernatural cosmic elements - Baya, rites of diagnosis, agricultural practices etc. Hence illness in this context does not restrict itself only to medicine/healing but cross cuts into meanings of other domains of social life.

EPISODE NO. : 32

Aim

To understand and explore the ritual healing which follows a snake bite in the Thakur tribe.

Background

Ambo Javgi Padir, married male, resident of Khondewadi, narrates the experience when his grandson was bitten by a snake.

Course of Events

Ambo's grandson, Bhika was bitten by a snake during January 1991. Bhika was then 18 years old and was returning from the fields. By accidentally he stepped on a snake and was bitten on his heal. He rushed home and told his grandfather who immediately rushed to the Bhagat of Khondewadi. The Bhagat applied charmed ash on Bhika's forehead and instructed Ambo to take Bhika to the Mantrik (snake bite and scorpion sting specialist) in the next village. He also instructed Ambo yo tie Bhika's leg with a rope.

The mantrik Bhika questions related to the length and colour of the snake. He also examined the bitten part. It was 8 p.m. by now. The mantrik asked Bhika to lie down and applied a medical herb on the bitten part. Taking a metal pot with him, the mantrik went to the well, jumped into the well, brought the fresh water. He told Bhika to face him. Then the mantrik faced east, chanted a prayer and bowed down. He then splashed the charmed water from the metal pot on Bhika's face five times. Bhika was then asked to light an incense stick facing east. Within a week Bhika recuperated completely. During the week, he visited the mantrik thrice.

Analysis

The belief that poison (zer) takes control over the soul (atma) is very common among the tribe. All medical efforts are directed to stop/prevent the poison from reaching the atma which is situated below the sternum in the rib-cage (pinjara). Methods followed are tying a rope, blood letting, consuming medicines which induce vomiting etc. In spite of these methods the patient still harbours the fear that the poison must have reached the atma.

To relieve him psychologically, the Thakur culture has designed a ritual of cleansing the atma(soul) so as to get rid of the poison. The jumping of the mantrik into the well to fetch the pure and holy water symbolizes water as an object of purification. In the hierarchy of body openings, the atma occupies the fifth position, hence the water is splashed five times as a symbolic gesture to get rid of the poison. Reciting a prayer facing east is symbolic of inviting the life giving and healing power of the sun to cure the patient.

When Ambo was asked whether the snake was poisonous, he replied that he did not know but his fears were allayed as the mantrik told him that the snake was not harmful. Ambo was asked why was water splashed, he replied this act removes the fear of the patient.

EPISODE NO. : 33

Aim

To explore the Thakur's concept of infant mortality as a result of failure to perform divine duties and rituals during pregnancy and during the post-delivery period.

Background

Kamli Ambo katwara, widow, 47 years, midwife (suine) by profession attributes the cause of death of her five children to failure to perform divine duties and rites.

Course of Events

Kamli had totally nine children. She lost five of them when they were between one to two months old. Kamli was asked if she knew the cause of the death of her five children. She answered very assertively that she had failed to perform the 'Panchvi punjan' ceremony. Kamli was asked about the ceremony and its importance. She answered that this ceremony is performed on the fifth day after delivery. This is a thanks giving ritual and the Goddess of fertility and fortune - mother earth also known as satvai. A midwife performs this ritual. An image of satvai is sketched with five different powders on the west wall of the house, where the mother and child are bathed.

The powders are - 1. kunku - pink powder, 2. halad - yellow powder, 3. gulal - red powder, 4. abir - black powder, 5. shendur - orange paste.

Coconut, date, almond and betal nut are also offered.

The Thakurs believe that for five days after delivery satvai takes charge of the newborn. After the Panchvi punjan ceremony, the child for first time is shifted to a swing (Jholi) from a basket. The basket is symbolic of mother's (earth's) womb and the child symbolizes the life in it. On the same day (after the ritual) at midnight satvai comes in the form of any creature such as cat, dog, bird etc and writes the life-span on the forehead of the newborn. Kamli failed to perform this important ritual so she believes that mother earth got angry and killed her five newborns.

Analysis

The fertility of a Thakur woman is because of the blessings of mother earth. All life on earth is nurtured by mother earth and hence she possesses the right to write the life span of the newborn. The Thakurs consider humans to be part and parcel of universe and the elements in it. Hence it is the duty of mankind to offer their newborns to mother earth so that she can write their life span. This is reason for performing Panchvi punjan.

There are a number of taboos associated with the behaviour of the mother, after delivery. If she breaks any then satvai kills the newborn. Most case of death of newborn are associated with or attributed to the wrath of satvai. Over 90% of such deaths are attributed to wrath of satvai and failure to perform her duties. Still-births and natural abortion are also attributed to the wrath of satvai.

EPISODE NO. : 34

Aim

To understand the Thakur's concept of causation of migraine and to explore the healing ritual.

Background

Damu Mahadu Padir, married male, aged 45 years, resident of Borwadi, Pathraj grampanchayat narrates his experience when he suffered from an attack of migraine.

Course of Events

Damu suffered from migraine attacks in the month of May 1992. He had a terrible headache which continued from 7 am to 12 O'clock in the afternoon. He tried a number of home remedies. Initially he applied lime of the forehead but this remedy did not work. He then applied the fluid of Biba seed (semicarpus anacardium). Due to this sores developed on his forehead. He also tries another remedy, he thrust the hard petiole of a mango leaf into his left nostril until almost half a cup of blood oozed out. Using this technique 2 to 3 times Damu was cured.

Analysis

The Thakurs believe that migraine attacks are due to the accumulation of spoilt blood which is dark in colour. Anything which is spoilt is a hindrance to the body and logically it should be removed from the body. Hence maximum efforts are made to achieve this end. The Thakur's concept of migraine thus reflects accumulation of morbid matter and its removal as being the body back from the state of ill health.

Tribhuwan Robin (1988) has reported that the Bhils (tribe) treat migraine by making an incision on the forehead of the patient with a piece of glass so that the spoilt blood flows out of the body.

EPISODE NO. : 35

Aim

To investigate the cause attributed by the Thakurs to blindness caused by small pox.

Background

Dehu Hari Darwada, 24 years, blind, resident of Borwadi kikuri village, has been blind since his childhood.

Course of Events

Dehu got an attack of small pox when he was 3½ years old. His mother suspected it to be small pox when she studied the early symptoms. She took Dehu to her sister's father-in-law who is a Bhagat. The Bhagat confirmed it to be a case of small pox. He put 2-3 drops of crab water (water extracted from the crab) into Dehu's eye.

That night Dehu slept, but the next morning he had completely lost his vision in the both the eyes. The Thakurs call such a phenomenon as 'gara padane' (eye balls have fallen down). Dehu's mother who is a midwife got very upset and took him to another Bhagat who interpreted the blindness as failure to adhere to the rules associated with the ritual of healing small pox. According to the Thakurs small pox is caused due to the visitation of Phodyadevi (planetary spirits). These devis are vegetarian and the first Bhagat had put into Dehu's eyes the fluid from the crab. Crab is non-vegetarian, this action of the Bhagat made the Phodyadevi angry and hence they had made Dehu blind.

Analysis

Dehu does not remember much of what happened. he has only heard from his mother the incident. he attributes the cause of his blindness to the failure of the Bhagat to adhere to the healing ritual.

The episode highlights the Thakurs concept of cause of small pox as the visitation of planetary spirits (devi mandal / Baya) who are believed to be the sisters of mother earth. The sun is believed to the husband of mother earth who infertile and gives birth to life, the planetary spirits are barren and express their wrath in this way because they are believed to be sexually frustrated.

EPISODE NO. : 36

Aim

To study the Thakur conception of the origin and cause of Leucoderma.

Background

Nanu Nama Dore, a married male, aged 48 years, resident of Thakurwadi narrates his experience of Leucoderma.

Course of Events

When Nanu was 40 years old he observed two-three pinkish white spots on his left foot. Later these, spots slowly started spreading on the right foot, then on hands and lips. His father Nama tried some herbal medicine which did not cure Nanu. A vaidu of Lobhie wadi was consulted but he also failed. Nanu gave up consulting any medical practitioner.

On enquiring from Nanu, what was the cause for Leucoderma. He replied my father Nama (baba) says that, "I must have consumed a wrong diet". "What diet, Nanu ?". He replied, "fish and milk. I must have been drunk at that time as it is my habit and I must have eaten fish along with milk. Fish and alcohol being very hot and milk very cold in nature must have caused an adverse effect on my blood and therefore some parts of my body have got these patches".

"Is wrong combination the only cause of Leucoderma ?". He said, "My father says that disease is because of wrong combination of food but the Bhagatin of Kotimba tells me that it is due to sorcery. I fully agree with her". Nanu said, "there are two kathkari men in the next hamlet who have this problem. They must have casted magical spells on me and therefore I have got Leucoderma - saphed kode, therefore I have given up consulting medicine men".

Analysis

Nanu was convinced by the Bhagatin's statement that his disease was due to sorcery and that there is no cure. Besides Nanu's narration of this illness, other three Thakurs were consulted for their experience of Leucoderma and the responses for causation were as follows,

1. Leucoderma - as a wrong combination of food.
2. as a result of sorcery.
3. as a result of God's curse.

Thus the interpretation of Leucoderma differs from situation to situation in which the disease has occurred.

EPISODE NO. : 37

Aim

To understand the Thakur concept of the cholostrom milk (from the mother) being the cause of dysentery and diarrhoea and to explore the symbolic aspects associated with it.

Background

Kamli Balu Shid, married female, aged 45 years, narrates the illness experience in which he grand-daughter suffered because she was fed cholostrom containing milk, Kamli is a resident of Saraiwadi.

Course of Events

Kamli's daughter, delivered a girl child in the winter of 1991 in Saraiwadi. On the seventh day after the delivery the child was suffering from dysentery and diarrhoea. The child was dehydrated. Balu (the grand-father) rushed his grand-daughter to the PHC where she was put on intra-venous. The PHC doctor prescribed some medicines. These were given regularly to child who soon got cured.

On enquiring from Kamli what was the reason of the child's suffering. She was very emphatic and said that the child was fed "naska dudh" - cholostrom milk. "Kamli is this milk bad and why ?". Kamli answered. "Yes, it is thick and cheese like and cannot be digested by the child and therefore causes diarrhoea". "Kamli, why is the milk thick ?". hearing the question Kamli smiled and said, "You ask my husband the reason" and she went into the house. Balu who sitting there replied, "For nine months during pregnancy a woman does not menstruate. The child feeds on her menstrual blood. The effect of menstrual blood remains in the mother's body along with the spermatic fluid. These thick fluids get mixed with mother's blood which turns into thick milk (cholostrom milk) which is known as Naska dudh.

"What is the child's diet for these five days ?". Balu replied that the child is given cow's/goat's milk, water and honey. "What is done with the mother's naska dudh ?". Balu said it is squeezed out on a piece of cloth and that these clothes are washed by the midwife in the river. Care is taken not to throw away these pieces of cloth to prevent them from becoming objects of sorcery/witchcraft to harm the mother and the child. The child is fed breast milk on the sixth day.

The naska dudh is squeezed out to remove the impurity from the mother's body. The midwife also takes great effort to let out blood from the mother's body as it is believed to be impure.

Analysis

The scientific explanation encourages breast feeding immediately after birth as it develops immunity in the child. At the same time the Thakurs believe that consumption of this milk causes dysentery and diarrhoea in the child. They associate the thickness of the milk with the menstrual blood and the spermatic fluid's effect. Whatever is impure should be let out so the 'naska dudh' is squeezed out and the blood from the vagina is also let out. Beliefs are meaningful among the Thakurs hence this practice continues as it is part and parcel of the Thakur culture. Thus to implement maternal and child health educational programmes it is very necessary to have a thorough knowledge of their belief system.

EPISODE NO. : 38

Aim

To explore the Thakur's concept of effect of breast milk on the health of infants in a given cultural situation.

Background

Mrs. XYZ, aged 35 years, resident of Naldewadi, narrates the Thakurs concept of the effect of breast milk on the health of infants.

Course of Events

Mrs. XYZ has three children. She gave birth to the third child in June 1992. Two months after delivery she joined her husband in the fields. She used to go out to collect firewood and help on the form. The child was left in the care of the older children. She returned after every three hours and fed the child. The farm is close to her hamlet.

The child had diarrhoea for 3-4 days. She did not take the child to the hospital or any practitioner. On enquiring what could be the possible cause, she replied that she used to come back home in the hot sun due to which her blood becomes hot, this blood is converted into milk. Thus the child cannot digest this hot milk and hence suffered from diarrhea.

Mrs. XYS was asked what happens if the breast milk becomes too cold when the body is exposed to cold environment. She replied the child gets cold and cough. "How did you treat your child ?". Mrs. XYZ replied that she stopped going out in the sun and ate lukewarm food.

Analysis

Diseases such diarrhoea/dysentery/cold among infants are directly related (by the Thakurs) to the temperature of blood in the mother's body. The temperature is related to her being exposed to hot/cold environment or consuming a dominantly hot/cold diet. The Thakurs believe that the mother's blood is converted into milk and thus its temperature has effect of the health of infants.

EPISODE NO. : 39

Aim

To understand the Thakur's concept of causation of sore eyes.

Background

Ananta jaithu Pardhi, married male, 30 years, resident of Kautewadi narrates the Thakur's perception of the cause of sore eyes.

Course of Events

Sometime during the summer of 1992, Ananta suffered from sore eyes. More or less at the same time about fifty people in the same village were also suffering from the same. He said that the children were the first ones to get affected. They play in the hot sun. Too much of heat gets accumulated in the eyes and the person suffers from sore eyes. He also said that the infection was contagious and spreads very fast.

He said first his son was affected, then his wife and in the end he got affected. Ananta was asked what medication di he take. He replied that he put 4-5 drops of goat milk in the eyes before going to bed at night. Ananta was asked if there was any alternative medicine. he said, yes, the medicine is pivli rui - Argemone mexicana, the yellow latex is put into the eyes as a remedy for sore eyes. "How does the disease spread, Ananta ?". He answered, "Air is the carrier, the smell of the disease is carried by air from one person to another.

Analysis

Sore eyes are believed to be caused due to excess of heat that gets accumulated in the eyes because of which the eyes become red. Thus what is caused due to excess of heat is treated with cold therapy. The Thakurs believe that goat's milk is cold and also the latex of Argemone mexicana is cold in effect. Hence either or both are used to neutralize the hot effect. thus the cause and treatment of sore eyes cross cuts the Thakurs concept of hot/cold concept and wind or air being the medium of transmission of the disease.

EPISODE NO. : 40

Aim

To explore the causational concepts that the Thakurs associate with severe headache.

Background

Rama Dharku Thorad, married male, aged 55 years, resident of Khondewadi, narrates his experience when he had a severe headache.

Course of Events

In June 1992, Rama suffered from a very severe headache. During the rains he worked in the field. He caught a cold and also suffered from a severe headache. When Rama was asked about the cause of his headache, he replied that his head was exposed to the cold air due to working in the rains and had become wet. When the head gets wet and the cold air enters the head through the nostrils and affects the two 'worms' - kidas which reside in the forehead. When these kidas get disturbed they start biting the head (Doka Chavto Ha Kida) and therefore the head pains. the severity of the pains depends upon the degree of exposure (of the kidas) to cold air. "Rama, how did you get allright ?". He replied that he rested for two days and his diet consisted mainly of hot foods. "Did you take any medicine, Rama ?". "Yes, I squeezed the juice of ginger (zingiber officinalis) in the tea and took the tea for two days, thrice a day. This decoction restored the normal temperature of the kidas.

Analysis

Headache is understood as a symptom and not a disease in scientific medicine, but the Thakurs know it as a disturbance of the worms which when exposed to excess cold or hot, start biting the head thereby causing pain. Thus the biting is associated with pain. It is thus evident that a symptom such as headache is so meaningfully interpreted in the Thakur culture.

EPISODE NO. : 41

Aim

To study the beliefs which the Thakurs associate with repeated abortions.

Background

Bhagi Nama Dhole, widow, midwife by profession, aged 58 years, narrates the tragic experience of her daughter Tambdi who had five consecutive abortions.

Course of Events

Bhagi, a widow, has four sons and two daughters. her youngest daughter Tambdi was married off at the age of 15 years. She conceived, but all the five times had natural abortions. Both, Tambdi and her husband Pandu were worried. They consulted many Bhagats but did not visit the doctors at the PHC.

Finally, Tambdi's mother Bhagi consulted Ambo Thorad, the Bhagat of khondewadi. He diagnosed the cause and interpreted, Tambdi's womb - 'oti' had become an object of black magic. Some person/s from the community had used the power of clan God to harm Tambdi's womb.

He applied charmed ash on Tambdi's forehead but did not reassure her that all would be well. he said that the person who had harmed her, had used good power (power of clan God) and hence nothing could be done.

Accepting the Bhagat's advice, Tambdi stopped approaching medical practitioners. Bhagi advised her son-in-law to remarry so that his generation could be continued but requested him to take care of Tambdi too.

Analysis

Repeated abortions are usually attributed by the Thakurs to the wrath of the satvai - goddess of fertility and fortune or witchcraft/sorcery. They are ignorant that early marriages and hard work during pregnancy lead to abortions. they strongly believe that unless and until someone harms the 'oti' - womb there will not be abortion/still births.

Scientifically abortion would be health disorder but in the Thakur culture itis meaningfully interpreted as being related to fertility cult, pathogenic agents such as witches/sorcery or wrath of divine being like satvai. these are believed to cause repeated abortions and even still births. Thus this episode symbolizes the social conflict, grudges, hatred and jealousy which prevail at social level among the Thakurs but are exposed at the spiritual level.

EPISODE NO. : 41

Aim

To investigate the cause of leucoderma as perceived by the Thakurs.

Background

Mr. MD, married male, aged 47 years, resident of Thakurwadi, narrates his experience.

Course of Events

Mr. MD has a pinkish spot on right foot since the last three years. He says that he had this disease since birth and it was manifested only since the past three years. (Janmacha rog). The Thakurs term leucoderma as 'kode'. MD has been to PHC at Kashale and also the Ayurvedic dispensary run by the Academy of Development Science, but in vain. He believes that the spot does not harm the body nor it is painful. When the spot is pierced red coloured blood oozes out and this is the sign of health. If the colour of blood were different then MD would have been worried. Colour of the blood is an indicator of health.

Analysis

Thakurs believe that 'kode' (leucoderma) is a disease present since birth and may be manifested anytime during the patient's lifetime. Hence it is not harmful and no social stigma is attached. A leucoderma patient has no difficulty in finding a life-partner.

Another view is that leucoderma is caused due to the intake of wrong combination of food.

Thus two types of beliefs as far as Leucoderma is concerned are that,1. Leucoderma is a disease present since birth and starts showing up as a person grows.

2. it is caused due to intake of wrong combination of foods.

EPISODE NO. : 42

Aim

To understand the Thakur's concept of the effect of excess alcohol on their health.

Background

Mr. DL, married male, aged 60 years, resident of Naldewadi, narrates the episode of his son who died due to excessive consumption of alcohol and smoking.

Course of Events

Mr. DL's son Mr. M. was a compulsive drinker. He would drink more and eat less food. Gradually his intake of food decreased. He would drink upto three to four bottles, approximately 3000 ml or even more in a single day.

Once, as per the information of the liquor owners, Mr. M had six bottles of liquor and went off into the jungle all by himself. He had been drinking from 9 am to 1 pm. He did not return home that day. His father, Mr. DL went into the jungle with the dog at night. He searched for his son (Mr. M) for two-three hours. He then finally returned home dejected. At home Mr. M's wife and children were worried about him.

The following day, one of Mr. DL's friends informed him that they had seen Mr. M lying under a tree in the jungle. Mr. DL rushed there with a friend and found the dead body of his son. The body was buried on the same day.

Mr. DL was asked what was the reason of his son's death. He replied that since his son drank too much and ate very little food , the liquor (daru) burnt up the blood due to this corrosive action Mr. M was very thin and the water content in the body became very less. Thus the atma (soul) does not have a favorable place to dwell in the body as there is little water, burnt blood and too much heat and hence leaves the body. Mr. DL voices that his son died due to this. He further adds if one wants to drink, he should eat well and then go to sleep as the liquor relaxes his/her muscles and one sleeps soundly.

"Mr. DL why do people lose their balance after drinking ?". Mr. DL replied, "there are two kidas (worms) in the head just below the forehead (fronto-nasal suture). When a person drinks alcohol it creates hot air in the stomach (potali), when this hot air reaches the two worms in the forehead, they start moving round and round and therefore one gets the giddy feeling and looses his balance. If one continuously drinks in excess, without eating food then the kidas die and the person is also dead".

Analysis

The concept of consumption of excess alcohol on the health in this episode reveals the Thakur ideology of body physiology and how its excess consumption affects health of the drinker to the extent that the soul (atma) which is nurtured in the body's physiological environment along with water, air, light, fire, food etc. leaves the body due to an unfavourable environment i.e. the body physiology of the drinker.

EPISODE NO. : 43

Aim

To highlight the symbolic elements that the Thakurs associated with object intrusion leading to the state of ill health.

Background

Mrs. X Married female, aged 27 years, resident of Borwadi, hurt her right hand little finger while cutting the firewood (fatya).

Course of Events

Mrs. X was cutting firewood for household use in the winter of 1991. She cut her finger, the cut was quite deep. She did not realize this. To stop the flow of blood she used a piece of her sari. When she reached home, the finger was swollen. Her mother-in-law applied some Mahua (Bacia latifolia) seed oil and tied up the wound.

A week later, the wound worsened. She consulted a vaidu but the medicines did not work. Finally her father-in-law consulted a Bhagat from Kharbachi wadi who used the metal pot technique of diagnosis. He spun the metal pot in clockwise direction while chanting. The metal pot came to a stop when he was chanting a line related to witchcraft and sorcery. He was then convinced that Mrs. X had become a victim of witchcraft. He interpreted Mrs. X's severe pain saying that dog's meat was filled in her wound hence the excruciating pain. The Bhagat did not tell Mrs. X the name of the woman relative who had performed witchcraft on Mrs. X. He said if he told her (Mrs. X) the name there would be fights and ill-will.

"Mrs. X was the Bhagat able to cure you ?". "Yes, he applied chanted ash on my forehead and also packed some of it and gave me. he then gave me some herbal medicine to apply. I went to him twice to apply the medicine and within ten days I was cured".

Analysis

The longer the period of illness, greater are the chances of searching for meanings related to the origin and cause of the illness. This episode highlights the expression of illness and its healing (in this context) as the disruption of man's relationship with his fellowmen. Social conflicts expressed through illness are solved at spiritual level. The concept of using dog's meat, goat's meat, bones, nagli grains (Eleucine coracana), vari grains (Panicum species) in witchcraft as objects of intrusion to cause ill-health is very common among the Thakurs.

Thus the action of object intrusion to hunt a person is symbolize of the community's (Thakur) expression of grudge, hatred, jealousy and other social conflicts with their fellowmen who could be family members, clan mates, members of the same tribe or other social groups.

EPISODE NO. : 44

Aim

To investigate the Thakur concept of guinea worms (naru), thread worms, round worms and their effect on the human body.

Background

Mr. MN, married male, aged 35 years, resident of Khondewadi narrates the concept of guinea worms.

Course of Events

Mr. MN recalls the monsoon of 1980, cultivation was in full swing. Mahadu was ploughing his field, he was barefoot in muddy water. While ploughing he hurt his left food with a nail. Mr. MN felt the pain. Not heeding to it, he continued ploughing. When he returned home, he washed his foot and found his foot was swollen. He applied some herbal medicine and with a piece of cloth tied his foot. Next day he went back to work in the muddy field. After a week Mrs. MN's foot worsened. One fine morning while going to work, he notice a guinea worm coming out of his wound. Taking a small stick he started rolling the worm till he was successful in taking out the complete worm.

"Mr. MN, how did the worm enter your body ?". Mr. MN was a bit sarcastic and first laughed then pointing to a tree said that even the tree is attacked by worms (kid lagte). So also the body is attacked by small organism (Jantu). Some live on the blood and some on the food which is eaten.

Mr. MN was asked what did the guinea worms (Naru) live on ?. Mr. MN said that they feed on blood and grow in the body and when they grow big they come out. "Are there worms in the stomach ?". Mr. MN replied, "yes, there are jantu (worms) and they feed on whatever food we eat". "Mr. MN, is it good to have worms in the stomach ?". "No, they are harmful and to kill the worms we have to take bitter medicines or karla (bitter gourd) as a result of which the developing worms die. When asked if all the worms die after taking bitter medicines, Mr. MN replied that all do not die, the body is just like a tree which is also constantly attacked by the worms.

Analysis

Just by probing into the Thakur concept of guinea worms has unveiled concepts of physiology, image of human body which is compared to a tree attacked by worms, growing on the food and blood in the human body and more significantly the therapeutic measures of taking bitter diet and medicines to get rid of the worms. Their ignorance about the scientific causational factors associated with guinea worms is the reason why the Thakurs accept the concept given by their cultural system.

EPISODE NO. : 45

Aim

To highlight the cause of jaundice and explore the treatment given by the Thakurs for the same.

Background

Mr. BC, married male, aged 50 years, narrates his illness experience as a jaundice patient.

Course of Events

In May 1991, Mr. BC suffered from jaundice. He says that week before getting the disease he ate a lot of mangoes and drank plenty of water therefore he got jaundice. Mr. BC was asked how do mangoes cause jaundice. He answered if a person eats sour foods or fruits such as pickles, raw mangoes, sour mangoes, lime, tamarind, badi sauf (Foenicum vulgare) he suffers from jaundice (kamin). On being questioned how do these cause jaundice, MR BC replied when one eats sour food the blood becomes yellow in the 'kalij' (liver) and from there this yellow blood is distributed to the whole body and the body becomes yellowish, eye, nails and urine also turn yellowish in colour. Thus according to Mr. BC citric fruits cause jaundice. Interviews taken with other Thakurs also reflects the same concept.

Mr. BC was asked what treatment he took and who treated him. He replied the vaidu (herbalist) treated him by giving him some medicines which he never reveals to anyone and after the treatment the green and bitter medicine is given, which got rid of the yellowish colour of the blood and brought it back to the original red colour.

Mr. BC was asked if he had green medicine, why didn't the blood become green. He replied nothing should be consumed in excess otherwise the colour of the blood will change. The blood gets the red colour because the food that is consumed is digested into juice and this juice gets boiled in the Agni (fire) in the stomach and hence gets the red colour.

Women eat "dudh kand" (dioscorea indica) to increase the breast milk. The juice of dioscorea is whitish hence the women get milk (white in colour). He also added that if a person is bitten by a cobra his blood turns blue because the poison is bluish black in colour. Similarly leprosy patient's blood is greenish in colour because when they are cremated the smoke arising is greenish yellow in colour.

Analysis

Jaundice, scientifically speaking is water borne disease but is interpreted very differently by the Thakurs. this interpretation is not due to their superstitious ignorance or illiteracy but their understanding about diet and its effect on body physiology. Their beliefs regarding health and disease are meaningful. Thus causation of jaundice penetrates into the Thakur's concepts of colour symbolism of blood, ethnophysiology and dietary concepts.

EPISODE NO. : 46

Aim

To highlight the effect on Thakur health due to intervention of evil spirits believed to belong to members of other caste and tribes residing near Thakur settlements.

Background

Mr. NP, married male, aged 45 years, narrates his son's illness experience who was possessed by an evil spirit.

Course of Events

Mr. NP's son Mr D was returning back from the farm to his home in the Thakurwadi. it was getting dark and the boy walked faster. He had to pass under the pipal (Ficus religiosa) tree. As he neared the tree the rustling of the leaves grew louder. Cold wind was blowing and when he passed under the tree two or three leaves fell on his head. Mr. D. got scared and ran all the way home.

When he reached home he was sweating profusely and had a very frightened look on his face. His father Mr. NP pacified him, Mr. D ate very little and went to sleep. In the night he was awake and behaving very neurotically, he had high fever and was shivering. Mr. NP suspected that his son was possessed. He rushed to the village bhagatin, who came and saw Mr. D. She brought along her articles of worship and after setting them, she got into a trance and asked Mr. D, who he was. The reply was that he was a kathkari (a tribe residing nearby) and wanted a blood sacrifice. the bhagatin whipped Mr. D and commanded the evil spirit to leave and assured it that the demand would be met.

She then put charmed ash on Mr. D's forehead and instructed Mr. NP to sacrifice a black cock near the tree where Mr. D was possessed. The next day after sacrificing, Mr. NP invited the bhagatin for a feast and offered her a bottle of liquor.

Analysis

On enquiring why the evil spirit was a kathkari. He replied, "the kathkaris are lower in status than us". They eat unclean foods such as monkeys, owls, crows, rats, bandicoots etc. They are not on good terms with the Thakurs and hence cause trouble by possessing a Thakur. Mr. NP was asked if the Thakurs are possessed by Brahmin. He immediately replied in the negative and said that the Brahmins come under the 'Devjatis' (Gods Jati). He added that kathkaris, Muslims, Chamars, Mahars, Mangs and even the Thakurs come under the Davan Jati (evil, giant like jati). All the above mentioned communities are lower in hierarchy than the Thakurs and these generally practice witch craft and sorcery. He said that the castes coming under the Dev jatis (God like jatis) are as follows :-

1. Brahmans	- Priests.
2. Gujratis	- Business caste groups
3. Marathas	- Warrior caste
4. kunbis	- Agriculturists
5. Agris	- Agriculturists
6. Sonar	- Goldsmith
7. Mahadev Kolis	- Tribe
8. Dhangars	- Shepherds
9. Sutar	- Carpenters
10. Lohar	- Blacksmith
11. Wani	- Business caste
12. Nhavi	- Barber
13. Kannadi	- Nomadic caste.

Mr. NP was asked if the above mentioned jatis practiced witchcraft and sorcery. He answered negatively and added that these jatis take the form of planetary spirits, Baya and visit the Thakurs to keep a check on their deviant behaviour and to bring back order into the society and that the Thakurs worshipped them.

Moving ahead with the analysis one infers that the illness episode highlight the Thakur conflicts with the other lower/Davan jati members and also the high regard and respect they have for the Dev-jati members. Also their concept of social hierarchy and interaction is highlighted.

EPISODE NO. : 47

Aim

To highlight the cause of fits as perceived by the Thakurs, in a particular cultural context.

Background

Mr. HJ married male, aged 57 years, resident of Naldewadi, narrates his experience when he suffered from an attack of fits.

Course of Events

Mr. HJ suffered from epileptic attacks for the period 1989-1991. He got these attacks all of a sudden and would start foaming at the mouth. His wife was very worried. She consulted the female shaman - bhagatin of Nagyachiwadi. The bhagatin come on a Tuesday and after having arranged the worship articles on the floor, she lit a lamp and an incense stick. She let her hair loose and rotating in clockwise direction got into a trance inviting the 'Baya' - planetary spirits to take control of her atma and her body.

While she was in a trance she shouted at Mr. HJ and said that the Baya were angry with him. Mr. HJ bowed down before the bhagatin (the Baya) and asked what was his fault. The Baya said (through the Bhagatin) that he had stepped on their idol which is near the well and hence they were angry. Mr. HJ asked the Bhagatin (Baya) what should he do to appease them. He was told to offer a coconut near the idol.

Mr. HJ offered the coconut near the idol and also to the bhagatin. The bhagat went back to the village. Ten days later Mr. HJ again had a epileptic attack, these attack continues from time to time. Mr. HJ grew tired of the magico-religious therapy and approached the local PHC doctor who cured him by giving allopathy medicines.

Analysis

The cause attributed to the epileptic attack was the wrath of the Baya hence a spiritual curer was approached. The societal pressure was so great that in spite of being tired of magico-religious therapy and the physical suffering Mr. HJ had to continue the same for two years. Finally gathering courage he went to the local PHC and was cured. It was not easy for Mr. HJ to break the cultural norms and meanings and seek relief and cure in allopathy.

EPISODE NO. : 48

Aim

The episode highlights the cause of illness, pain and discomfort suffered by a young male talented Thakur (kirtankar, singer and drummer) which eventually led to death.

Background

This episode was narrated to the researcher by Nambai, Ganpat's mother. Nambai Lachak is a married woman of 45 years, a resident of Borwadi, Pathraj village. By profession she is a potdhari (helpmate to midwife) and the mother of the talented young man, Ganpat. She narrated that Ganpat had the talent of composing bhajans and kirtans. He was also a very good dancer and a drummer. As Ganpat worked in tamasha (drama party/group) he was an extremely popular artist. He always told his mother that he wanted to stay unmarried and become a true devotee of God.

Course of Events

It was in the summer of 1979 that Ganpat was to perform in a kathkari hamlet of Kotimba village along with the other members of his group. The show was to go on for two days. The audience was large and included many kathkaris.

The show on the first night got over at about 11 O'clock. After the show many people came and congratulated Ganpat on his performance. A young kathkari girl also congratulated and praised him. The following day, Ganpat was resting in his tent after lunch when the same kathkari girl came to meet him. She spoke to him and in the course of their conversation told him that she liked him and would like to get married to him.

Hearing her, Ganpat was greatly angered and told her in no kind words to leave his tent. That night he performed and left with his troupe.

A week later, Ganpat suffered from a severe stomach problem. His stomach was swollen up and caused him great pain. He was taken to a doctor but his condition did not improve. Two bhagats were consulted and both diagnosed that Ganpat had become a victim of witchcraft. His suffering lasted two weeks after which he breathed his last. Ganpat's parents made no effort to trace the kathkari woman who resorted to magical spells and had planted a dholki (a small drum) in Ganpat's stomach as he had refused to marry her. Nambai till today regrets the untimely death of her talented son who became the victim of witchcraft.

Analysis

The Dholki (a small rhythm instrument) was used as a magical object to be planted in Ganpat's stomach as it was associated with his talents of a dancer and a drummer. Ganpat was talented, popular, handsome, unmarried young man who refused to marry the kathkari girl.

Thus jealousy, hatred and revenge got the better of her and she cast a powerful magic spell which first made Ganpat ill, caused him severe pain and suffering and finally killed him. This incidence also highlights the inter-group conflict between the Thakurs and Kathkaris at a spiritual level. Emotions such as jealousy, hatred, group conflicts as reflected in the illness episodes remain unsolved at social interactional level (between the Thakurs and Kathkaris) and are solved through healing rites at a spiritual level.

EPISODE NO. : 49

Aim

To investigate the role of animal spirits that intervene the health of the Thakurs.

Background

Mr. ZX, a married male, aged 46, resident of Nagyachi wadi narrates the experience of his son Mr. TX who was possessed by the spirit of fox (Kolha Bhut).

Course of Events

It was 'Holi Festival season', i.e. somewhere in the month of March 1991 when Mr. TX had been out in the woods for hunting rabbits with his friends. When he returned back in the evening he had fever. His friends were asked why Mr. TX had fever. They said they don't know. Mr. TX was taken to a Vaidu (herbalist) who told TX's father that the illness is caused by some spirit and that the patient has to be taken to a shaman (Bhagat).

The patient was hence taken to Walku Thorad - the shaman, Walku washed himself first, lighted an incense stick, took a metal pot with water, put a pinch of ash in itand underneath it and spun it in clockwise direction to diagnose the origin and cause of TX's illness. He recited the 'Mantra' (chant) of diagnosis and found out that TX was possessed with a spirit of the fox. The shaman asked the spirit what he wants from the boy. The reply was blood! The Bhagat agreed that he would offer him a cock. The next day as instructed by the Bhagat a cock was offered. The Bhagat then applied the charmed ash (Ibut) on the forehead of TX.

Analysis

The belief that animal spirits besides human spirits also cause illness is very common. Spirits of foxes, owls, tigers, snakes, peacock etc. are believed to attack human beings in person or in dreams. When it was was enquired of Mr TX why the spirit must have attacked him, he said he unknowingly urinated near a fox den. Therefore he was possessed by the spirit of the fox (Kolha Bhut).

Fox is classified as doer of evil work among the spirits by the Thakurs. Howling of Jackals and foxes during an auspicious occasion is considered to be a bad omen. Secondly foxes are consumed by the Kathkaris who are lower in status than the Thakurs and therefore foxes are believed to be evil.

EPISODE NO. : 50

Aim

To explore the intervention of deities of the untouchable caste groups (Bhavani, Mariai etc.) in Thakur health.

Background

Mrs. ND, a married female, aged 38, a resident of Chaphe wadi narrated her illness experience when she was troubled by Goddess Mariai, the Goddess of Mahars (Lower caste group).

Course of Events

Mrs. ND once passed by a Mariai Goddess's shrine during her last day of menstruation period when she was going to the river to wash herself. Mrs. ND fell ill that evening. She had fever. She was taken to a local Bhagat who diagnosed and confirmed that she fell ill because she passed the shrine during her menstrual periods. Mariai therefore got angry and brought about sickness. Bhagat then instructed Mrs ND's husband to offer a coconut to Mariai Goddess. After 3-4 days Mrs ND was allright.

Analysis

The Thakurs consider Mahars, Mangs, Chamars and kathkaris lower to them in social status and hence deities worshipped by these social groups are considered to be dangerous. Illness are caused by these deities is very commonly believed. Mrs ND passed the Mariai shrine with polluted blood (Menstrual blood) and aggravated her wrath. The Goddess therefore demanded the holy water of the coconut. Other respondents have revealed that Thakurs fall ill most of the time due to the attack by the deities of lower caste groups.

❋❋❋

CHAPTER V

BODY SYMBOLISM

Body Image

Use of human body as a symbolic material has been discussed by anthropologists and analyzed in allied disciplines (Joshi 1992:9). As a symbolic instrument a person may use his body as means of communication, to indicate by bodily actions or with reference to some more abstract idea which is meaningful to him. As Mauss puts it, 'the human body is the first and most natural instrument of man.' (1950:372). Human body as a symbolic instrument conveys meaning and is used as means of communication. Meanings of bodily symbols are situationally defined and expressed within cultural contexts.

As rightly pointed by Mary Douglas (1970:65), 'the social body constraints the way the physical body is perceived. The physical experience of the body, always modified by the social categories through which it is known, sustains a particular view of society. There is a continual exchange of meanings between two kinds of bodily experiences so that each reinforces the categories of others.

Both Turner (1966) and Douglas (1970) have discussed the use of body and bodily emission as non-verbal categories in society. Following the interest sparked by Levi-Strauss in dual organization and the work of Robert Hertz on right hand symbolism and the relationship of such dual model, based on the natural proclivity of the body to other spheres of social behaviour. (See Needham 1973).

Devisch, Renaat (1985:693-70) has shown how the northern Yak, construct a meaningful world by reference to the human body. They understand the socio-cultural domains in terms of bodily exchanges such as ingestion, excretion, sexual process or listening and speech. The physical body as the tangible form of selfhood is the symbolic frame through which social, spiritual, cosmological paradoxes are expressed.

The Thakur body symbolism in ritual healing contexts unravels the entire cultural belief system through the domain of ethnomedicine. This chapter highlights the body as perceived by the Thakurs as natural, social, cosmological, spiritual and supernatural symbol.

A Thakur's knowledge of human body is based on the close observation and his study of animal and plant life in and around the forest. His ideas about the anatomy and physiology of human body are derived from what he knows about the animals he kills for food. His interpretation of human body on the whole reflects his ideology about universe. 'Khanda Sarkha pind' - meaning the human body is nothing but an image of the cosmos.

According to him, human body is a symbol ofnatural, supernatural, cosmological, spiritual and social elements. The first section of this chapter describes the Thakurs ideology of body image and the second part explains the natural, cosmological, social, spiritual and supernatural symbolic forms and meanings as expressed and communicated through human body during the process of ritual healing.

Chaphekar (1961:83) highlights the perception of Thakurs as far as main bodily organs are concerned. According to the Thakurs the body of a beast has following major organs - 1. Kalij (liver), 2. Phuphus (lungs). 3. Dil (heart), 4. Pitta (bile), 5. Aatadi (intestines), 6. Potala (stomach), 7. Pitha (spleen), 8. Yiv (neck), 9. Mutlani (urinary bladder), 10. Satputi (Deudonum).

Chaphekar has also reported a song which describes some anatomical and physiological aspects of human body in a question and answer form. The song is known as Dehabhanga-che-gane - songs concerned with human body).

The SongQuestions

In our body oh brother
where is the bone sixteen cubits ?

To our body oh brother
how many doors are there ?

In our body oh brother
which part is a cubit and quarter ?

In our body oh brother
where if the secret fire that ever burns ?

In our body oh brother
which is the small bone as seasum ?

In our body oh brother
where is the 'vital vein' ?

In our body oh brother

where is the flowing Ganges ?
In our body oh brother
where lies the dry ocean ?

There are problems oh brother
please explain me oh brother

The Answers

The bone sixteen cubit long is the
vein of our body oh brother

In our body oh brother
there are nine doors oh brother

The place a cubit and a quarter long
is the circumference of our head

In our body oh brother to the left
is the second fire that burns

To the bone as small as seasum
is in our penis, oh brother

And the vital vein oh brother
is our throat oh brother

And the dry ocean is our
throat oh brother

At another village Chaphekar reported a different version about the doors of human body (1960 : 82)

To our body, oh brother,
How many doors are there ?
There are ten doors oh brother
How many are open ?
Nine are open oh brother
and the tenth one is secret.

Chaphekar (1961:82), further points out that the 'secret door' is supposed to be the apex of the scalp. The song continues to say that the key to the secret door is with the Sadguru, the spiritual teacher and opens the door when the soul (atma) leaves its tabernacle (body) for good.

Chaphekar's brief account on the Thakurs ideology of body image was an incentive for the researcher to probe into their concept of body symbolism and ethnophysiology from an emic perspective. Interpretations regarding how thebody functions, what makes it exist, what fluids and elements does it constitute, how the various systems of the body function, their concept of life and a detailed analysis of body symbolism is discussed in this chapter.

Bodily Fluids

A Thakur classifies human bodily fluids in to two categories, namely,

i. The fluids of life - meaning the fluids such as water, blood, breast milk, sperms, vaginal fluid etc. which sustain and create life.

ii. Excretory fluids - fluids such as urine, sweat, menstrual blood, tears, pus, mucus etc. which are excreted or thrown out by the body fall in the second category.

Their knowledge of both fluids of life and excretory fluids is vast. They interpret healthy and unhealthy conditions of the human body based on the colour, production, type, the contribution of these fluids to the body, symbolic aspects of the bodily fluids and so on. The Thakur knowledge of the above said categories of bodily fluids was assessed in the light of health behavioural aspects.

A. The Fluids of Life

Fluids of life according to the Thakurs have two types of functions -

a. Fluids that create life.

b. Fluids that nourish and sustain life.

The Thakurs believe that sperms (virya) are stocked in the forehead, just above the fronto-nasal suture. Sperms are produced by two worms (Kidas) which are situated in the forehead. During the sexual intercourse these sperms travel down from the forehead touching the atma (soul) which is situated below the sternum and comes out through the urethra. Presence of testes is just a sign of being a male species. (Chaphekar 1960).

A Thakur believes that 40 morsels (ghas) of food produces 1/2 ml of semen and just one small speck or drop of it fertilizes the flower (egg cell) of the female. Just as the flower produces fruit, so also a woman liberates flowers which are stocked in her worms of forehead and produces a child.

This concept of reproduction, very much resembles plants. In plants pollen grains fall on the stigma and fertilize and hence a fruit is produced. A woman liberates a flower which is fertilized just by one drop of semen and therefore child (fruit) is produced.

A sterile/barren woman does not liberate 'flower' (in this case egg cell). A man whose semen colour is yellow is believed to be sterile. The status of both sterile men and women in the Thakur society is very low. They are prohibited from participating in fertility rituals such as puberty rite, wedding, turmeric ceremony, panchvi punjan (worship of mother Earth) and so on.

Thus semen and vaginal fluids are the main sources of producing life. The combination of these two results into an offspring and therefore they are classified as life fluids - that contribute in creating life.

B. Fluids that Sustain Life

Blood, breast milk and water are some of the major fluids which according to Thakurs sustain life. Their perceptions of these major fluids revealed following facts -

Blood

Blood (Raghat) is the most important fluid in the human body that contributes to its survival. Blood contributes to the production of breast milk, sperms, vaginal fluid and strength.

They judge a person's strength and stage of growth, ill health conditions based on the colour of his/her blood. The table given below shows their concept of colour symbolism associated with human blood.

Table V : 1. Concepts of Blood Colour and Illness

Sr.No.	Colour of Blood	Concepts
1	Red Blood	a. children and teen-agers have red blood. b. Red blood is a sign of healthy body. c. It also symbolizes power or strength a child or teen-ager has which is fairly good.
2	Reddish Orange	a. Adults have Reddish orange blood. b. Symbolizes higher degree of strength. c. Sign of healthy body.
3	Black Colour	a. Old people have black colour blood. b. Symbolizes lowest degree of strength. c. Sign of ill health.
4	Reddish black	a. Menstruating women have this blood. b. It is hot in nature and has a foul smell. c. Is is evil and brings about diseases such as leprosy, STD etc.

5	Yellow	Yellow colour blood in some parts such as eyes, nails and if seen on the skin is a sign of Jaundice Blood which turns into yellowish green colour is 'pus' again a sign of ill health.
6	Greenish Yellow	Leprosy patients are believed to have this colour. When they die they are cremated and the smoke that comes out is greenish yellow colour.
7	Bluish colour	When a person is bitten by a cobra his/her blood turns bluish in colour because of the effect of poison. Its a signal of death.
8	White	White discharge among the women is con sidered to be a sign of ill health as it is against the orderly routine of menstrual flow.:

Blood according to the Thakurs must be utilized by doing work so as to dispose it in the form of energy. It should be utilized for the production of breast milk, semen, vaginal fluid etc. but never must be accumulated in the body. A person who do not work hard accumulates blood in the body and invites diseases (rog). Blood circulates in the body in an anticlock manner (the auspicious manner). The Thakurs believe sun, moon, clouds, winds etc. move in an anticlock manner. These cosmic entities being divine move in an auspicious direction. Hence air, agni (fire), water (pani), blood (raghat), light (tej) move in an anticlock fashion.

All the Davan Jatis (evil social groups), including the Mahars, Mangs, Chamars, Thakurs, Kathkaris etc. believe that anticlock movement is an auspicious movement. While the Dev jatis (god) like Brahmans, Marathas, kunbis, Mahadev Kolis, Gujratis etc. believe that clockwise movement is auspicious and anticlock is inauspicious. Thus all auspicious rites performed in the Davan (evil) jati show anticlock movements or actions while it is exactly opposite with the dev (godlike) jatis.

Breast Milk

The belief that breast milk is produced from woman's blood in her breast is a very common belief among the Thakurs. An infant survives on breast milk nearly for a year. Milk of a mother is a medium through which her strength (blood) is passed on to the child. Yet another phenomena regarding breast milk which is directly connected with the child's health is their concept of 'Naska Dudh' (spoilt milk).

The Thakur mothers do not breast feed the child for the first five days.

They believe that the mother's milk is thick and is harmful as it causes indigestion in the child. The word 'Naska' means spoilt. For nine months and nine days the foetus is in the mother's womb and the mother's body internally gets polluted with spermatic (sticky) effect due to menstrual blood which according to the Thakurs is evil. Due to the thickness of menstrual blood which is inside the body for nine months and the spermatic effect the normal blood of the woman also gets slightly thick and hence cheesed milk or 'Cholostrom milk' (spoilt milk) is produced. For five days the cholostrom milk is squeezed out and the child is given goat's milk, honey and water.

Water : The King of Bodily Fluids

The source oflife giving fluids is water. Thakurs believe that blood, breast milk, vaginal fluid, mucus, sweat, semen, pus, tears, urine etc. are produced because of intake of water. Blood is of course produced as a result of watc and food together which turns into juice which is acted upon by agni (heat) in the stomach and then converted into blood. The human body has life only because of intake of water and food. Even the atma (soul) which is situated just below the sternum is nourished by water, wind, fire and light.

Thus, whatever water and food is taken in it contributes to the production of blood first - blood then turns into breast milk. Vaginal fluid and semen are produced in the respective worms (kidas) of males and females in their foreheads.

Water is considered as God. Water is believed to be the brother of Sun and Moon. Therefore water is used in many auspicious occasions by the Thakurs, healing rites, marriage and turmeric ceremony rites, purification rites, fertility rites and so on. Water is very scarce in Karjat tribal areas. The tribals have hard times during summer. Most Thakurs do not use water after defecation. They use stones or leaves. They believe that it is an insult to their God and his brothers Sun and Moon.

ii. Excretory Fluids

Fluids such as urine, sweat, tears, mucus, pus etc. are believed to be residual fluids of water. Water and food which is consumed gets converted to blood and waste products such as urine and excreta. Fluids such as pus and menstrual blood are spoilt products of good blood and hence are eliminated out of the body naturally. Tears are produced in the eyes. Mucus is believed to be the excreta of worms (Kidas) which are situated just above the fronto nasal suture.

The state of health and ill health is judged on the colour and abnormality of the excretory fluids. Thus when mucus is very watery it is believed that the forehead has been overexposed to cold water and wind. When the colour of urine changes to yellow or red it is a sign of ill health.

The Thakurs believe that if a person walks or works in the Sun (heat) for long time his blood gets burnt and comes out of his body in the form of sweat (gham). To substitute the loss of blood one needs to then take water. One feels thirsty and drinks more water which again turns into blood and blood into sweat. The movement of these fluids in the body and their elimination is done with the help of wind in the body. Blood circulation in the body is because of the flow of wind in the body.

Physiology of Bodily Systems

Indigenous knowledge of body physiology very much differs from the scientific knowledge of the physiology of various bodily systems, namely, respiratory system, circulatory system, nervous system and so on. The science of ethnophysiology as a sub-discipline of medical Anthropology deals with beliefs, values, perceptions, knowledge and understanding of a community regarding the functioning of various bodily systems and organs and their contribution to body survival.

It is very necessary to understand people's concept of body physiology, dietary behaviour, illness etiology, ethnnomedical therapy, preventive medicine, etc. in order to implement culturally acceptable health education programmes.

Nitcher and Nitcher (1981:75) have pointed out that the elaborate and detailed belief systems and underlaying food habits in traditional societies are often overlooked. Sometimes they are dismissed as unrelated and haphazard collection of superstitions and customs based on ignorance.

Today especially in a developing country like India where 80% of the population resides in the rural and tribal areas food traditions and related concepts of ethnophysiology still continue to play an integral part of many societies. They often help to maintain cultural identity and traditional values in the face of destabilizing influences.

In order to educate people on health it is very necessary to understand what they have. Study their belief system and build on what is available. The Thakur concept of ethnophysiology of bodily systems reveals following facts -

Concept of Reproduction

Thakur concepts of reproduction resembles theplants. Just as a plant produces fruit from a flower after having fertilized by water, so also human beings both male and female produce an offspring (fruit) after sexual intercourse.

Semen according to the Thakurs is stocked in the forehead. In the forehead i.e. just above the fronto-nasal stature dwell the 'worms of life' (kidas) which produce semen. Thus sperms as believed by Thakurs are liberated from these kidas and come out through the urethra touching the soul (atma), carrying the element of life with it. One drop of sperm fertilizes a flower (phool) which is liberated by a woman's 'worms' from the forehead and come out in the form of vaginal fluid in the vagina, where a drop of sperm fertilizes it and is nurtured into a fruit (foetus) into the mother's womb. Thus if two flowers are released by a woman during sexual intercourse and if they are fertilized by two drops of sperms twins are born.

The Thakurs believe that for nine months and nine days a pregnant woman does not menstruate. The foetus lives on her menstrual blood. Besides this the foetus gets sufficient warmth, air, water, blood, light etc. from the mother's body. Thakur'sconcept of reproduction is thus symbolic and expresses the natural fertilization concepts which they observe in plants.

Concept of Digestion

Digestion of food according to Thakurs starts in the mouth where food is ground and pushed in the stomach (potali) with the help of wind. In the stomach fire (heat), light, water convert the food into liquid form. This liquid food is filtered and separated into blood and excreta in the intestines. Excreta comes out from the anus (Gupta Darwaza or secret door), spoilt water (urine) comes out from urethral/vaginal opening.

The Thakurs believe that for digestion of two bhakars (coarse bread) two glasses of water are required, if one bhakar is consumed on must drink one glass of water. The proportion should be equal. Bread (Bhakar) prepared from wheat or bajra (millet) needs more water for digestion as they are believed to be heavy. Thus one bhakar of bajra requires 2 1/2 glasses of water. On enquiring from Thakurs what happens when one does not drink water after food. The reply was 'stomach upset'. No water, no digestion. Over eating, wrong combination of foods, too hot or cold foods cause indigestion.

The digestive power of an adult and a youth is greater than a child and a old person. The ability to digest food varies at different ages. It takes at least three hours for food to be digested to blood. Food helps body to grow and survive.

Concept of Respiration

Thakurs believe that air is one of the most important constituents of the human body. It is inhaled from the atmosphere and circulated in different parts of the body by the phuphus (lungs). Air in the body contributes to circulation and digestion processes. The concept of oxygen and its role etc. is absent among Thakurs. They classify auspicious and inauspicious air (vara). The auspicious air is one that flows from east to west and from north to south. Human beings breath air from North, west and east. The air or wind flowing from South is inauspicious and causes illness and brings about death. South is the direction of death and evil. While east is from where rises the 'Sun' the creator, west - the direction of mother Earth and north the dwelling place of Gods.

Concept of Nervous System

Atma (soul) is the seat of thinking. It is situated right below the sternum in a cage of ribs. Human brain is termed as 'mun' which also helps to think but all sensory actions are co-ordinated by the atma. Most informants said that all nerves are linked with the atma. A bad atma allows bad thoughts to enter human body and vice versa.

Nerves are attached to muscles and bones and hence make the body flexible. Movement of body is possible because of nerves. Thus all biological actions of desire for having sex, food, water etc. is governed by the 'atma' (soul).

Concept of Excretion

The Thakurs concept of excretion to certain extent resembles to the 'foreign matter theory' of Louis Kunhey - a Naturopath. They believe that un-utilized and waste matter in the body must be eliminated through excretion, blood letting, surgery, suction methods etc. The presence of waste matter in the body causes diseases. Efforts must be made to eliminate these matters. Of course their interpretation is not that scientific as Kunhey's. They do believe in elimination of waste products from the body.

Thus sweat, excreta, urine, menstrual blood, spoilt blood, mucus etc. are waste products that the body throws out. Sweat is thrown out through skin, excreta by anus, spoilt blood by blood letting and through natural menstrual flow.

Circulatory System Concepts

The Thakurs believe that blood is circulated in the body in an anticlock manner with the help of wind (vara) that is present in the body. The anticlock movement of blood is associated with movement of cosmic objects such as sun, moon, clouds, etc. Anticlock movement of blood is a symbol of auspicious movement in this context. Blood is situated in veins (nadya). While a person is sleeping the blood keeps on circulating.

Atma (Soul) : The Co-ordinator of All Bodily Systems

Atma (soul) of a human being is situated just below the sternum according to the Thakurs. It is associated with life (jeev) of a person. It exists in the human body, to keep a person alive depending on the number of days destined by mother Earth, who writes the life span of a child after its birth on its forehead.

Atma according to Thakur constitutes fire (agni), water (pani), wind (vara) and light (tej). It is situated in the cage of ribs. It gets light and fire from the sun and moon, wind from the cosmos and water from man. Thus an atma needs a regular flow of water, light, fire and wind which it gets from cosmos. A person is alive because atma dwells in him.

A Thakur song on the atma goes on to state :

Pinjara banivala Patichare
Aatmadhi Ragho motyachare
Pinjara akashi dulere
Aatmandhi Ragho bolere
Pinjara gela tutunire
Raghoba gela udunire
Gela swargachya vatire
Tethe anandachi madire
Tyachi anandi madire

The Song

In the cage of flexible sticks
there dwells the parrot,
the parrot speaks sweetly
as the cage swings in the sky

It so happened oh brother
the cage was broken
and as the cage broke away
the parrot got ready to fly away
he flew towards heaven
where exists a place of happiness.

Meaning of the Song

About seven to eight Thakurs who were singing this song during a healing ritual were asked to give the meaning of the song. They explained that the cage symbolizes the ribs of the human being. In which dwells the atma or soul (parrot). Every cage breaks some or the other time in life.

breaking of the cage symbolizes death. The parrot flies away, meaning the soul leaves human body for heaven where always happiness reigns.

On enquiring from the respondents, how does a soul leave human body ? They said, we get to know of this by looking at the corpse. If the mouth of the dead body is open it means that the atma has left the body through the mouth. So is the case if eyes are open. If both eyes and mouth are closed the Thakurs believe that the atma has left the person's body either through ears or nose and through the scalp of the apex as reported by Chaphekar (1961:82).

On the ninth day, in case of married women, tenth day in case of married men and seventh day in case of bachelors and spinsters after their death the Thakurs perform the ritual of soul migration. The aim of the ritual is to send the soul of the dead person to heaven. A palas leaf (butea monosperma) is taken on which a stone studded in rice flour is placed and ritually left in the water along with nine other flour balls with no stone in them. (See diagram V : 1).

The leaf symbolizes the body of the dead person, the rice flour ball the cage and the stone (jeev khada) symbolizes the soul of the dead person which is left in a running river water facing the east for it is to merge with the cosmos and go back to heaven which is towards the east. The other nine rice flour balls symbolize the ten bodily openings in which dwell the planetary spirits. These are also left in the water to merge with the cosmos.

A Thakur riddle goes on to say 'Manev pind banavito _pun parmatma atma banavito', meaning man makes the body (foetus), but the soul (atma) is the foetus is created by 'Sun God'. Atma according to the Thakurs is the co-ordinator of all the systems of the body and controls all the physiological and nervous functions of the body. What the human body symbolizes in different ritual healing contexts or situations is explained in the second part of the chapter.

Human Body as a Natural Symbol

The Thakurs associate their body morphology, anatomy and physiology to that of a tree. It is their belief that the human body is very much similar to the natural elements which a plant comprises of.

i. Bones

The skeletal framework of the human body is associated with the trunk and branches of the tree.

ii. Flesh And Skin

The flesh and skin of the human body is associated with the bark.

(covering of the trunk and the branches).

iii. Blood

This red fluid in the human body is associated with the sap, the latex and/or water content in the tree.

iv. Soul (Atma)

The human beings have soul (atma) which is situated just below the sternum so also the trees have atma in the roots. The atma is believed to be the seat of intelligence and co-ordinates all the systems and also controls the thinking process. There is no concept of nervous system.

v. Veins/Arteries

The human body has blood vessels like arteries, veins and capillaries which are a part of the circulatory system. In a similar manner the atma of the tree which is present in the roots pumps the water and food to all the parts of the plant body through the vascular tissues xylem and phloem.

vi. Hair

Just as human beings have hair on their body so also the plants have hair on the leaves, branches and on trunks, according to the Thakurs.

vii. Feelings

Akin to human beings plants also have feelings and emotions and are hurt/wounded when they are cut.

viii. Concept of Death

Plants die or are killed when they are uprooted or destroyed from the roots. This is similar to the human body which becomes a corpse once the atma/soul leaves it.

ix. Human Body and Plant Body Become Mud AfterTheir Death

Both the human and plant body after their death return back to the earth and turn into mud. (Human body : pind).

x. Reproductive System

The flowers of the tree are turned into fruit after fertilization. The female reproductive organ of the tree is its flower and the male reproductive organ is the water. The water drop (fertile water) from the atma situated in the roots fertilizes every flower of the tree which bears fruit.

Male and Female Reproductive System

The Thakurs differentiate between a male and a female on the presence of testicles among the males and breasts among the females. The Thakurs believe that males have two worms (kidas), white in colour present in the head above the fronto-nasal suture and when the kidas excrete mucus flows out of the nose.

If a person drinks liquor, he becomes intoxicated and loses his balance. An intoxicating drink makes the kidas swirl due to which the person feels giddy and loses his balance.

A person is believed to suffer from a headache when these worms (kidas) start biting the brain.

The kidas are also believed to have a reproductive function. The kidas produce sperms which flow down from the head during intercourse and flow out of the penis. One drop of semen is capable of fertilizing a flower which is produced by the female kidas and also flows down during intercourse.

sperm (water) + flower (egg) = child (fruit)

When two flowers are contributed by the female kidas, these flowers are fertilized by two drops of sperms and results in twins.

a. 2 flowers + 2 drops of sperms = twins.

b. 3 flowers + 3 drops of sperms = triplets.

a. 4 flowers + 4 drops of sperms = Quadraplets.

It is believed (by the Thakurs) that the flower (egg contributed by the woman) opens up and receives the sperm drop to produce the fruit (child). Flowers are produced in a woman after menstruation.

xi. Classification of Male/Female Aspects Among Plants And Its Significance

The Thakurs have a peculiar fashion of differentiating male from female plants. Some plants and trees are given male or female status and have integral socio-cultural meaningful functions within the Thakur culture. Listed below are some plants which are classified as male or female.

Male Plants

1. Mango - Mangifera indica
2. Mauha - Madhuca indica
3. Teak - Tectona grandis
4. Amla - Embelica Officinatis
5. Fig - Ficus Glomerata
6. Coconut with water - Cocos nucifera
7. Hirda - Terminellia chebulla
8. Banana - Musa paradisica

9. Drumstick - Moringa olifera
10. Shid - Bauhinia racemosa

Female plants

1. Halad Turmeric - Curcuma domestica
2. Kharik - Phoenix species
3. Papaya - Carcica Papaya
4. Cotton - Caltropis gigantea
5. Jamun - Eugenia jambolina
6. Palas - Beutea frondosa

Thus according to the Thakurs each plant, animal (including man) has male and female elements in their respective bodies.

xii. Concept of Age/Growth

Plants also go through various stages of growth during their lifetime like the human beings. Plants are green and healthy when young just like youths.

xiii. The Worm Attack

Worms and white ants attack plant and more often than not cause decay and disease in plants. The human body is also believed to be attacked by worms (Kide) which cause disease. Eg. Scabies is believed to be caused by the Jantu (germs) which suck blood (Raghat) when it becomes sweet. Therefore to neutralize this sweetness bitter plants are taken as medicines. Thus scabies is perceived as an internal rather an external disorder and the Thakurs therefore mock at the PHC doctors who advise them to use soap on the infected parts.

xiv. Manure Vs Food

The plants obtain nutrition from the manure like compost, farm yard manure. This manure helps plants grow. In a similar way the human body obtains nourishment from food. Lack of manure and food in the plants and humans respectively leads to weakness which at times is fatal.

xv. Survival

The survival of the human body, plant body and atma depends on a continuous proportionate supply of water, sunlight/moonlight, air, fire or heat (Agni) and food.

The above mentioned elements have their sources in, 1. Sun, Moon (Male Gods) - light, 2. Wind (Female God)- wind, 3. Sun (Male God) - fire, 4. Water (Male God) - water, and 5. Natural environment - food,

The morphology of human body is made up of mud (mother Earth - female).

Inter-relationship Between Plant Symbols and Human Body

Plants have profoundly influenced the culture and civilization of man (Choudhari 1981). Traditional tales, mythological stories, events in epics, religious worships, festivals, rituals of births, puberty, marriage and death, in many cultures have references to plant symbols and their meanings in human social system.

Plants have been the oldest associates of man and therefore form a integral part of human culture. The fact that plants have found usage in rituals and ceremonies proves that they have symbolic and meaningful values.

An attempt is made to -

a. highlight the plant symbols in the Thakur culture and their association with the human body.
b. to demonstrate the manner in which the Thakur's interpret human body as a part of the universe and nature (i.e. plants).

i. Butea Frondosa (Palas) Family : Papilionaceae

This plant is classified by the Thakurs as belonging to the feminine gender. It is used in many rituals and ceremonies where it symbolizes or is associated with human body.

a. Birth Ritual

Soon after birth of a child, the midwife (Suine) cuts and buries the umbilical chord (nal) and the placental waste (var) as a preventive measure, so that the chord and the waste may not become an object of sorcery and witchcraft.

The midwife takes a palas leaf, places on it the umbilical chord in the centre with some rice, gulal (red powder), a coin and a wick. Th leaf is then buried (along with the things placed on it) on the outside of the western wall of the house. A temporary bathing place is made for the mother and the child to bathe. Thus the used bath water is allowed to flow over the buried palas leaf as the water helps the chord to decay and perish.

Diagram V : 1. showing symbolism of the burial of umbilical chord.

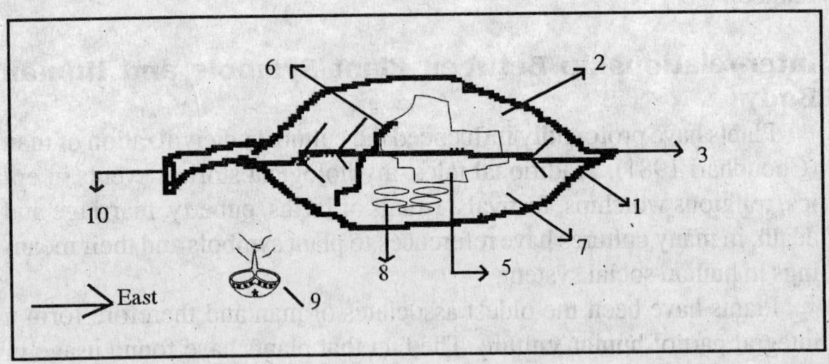

Meanings

1. **The Palas leaf** - symbolizes the woman.

2. **Leaf placed with its dorsal side upwards** - this symbolizes the sexual position of the fertile woman.

3. **Apex of the Leaf** - symbolizes the woman's head.

4. **Central part of the leaf** - is symbolic of the womb.

5. **Var (Placental waste)** - placed in the central part of the leaf is symbolic of the uterus in which the child is nurtured.

6. **Umbilical Chord** - Symbolizes the child.

7. **Gulal (red powder)** - symbolizes the menstrual blood of the woman, her fertility.

8. **Rice** - the rice is symbolic of the continuity of fertility.

9. **Wick (Wat)** - symbolizes the presence of the sun (masculine nature). It is believed that the light of the sun and fire help the atma (soul) of the mother and child to survive.

10. **East-west placement of the leaf** - is symbolic of two aspects -
    a. Delivery posture of the woman.
    b. Sexual posture of the woman.

11. **The base of the petiole** - symbolizes the vaginal opening. The dorsal placing of the leaf signifies the woman's desire for having more children.

The Turning Over of the Palas Leaf

Chaphekar L.N. (1960:45) states that a Thakur woman who does not wish to bar anymore children buries the placenta of her child in an inverted position. The meaning of this action according to the Thakur midwives and elderly women meant the concerned family must put an end to producing more children. The symbolic elements associated with this action are related to social control designed culturally through spiritual media i.e. 'Satvai' (mother Earth's desire or wish for the family to stop producing children). This ritual expresses or symbolizes a cultural check on population growth.

The Cosmic Elements Associated with the Burial Rite of the Umbilical Chord

The fertility of a woman, her sexual behaviour, her feminine nature etc., is on the whole linked to mother earth by the Thakurs. They believe that the dorsal side of the mother earth faces the sun - her husband and all life on earth are their offsprings.

At the time of the burial (of the palas leaf) a wick is placed on the palas leaf. The wick is symbolic of the sun's posture during sex with the mother earth. The water which flows on the buried leaf symbolizes the flow of spermatic fluid of the sun into the mother earth. This sexual union of the sun and the earth at cosmic level is prevalent in the Thakur culture.

Marriage Ritual

The palas leaf is also used in the wedding rituals by the Thakurs. During the wedding, the bride is separated from the groom by a curtain, while the Brahman (priest) chants the scriptures.

The bride places her left foot on the palas leaf and the groom places his right foot on another palas and apex of the two leaves point towards the east in case of bridegroom and west in case of the bride. As soon as the chanting of scriptures is completed the curtain falls.

The falling of the curtain symbolizes the union of these two leaves, thereby uniting symbolically two physical bodies into a social unit (family). The overlapping of the male (bridegroom's) leaf over the female (bride's) leaf symbolizes the social sanction given by the Thakur society for these two to have sexual relationship, to be fertile and fruitful.

Diagram V : 2. Showing sex symbolism of a wedding ritual.

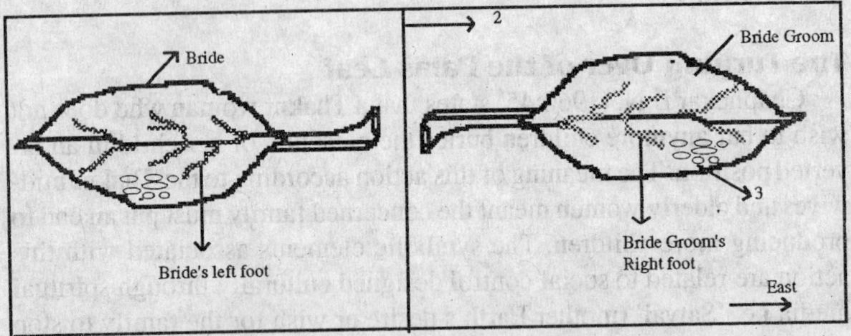

Meanings

The two palas leaves used in the context of marriage ritual are associated with sexual union, physical bodies of the bride and the bridegroom, fertility, the establishment of family (social unit) and rules of sexual behaviour. The meanings are as follows -

1. The two palas leaves symbolize the physical bodies of the bride and the bridegroom.
2. The falling of the curtain symbolizes the union of these two into a family and a socially sanctioned and recognized liberty for them to live together and sex inorder to help the Thakur society multiply.
3. The rice grains on these two leaves symbolize the people's blessings and desires for the couple to be fertile and be fruitful.
4. The right foot of the groom and the left foot of the bride on the leaves facing each other symbolizes that when the groom's leaf (physical body) fall on the other leaf the man's right foot is over her left foot and right hand over left hand during the sexual intercourse.
5. The male leaf falling over the female leaf symbolizes the man's authority, dominance and superiority over a woman.

In another marriage ritual the Thakurs again associate plants with human body. Given below is the diagram with explanation of meanings of every object (plant) used in the ritual. A pot filled with water is kept near a pole with a twig attached to it as shown in the diagram. On the neck of the pot leaves of rui (calotropis procera) are tied. This pot rests on the palas leaf again.

Diagram V : 3. Showing symbolic aspects of fertility.

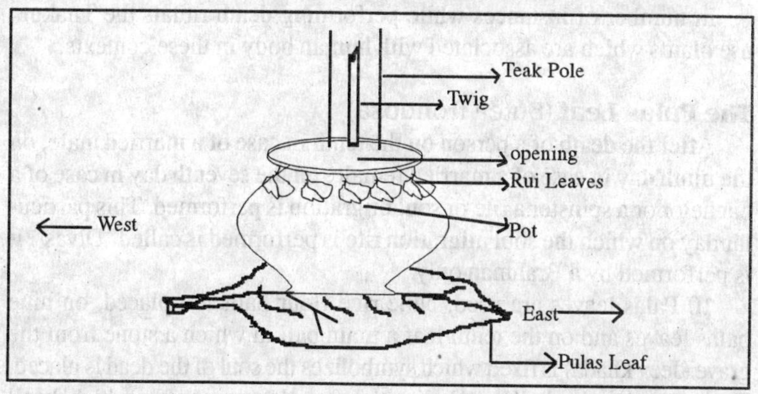

Meanings

This ritual symbolizes the human body as nothing but a part of the universe. The teak pole (male) symbolizes the Sun's body isof course associated with the groom. The palas leaf (female) symbolizes the mother Earth's body again associated with a bride. The twig on the wooden pole symbolizes the urethra of the male (groom) showing the penis. The pot symbolizes the mother's womb. The rui leaves symbolize the children. The rope with which the leaves are tied symbolize the placenta (the attached relationship of the child with the mother).

The male body on the top again symbolize the man's superiority, authority and dominance over the female (woman). The leaf pointing towards the east is the sexual posture during intercourse. The closeness of the male (teak pole) with the palas leaf symbolizes the union of the two families and also the husband and wife relationship of the sun with the mother earth.

The pot opening symbolizes the vaginal opening of the bride, ready to accept the water of life (sperms) to be fertile and fruitful. The facts interpreted about this ritual show that human physical body is symbolically related to cosmic objects (sun, earth & plants). The Thakurs believe that mother earth and the sun are the life giving sources. The Sun gives life which the mother nurses and nurtures.

The physical bodies of the bride and groom are socially perceived as cosmological entities forming a union there by creating happiness in the universe as it were. The Thakurs take pride in performing this ritual for it symbolizes the presence of their divine or supernatural powers (sun & earth) participating in this auspicious ceremony or event. This is how in reality the physical body is not physical body but a representation of the cosmos.

Plant Symbols and Death Ritual

In number of instances while performing death rituals the Thakurs use plants which are associated with human body in these contexts.

The Palas Leaf (Butea frondosa)

After the death of a person on the tenth in case of a married male, on the ninth day in case of a married female, on the seventh day in case of a bachelor or a spinster a rite of soul migration is performed. This particular day on which the soul migration rite is performed is called 'Divas'. It is performed by a Brahman only.

10 Palas leaves are used. Nine rice flour balls are placed, on nine palas leaves and on the tenth leaf a main ball in which a stone from the grave (Jeev khada) is fixed which symbolizes the soul of the dead is placed. The other nine rice balls symbolize the nine planetary spirits which dwell in the nine openings of human body namely eyes, ears, nose, the wrist pulse, the naval, the urethral or vaginal opening, the pulse of the feet and the anal opening.

Mango Leaves

In yet another soul migration ritual which is performed in the house, a twig of mango leaves is tied at the door post by the head of the house. This is the last act of performing the soul migration ritual. In the case of a male mango leaves (Mangifera indica) are used and in case of a female. Jamun leaves (Eugenia jambolina), are used.

Mango symbolizes the male soul and jamun female. The Thakurs have their own system of classifying male & female plants. The action of tying the mango twig on the door post means the soul is fully satisfied through the performed rituals and can leave the house peacefully.

The Human Body as Cosmological System

The Thakurs describe the human body in one of their riddles as an integral part of the universe stating, 'Pinda sarkha khand'. Here Pind (human body) is referred to as khand (universe). Another riddle goes as follows -

In our body oh brother
how many doors are there ?
In our body oh brother
where is the sacred fire that forever burns ?
These are my problems please explain to me oh brother
The answers are
There are nine doors oh brother and

the tenth one is secret door (gupta darwaza) oh brother
And in our body oh brother
to the left is the second fire that forever burns.
Chaphekar (1960:180-81).

At another village Chaphekar (1960:82) reports a different version about the bodily doors or openings.

To our body, oh brother
how many doors are there ?
and how many door are open ?

Answer -

To our body oh brother
there are ten doors, nine are open
and tenth one is secret

Chaphekar points out that the 'secret door' is supposed to be the apex of the scalp. The song goes on to explain that the key to the secret door is with the spiritual teacher (sadguru). The secret door opens when the soul leaves its human tabernacle for good (Chaphekar, 1961:82).

The meanings and explanations of the above riddles and songs point towards the Thakur concepts which co-relate the human body with the universe. To continue further and explore their concept of body symbolism is the aim of this present study.

The Ten Doors of the Body Compared to the Ten Planets

The Ma Thakurs of Kashale and Pathraj villages of Karjat Tehsil classify the ten openings of the human body in a hierarchial manner as follows :

Ten Openings of the body

The Thakurs classify hierachially the ten body openings as follows - 1. The eyes (Dole), 2. The Nostrils (Nak), 3. The mouth (Tond), 4. Ears (Kan), 5. Atma or soul, 6. Wrist pulse (Hatachi nadi), 7. Navel (Bembi), 8. Urethral or vaginal opening, 9. Pulse of the feet (Payachi nadi), and10. Anal opening (Gupta darwaza).

The Thakurs co-relate these ten openings of the body with the ten planets (nav nath) which have a definite order and hierarchy in the cosmos. The earth (Dantari) is the main planet situated in the fifth position and is the centre of the universe and holds a very important position in the

Thakur cosmological conceptions.

The atma (soul) also is placed at the fifth position (hierachially) like the mother earth and is considered to be the opening of life. Every bodily opening has a spirit which is directly linked with the respective planets in the cosmos.

Life (atma) is believed to be a combination of light (tej), fire (agni), wind (hawa). Water and mud (mother earth) along with the ten spiritual forces (from the ten planets) from the human body.

A human being exists or survives when these cosmic elements are present in the body. A person dies when life (atma) leaves the body (human tabernacle). A person falls sick or suffers from ill-health when his atma, body and mind malfunction or when there is some disturbance. caused by pathogens. The pathogens are believed to enter into the body through any of the ten openings. The Thakurs classify the ten pathogenic agents or beings within their natural, supernatural, cosmological, ancestral, social and spiritual world that exist within their cultural framework.

The Planetary Spirits and the Bodily Openings

The Thakurs believe that each body opening is linked to every planetary spirit (the spirit of life). When these ten planetary spirits leave the body the human beings dies. After this there is no relation between the dead person and the cosmos as the planetary spirits have left for their respective planets.

These beliefs are symbolically expressed during the ritual connected with soul migration. This ritual is performed on the tenth day (after death) for the married males, on the ninth day for married females and on the seventh day for bachelors and spinsters. This ritual is performed so as to ensure the migration of the human soul to its heavenly abode and the migration of the planetary spirits to their respective planets.

It is believed that life (i.e. soul and the planetary spirits) and the khand (i.e. universe) merge with one another, and the pind (i.e. body, made up of soil) merges with the earth on the death of a person.

The Soul Migration Ritual (Divas)

As stated earlier this ritual is performed on different days according to the marital status and sex of the dead person.

Ten rice flour balls are made, one of them is bigger in size than the others. Inside this ball there is a small stone. This rice ball is placed on a palas leaf (Butea frondosa) and this ball is known as jeev khada. The stone in the rice ball is collected from the grave of the dead person and symbolizes the atma (soul) of the person.

The other nine rice balls symbolize the nine planetary spirits of the cosmos which are linked with the openings of the human body. These rice balls are thrown in the river facing east by the eldest son of the deceased. In case, the deceased is a bachelor or a spinster this rite is performed by the elder brother. If the deceased is a male the balls are thrown in such a way that the ball touch the thumb while being thrown. If the deceased is a female the balls are thrown into the river with the balls touching the little finger.

The thumb and the toe symbolize masculinity while the little finger and the fifth digit of the foot symbolize femininity.

The red powder (gulal) sprinkled on the ten rice balls are symbolic of the blood of the deceased. The ten incense sticks which are burnt represent the departure of fire and wind from the body of the dead and their return to the universe. The body (pind) merges with the soil. The river water is believed to transport these spirits back to the planets. The act of dropping rice is symbolic to the departure of the atma and the planetary spirits into the cosmos.

Alongwith the red powder, a black coloured powder is also sprinkled on the rice balls. This black powder symbolizes the sins of the human beings which they commit while they live. To purify the sins of the atma a solution, which has five constituents is sprinkled on the rice balls. The five constituents are water, coconut water, milk, honey and cow's urine. The Thakurs believe that when the soul leaves the body and merges with the cosmos, the almighty God (Sun) questions the atma and asks 'What did you bring from the earth ?' The atma replies 'Panch amrut'.

The Mother Earth and Her Sisters (Mothya Baya)

The Thakurs place mother earth (Dantari) on the fifth position on the planetary hierarchy. Earth is the most important of all planets (khand) and she gives birth, gives life and also writes the life span of human beings. The other nine planets are her sisters and are locally known as 'Mothya Baya'. The word 'Baya' refers to a group of women.

The 'baya' have a direct control on the human body. If the Thakurs fail to perform some religious rite or duty the Baya bring skin disease such as small pox, chicken pox, boils, body sores etc. They enter the human body in the form of hot wind through the nine openings. This heat in the body results in the eruption of sores. The Baya are believed to be spinsters while Dantari (earth) has a husband, the Sun. Their entry into the human body symbolizes their desire for sex with the male cosmic forces and hence the heat in the body is symbolic of their sexual desire.

Sexual Satisfaction at the Cosmic Level

The Shaman (Bhagat) diagnoses and interprets the origin and the cause of the chicken pox as the heat created by the 'Baya' in the body which results in the body breaking into sores. The Baya desires to have sex with a male cosmic object.

The Bhagat recommends that the patients go to the Umber tree (Ficus glomerata) and worship it. The (patient/s) relatives put red powder on the roots, dig a hole **under** the root so that a small pot can fit into the hole. Then a slash is made on the root so that the milky latex flows into the pot. This sweet, white and cold latex is consumed by the patient two or three times a day. This remedy cures the patient.

The Ficus glomerata tree symbolizes the moon (chandra). Its white latex, consumed by the patient symbolizes the spermatic flow which is believed to cool the heat created by the sexual aggravation of the 'Baya' and is believed to satisfy them. The patient is bathed on the fifth day. The act of bathing symbolizes the washing of 'Baya' after sex. There the bathing is always done by a woman. The physical sex is culturally perceived as a sexual relation between the moon (a male cosmic object) and the Baya (female cosmic planets). This relation is perceived, accepted and expressed through the human body during its state of ill-health.

Thus, visitation of goddesses 'Baya' is nothing but an expression of their desire for sex with the moon. This is symbolically expressed in the healing rite of chicken pox. The Baya are satisfied after the latex of Ficus glomerata is consumed by the patient and the bathing of the patient cleanses and satisfies the Baya after which they return back. During the five day period and the healing rite the Thakurs sing songs of praise in which they praise the cosmos and the ten planets.

A Song During the Healing Rite

The Thakurs sing special songs which are sung during the healing rites to appease the cause (Baya) of the disease. One of the songs sung during the healing rite is as follows -

The Song

Let us humbly bow before
the Baya oh brothers and sisters
To whom should I sing a song
of praise first oh brother
I will song for the mother earth
first oh brother
To whom should I sing the second praise
oh brother
I will sing to Mata (mother earth) and Pita
(father Sun) oh brother

To whom should I sing the third praise
oh brother
I will sing the third praise to the sky,
earth and other planets oh brother
To whom should I sing the fourth praise
oh brother
I will sing the fourth praise to the moon -
the husband of the fourth planet
To whom should I sing the fifth praise
oh brother
I will sing the fifth praise for the five Pandav
To whom should I sing the sixth praise
oh brother
I will sing for the sixth planet oh brother
To whom should I sing the seventh praise
oh brother
I will sing for the seven planets oh brother
To whom should I sing the eighth praise
oh brother
I will sing for the sun oh brother
To whom should I sing the ninth praise
oh brother
I will sing for the nav khand (nine planets)
oh brother
To whom should I sing the tenth praise
oh brother
I will sing for the tenth planet oh brother

Body Worship During the State of Ill-health

Body worship is very common in the Thakur healing cult. The Thakurs believe that the illness is caused by good and bad agents/spirits. When good supernatural spirits cause illness it is believed that they should be worshipped, so as to appease them and that they may then leave the patient's body. Bad spirits are ritually driven out by the Shamans (Bhagats).

In case of chicken pox the origin and cause is attributed to the visitation of the Baya, which enter in the body in the form of spirits through the medium of wind. Thus the physical (human) body in this context becomes the cosmological body, the home of the Baya. The Thakurs consider that Baya are good goddesses and cause illness only when a person deviates from the social norms. They visit the patient to wean him onto the right path.

Human body (patient) thus becomes a cosmic symbol for the Thakur society residing in the village. The other community members hence participate in the healing rituals by singing songs of praise to the goddesses asking them to depart from the patient's body. The patient's body in such a situation is worshipped by the family members and other villagers.

Human Body as a Social Symbol

Human body during the state of ill-health expresses or communicates signals of man's disrupted relationship with his clan members, close relatives, other clans member of other sect of the same tribe and other caste group members.

The analysis of the Thakur conception of body symbolism, illness ideology and ritual healing depicts that body becomes a victim of disease and illness due to a situation within social and inter social group conflict. The origin and cause of ill health is interpreted in terms of illness caused by the relatives, other clan members, members of other tribes or other caste groups through the use of good and evil means.

This chapter highlights the various good 'Social pathogenic agents' that bring about illness and which is symbolically expressed through the body. In other words it aims to show how human body reflects the social situation, social interaction, social hierarchy and conflict as part of the cultural whole. It is necessary therefore to understand what social system, interaction and relation is meant or perceived by the Thakurs. How do they view or look at their ordered set of social relationship which at one point (during the state of ill-health) gets disrupted.

The Social Setting

The tribal communities of Kashale and Pathraj region have been interacting with each other and with other caste communities for ages. There has been an exchange of economic,social and religious services among the tribal and caste communities. Although there exist social interaction there is yet a clear cut demarcation between these groups. This demarcation of social groups and their access to economic, political and educational resources have made it possible to categorize every group into a hierarchy to be recognized within that regional-cultural system.

There are a number of caste and tribal communities residing in Kashale and Pathraj village areas. Thakurs have been interacting with these communities for ages. The Thakurs have their own system of classifying and hierachially categorizing their jatis based on the socio-economic status, religious functions and dietary habits. These jatis are classified into two main social strata -

1. Devjati or Maratha jati
2. Davan, Rakshas or Musalman jati

Dev (God like) Jatis

A Thakur hierachially classifies the Dev or God like jatis as follows -

A. Brahmans	Priests & Teachers
B. Marathas	Agriculturists
C. Gujratis	Business groups
D. Sonars	Goldsmiths
E. Malis	Gardeners
F. Agris	Criminal agricultural community
G. Kolanis	Mahadev Koli tribe
H. Kannadis	A nomadic caste community
I. Lohars	Black smiths
J. Dhangars	Shepherds
K. Nhavi	Barbers.

Davan Jatis

A. Thakurs	Tribe
B. Mahars	Disposing of dead cattle out of the village
C. Mangs	Official hang men and rope makers
D. Chambars	Shoe makers
E. Wadari/Beldaris	Stone workers
F. Muslims	Religious groups
G. Kathkaris	Tribe

Origin of Jatis

The creation myth of the origin of life according to the Thakur states that, in the beginning there was no sky, mountains, no clouds, no trees, except that the mother earth was covered with water. An arrow (vayuban) of wind on the earth was shot by Rama (Sun). As a result of which 3/4 of water on the earth was removed.

The almighty (Sun) then to stir red the sea till a lot of foam was formed. The lord Brahma (Sun) took these types of soils, namely, Jaraj, Goraj, Naraj.

He mixed these with the foam of the sea and some water and made 'Pind' i.e. man's body. He made two statues of a man and a woman. Soon it was found that 'Ghungara' a black evil insect would come and break the pind. Then God Shaker (Sun) created a dog to watch over the statues and keep the Ghungara away. Later on Agni (fire), light (Tej) and wind (vara) were put into these statues to make them living man and woman. Once there was a great flood on the earth, water was rising on the mountain. These two human beings sat in a pumpkin and were saved after the flood subsided. The pumpkin rooted on the mountain which is still there known as 'Shid God'.

The man and woman later on multiplied and there were a lot of people on the mountain. Due to scarcity of food they then thought of going down to the plains as instructed by Sun God. The lord Sun then distributed the jatis and diet, assigned them occupation. This is how the devjatis and Davan jatis came into being. Ever since then till this date the Thakurs of Kashale and Pathraj classify the two categories of social groups living in Karjat tehsil.

The Thakurs categorize or classify the Dev and Davan jatis on the basis of -

1. Social hierarchy
2. Dietary habits
3. Occupational function
4. Religious duties and ritual functions
5. Rules of social interaction
6. Economic and social status
7. Language

The Devjatis as the name suggests are god like jatis, for many social function such as marriage, birth, death, house building, cultivation etc. the Thakurs have been economically dependent on the dev jatis. Other than economic reliability the dev jatis perform a number of life crisis ritual such as birth, marriage, death for the Thakurs. The Dev jatis have been a source of security for the Thakurs for ages. Irrespective of the constant of exploitation the Thakurs still respect the dev jatis because they live at their mercy.

The Thakurs believe that the dev jatis are the avtar (incarnation) of the Baya, the cosmic planets. The Baya take the form of social beings and live with the Thakurs to check them and their deviant behaviour.

On the other hand the Davan/Rakashas jatis, are classified at a very low status compared to the dev jatis and are socially degraded jati, economically poor, they have no role to play in life of crises rituals, their social interaction is limited, their dietary habits are non-vegetarian type like the giants. They are specialized in hunting and killing and also practice evil deeds such as witchcraft and sorcery to harm others. They are a part of the 'Rakshas or giant community' that resides towards the evil south direction.

Health and Social Relationship

The analysis of the qualitative data of Thakur illness ideology body symbolism, ritual healing and the symbolic meanings and their inter-relation within broader cultural frame clearly points out that there is a close relationship of one's health with that of the smooth harmony with other social beings such as relatives, clan members, other tribes men & other group members with whom the Thakur interacts.

An individual enjoys sound health when his social relationship with his fellow men and other groups is harmonious and in accord with the expected cultural norms of social interaction, purity and pollution concepts. Witchcraft and sorcery are very good examples of disruption of social relationship. The Thakurs and even the members of the devjatis believe that witchcraft and sorcery is practiced by the members of Rakshas jatis which include members of the Thakur and Kathkari tribe, the Mahars, Mangs, Chambars, Beldaris and muslims.

A. Sickness Caused by Dev Jatis

The Thakurs who are classified as members of the Rakshas jatis are inferior to the Dev jatis in social, economic, political, religious statues and are very much dependent on the caste groups of the devjatis. The total (cultural) livelihood of a Thakur has been dependent on the dev jatis. Despite the dominance in their interaction, and the exploitation by the dev jatis, the Thakurs depend on them because there is no other source to borrow loans for, cultivation, marriage, birth, death ceremonies and for festivals.

Illness episodes have revealed the 'Baya' - cosmic planets (sisters of mother earth) take the form of caste groups of the dev jatis and visit the Thakurs by causing illness/sickness. Cosmic spirits (invisible) take the form of social beings (visible) to check on deviance of the Thakurs as far as socio-cultural norms are concerned.

The visitation of the cosmic forces through social forms (dev jatis) is termed as visitation of (Baya) goddesses. Each 'Baya' is given a caste group name -

1. Brahmani Baya — Symbolize Brahman caste group.
2. Marathani Baya — Symbolize Maratha caste group.
3. Gujrani Baya — Symbolize Gujrati caste group.
4. Sonarni Baya — Symbolize Gold smith caste group.
5. Malani Baya — Symbolize Gardener caste group.
6. Agarni Baya — Symbolize Agriculture (agri) caste group.
7. Kolani Baya — Symbolize Superior tribe the Mahadev Kolis.
8. Kannadi Baya — Symbolize the nomadic caste group.

and so on.

Hence, sickness such as measles, body fever scabies, black spots on the body, boils etc. are caused by the Baya (dev jatis). This form of sickness which is interpreted by the Bhagat (Shaman) as caused by the social groups (dev jatis) symbolize the social dominance and authority that the dev jatis have over Rakshas jatis. The members must therefore be worshipped by the Rakshas jati so that they do not bring or cause trouble for the Rakshas jati.

The Healing Rite if the Baya

The sisters of mother earth 'Baya' or the planetary spirits of the cosmos take the form of the dev jatis and visit the body of the Thakurs there by causing illness. This symbolizes a transition of cosmological being to physical beings through social beings. When some supernatural force visits a human body, even if it has to cause illness it is an auspicious thing according to the Thakur. In such a situation the holy pathogenic agents are worshipped and appeased so that it takes away trouble.

The Two Types of Baya (Dev Jatis)

The Thakurs believe that the dev jatis that cause illness are of two types. This classification is done on the basis of dietary habits of jatis (castes) -

1. Ratya Baya -	Nonvegetarian dev jatis
2. Chokhya Baya -	Vegetarian dev jatis

The Ratya Baya - Include the Maratha, Agri, Kannada, Mahadev kolis, sonar and lohar jatis

The Chokhya Baya - Include Brahmans, Gujratis.

The Bhagat or Bhagatin (Shaman) are only in a position to tell whether the skin disease concerned is caused by a Ratya or a Chokhya Baya.

The Social Therapy

Having traced the social elements that cause illness in this case the 'lahan Baya or dev jatis' could be either Ratya (non-veg) or chokhya (veg). It becomes the duty of the Thakurs to pray and worship these social forces. The logic on which the social therapy is based is as follows. What (dir) comes socially (through dev jatis) has to healed socially using social therapy. It is at this stage of healing the deviated norms of social interaction area are recalled symbolically at the spiritual level.

Songs and Praises as Part of Social Therapy

Hya Ghari Baya Alya, Bayancha anand Zalare
Devincha anand Zalare
Baya alya aaichya satavan ghyaya
Bapachya chitwan paya.

The above song about visitation of Baya describes the situation as a happy one. They have come to console the mother (in this context) earth. Let us praise the father sun. Praise the Baya for having visited us.

For five continuous evenings right from 8 o'clock to 12 o'clock in the night worship 'the Ghat' a symbol of the Baya, singing and praising them for five nights so that they may take away the physical trouble which is caused to check the deviant behaviour of the Thakurs.

Diet as Part of Social Therapy

It is believed that when the social elements (dev jatis) visit the body the body in reality becomes a social symbol to be worshipped, praised to be looked upon as a higher social force of entities (baya) that has come to check on the deviant behaviour of the Thakurs. The supernatural which take the form of social beings (dev jatis) are 'guest' (pahune) who visit the Thakurs society. It therefore becomes a duty of the Thakurs to give the Baya food.

Depending on the socially prescribed diet which is consumed by the dev jatis the Thakurs make an attempt in reality to feed the patient. (representation of the jatis) their prescribed food. The culturally recognized forms of diet or dietary habits of the dev jatis with whom the Thakurs interact are symbolically reflected in this healing rite of the lahan Baya (dev jatis).

The diet given to the patient during the state of ill-health is as follows:

1. The Brahmani Baya - are only given veg food.
2. The Gujrani Baya (Veg. caste) - veg., milk, ghee & milk products.
3. Marathas (Non-veg caste) - veg, goat meat, chicken
4. Agris - veg, goat meat, chicken
5. Malis - veg, goat meat, chicken
6. Kannadi - veg, goat meat, chicken
7. Sonar - veg, goat meat, chicken
8. Mahadev kolis - veg, goat meat, chicken
9. Lohar - veg, goat meat, chicken

Depending on the Jati band of 'Baya' that visit the body they are given their choice of food which is socially prescribed as per the rules of dietary habits of caste groups existing in Kashale and Pathraj area. If the band of baya are Brahmani they are given any veg food and if Gujrani they are given milk, ghee, milk products and so on in the case of other band of jatis Baya.

The diet therapy administered to the patient during the healing rite the visitation of lahan baya is symbolic of the Thakurs gratitude, loyalty and willingness to worship, to be socially inferior to the dev jatis who have been a source of social, political and economic security for the Thakurs since ages. The appreciation of the same is shown at the spiritual level in the Thakur concept of illness ideology, body symbolism and ritual healing.

Norms of Restriction

During the healing rite (for five days) the family which is visited by the lahan Baya (dev jatis) has to observe a number of restricted rules. It is believed that if these rules are not observed strictly the suffering or trouble of the patient may be aggravated and at times may be fatal for the patient. To avoid the increase in physical suffering the Thakurs observe certain norms which are as follows -

a. Purification rite

For five continuous evenings the Thakurs, sing praises, playing drums (Dholki) for the Baya who visit a particular house. In order to participate in singing the owner of the house cleanses every person who attends the 'jagran ceremony' with gomtir (cow's urine). The Thakurs are well aware of the fact that a cow is worshipped by the Hindu caste groups, & hence its urine is given a satisfactory and divine status to clean the souls of the Thakurs before participating in the 'Jagran ceremony'. The Baya get angry if the purification rite is not performed.

b. Restriction For Menstruating Woman

The Baya (planetary spirits) who are sisters of the mother earth are sterile and hence not married. They take the form of social beings (dev jati) and visit a house. The Thakur believe that since the Baya are sterile they hate something that is fertile and hence a menstruating woman who later is ready to conceive is disliked by the lahan as well as the mothya Baya.

The Thakurs take precaution that no menstruating woman attends the 'Jagran ceremony' nor there is any menstruating woman from the concerned family. If there is one, she stays outside that room where the 'Ghat' (the symbol of Baya) is kept. In case there happens to be a woman who is menstruating and is attending the ceremony the Baya get angry and the sickness becomes worse.

c. Restriction for Drunkards

It has been observed that the rule of consuming alcohol is very less among the dev jatis. Especially the Brahmans, Gujratis, Sonars etc. do not drink at all. In instances where the Brahmani Baya or Gujrani Baya or Sonarni Baya visit a house, drunkards are prohibited from attending the Jagran ceremony. Even if by chance a person enters a house he is cleansed with 'Gomtir' - cow's urine and made to sit far away from the Ghat, which is the symbol of the Baya. This norm is observed again to guard the patient from becoming an object of the warth of 'baya'.

This norm expresses the Thakur loyalty to their authorities (dev jatis).

d. Restriction on Diet

If the 'Baya', the band of goddesses who visit the Thakur patient's body happen to be from a vegetarian caste, then the members of that family have to restrict themselves from eating non-vegetarian food, or else the suffering of the patient becomes worse. Similarly if the 'Band of Baya' who visit the patient are a non vegetarian caste group such as Marathas or even Mahadev Kolis the diet of their choice is given to the patient. It is believed by pleasing the patient the social demands of the caste groups (Baya) are fulfilled.

Gifts as Part of Social Therapy

There are various types of gifts which are given to the patient during the healing rite. The Thakur society has designed this scheme of giving gifts to the patient probably to satisfy a person's personal needs as well as the needs of the dev jatis.

Personal Gifts

During the healing rite the patient is gifted with cloth, ornaments, coconuts, fruits etc. In case of female patients a blouse, sari or some ornaments are given. The male patients are given a shirt piece, ornaments or a towel. Many a times these gifts are accompanied by eatables. This scheme exists to satisfy personal needs which are taken up at spiritual level and solved. By giving gifts to the patients it is understood that the Baya - divine forces are satisfied. Body decoration is also a part of this therapy.

Gifts are given to the patient on the suggestion of the Bhagat. Depending on the socio-economic status of the family the Bhagat (Shaman) advice's to offer gifts to the patients. Thus if a family is well off the Bhagat might suggest ornaments of silver, if poor inferior metal such as steel, copper or brass serves the purpose.

Gifts to the Community

There is yet another category of gifts given to the patient. These gifts are given to the dev jatis to satisfy them. For eg. the Malis (gardener caste) are involved in flower business and gardening, if a patient is visited by the Malani Baya (the gardener community) he or she is offered a small basket of flowers. The basket of flowers in this situation symbolizes the occupation of the Mali caste and is given to please the Malani Baya.

Similarly ornaments of silver are gifted to Sonarni Baya (goldsmith community). Metal ornaments are again associated with the goldsmith community. The offering of the gifts which are associated with occupational, dietary and social status of the caste is symbolic of fulfilling the rules of social interaction at spiritual level.

Pani Ghalne Rite

The last rite performed on the fifth day at 3 o'clock in the afternoon is pani ghalne rite, means ritually bathing the patient. The Thakurs believe that skin diseases such as chicken pox, scabies, measles, boils etc. are as a result of heat in the body which is created due to visitation of the sterile Baya.

Heat in this context is symbolically associated with the Baya'surge of having sex or to be sexually satisfied. Pani (water) Ghalne (to pour) means the Baya are satisfied by pouring pani or water (sperms) to be sexually satisfied. The coconut which has water in it is also offered to symbolize the same concept.

Body Symbolizing Political Pressures

Intrestingly it was observed that the Thakurs during the state of ill-health i.e. during the visitation of lahan Baya sing songs about the cunning rule of Britishers over the Indians. It was earlier believed that the Baya (planetary spirits) took the form of Britishers and brought the cruel and hard rule over the people of India. Thus during the state of ill-health the Thakurs sing about the cunningness of the British rule. One of the song sung during the healing rite is as follows :

The clever Britishers,
took the political charge over,
Made roads of mud and
invented electricity
They built the railway
on which trailed the train
The station was built of glass
The porter would ring the bell

The ticket collector too is here
Baya sat in the train and
were taken to Poona
The city of Poona so big
Buy Gond (ornament) for Baya
from Poona, Gond is hung
in the house for the Baya
to visit us.

Body Status in Healing Context

The data on the Thakur body symbolism has revealed the human body as a symbolic instrument and is expressed through culturally held conceptions of cosmology, nature, social structure, religion, their world of good and evil spirits etc. within a given ritual healing context.

Further depending on the entry of the type of the pathogenic agent or disorder in the body, the Thakurs assign a certain 'status' to the body. I would define bodily status as a particular place or position which a patients/medical practitioner's body occupies at a particular time, within a given ritual healing context, depending on the native's perception of the entry of pathogenic agent, will be referred to as bodily status with respect to that cultural system. Given below are certain instances where body is perceived to get a divine, spiritual, cosmological, natural, social etc.

a. Divine Status of Human Body

Both medical practitioners and heads of house holds reported that human body gets a divine status when a divine entity (Gods and Goddesses) enters their body. Entering the body according to the Thakurs means a divine spirit taking control of the person's atma (soul), where in the concerned person looses his identity with in that context, for certain time, i.e. as long as the divine spirit dwells in his/her body.

There are two types of persons whose body gets a divine status -

1. Medical practitioners especially Shamans.
2. Tribal folks who become patients (victims of divine warth).

When the Bhagats and Bhagatins get into trance the divine spirits of sun and mother earth enter their body. The Bhagat who is actually a social being looses his social identity and gets a divine identity if the spirit of God 'Sun' or the village god 'Waghoba' enters his body. This means God actually has come with in human body and hence the Bhagat's body gets the status of God. The Bhagat speaks like a God during the state of trance. People fall at his feet and worship him. So is the case with the Bhagatin when she gets into trance (vara yene). Spirits enter the bodies of

Bhagats and Bhagatins in the form of wind (vara) through their mouth or nose.

A patient's body is literally worshipped if the cause of his illness is interpreted as the wrath of a particular God or Goddess. His body gets a divine status and is appeased so that the sickness and suffering is taken away. A Patient's body thus gets a divine status. For example when Thakurs fail to offer a goat sacrifice to the village God, he brings about epidemics. During this ill-health period the patient's body is believed to be a reflection of the village God and hence is worshipped in order to please him.

b. Cosmological Status of Human Body

Diseases such as chicken pox, measles, body sores, boils etc. are believed to be caused due to visitation of 'Mothya Baya' - planetary spirits. Thus for seven - fourteen days the patient is worshipped and given good treatment. Every evening a 'Jagran' (singing) ceremony is performed to please the Baya to forgive them for their sins and wrong doing and to take away the suffering.

All life on earth including plants, animals and human beings belong to mother earth. Mother earth is the sister of other planets (Baya). These Baya hence come to visit their sister and enter into plants, animals and human beings. Baya enter the human body in the form of hot air which erupts the skin because their blood gets hot and hence results into body sores. When cosmic spirits take charge of the body, human body gets a cosmological status.

c. Spiritual Status of Human Body

Thakurs believe in two types of spirits, evil and good. The evil spirits Munja, Khais and Hadeli attack the human body to bring about trouble, sickness, suffering and so on. Thus during the possession of evil spirits, the patients looses his identity and tells the Shaman the name of the spirit/s which has attacked him and tells his dwelling place and why he has attacked the patient. During this context a patients body gets evil status (refer episodes 14, 15, 16). Efforts are made by th Shaman to fulfill the demands of the evil spirits and drive them out ritually.

In a like manner when good spirits such as ancestral spirits, spirits of clan gods etc. take charge of a patient they are given royal treatment and their demands are met inorder that they leave the patients body peacefully. (refer episode No. 9). Whether the spirits are driven out or pleased to leave the patients body, the fact remains that the patients body gets a spiritual status during the state of ill-health.

d. Social Status of Human Body

Besides divine, cosmological and spiritual pathogenic agents, human body also becomes victim of social agents. Illness episodes have pointed that the dev jatis (God likecastes) namely, Brahmans, Gujratis, Marathas, Kunbis, Malis, Kannadas, Agris etc. are worshipped during ill-health for they are believed to cause illness. These pathogenic agents are popularly known as Brahmani Baya, Marathni Baya, Kolani Baya, Malani Baya, Gujrani Baya, Kannadi Baya and so on. They are given a female status and are also known as the 'Lahan Baya'.

The Thakurs depend on the Dev jatis for their survival, jobs, clothes, ration, money, loans for certain rituals. The dev jatis or superior caste must be worshipped and if not worshipped they bring about troubles and sickness. (refer episode 31, 46). Depending on which caste has caused illness, the diet is given to them, either veg or non-veg. For instance if a patient becomes a victim of 'Gujrani Baya' (the Gujratis) he is given rice, dal, ghee, etc. the diet of Gujratis to please the pathogenic agent, in this context the Gujrani caste according to the Thakurs.

e. Natural Status of Human Body

The belief that human body is like a tree and that just as a tree is attacked by worms and insects so also the human body is attacked by 'Kidas' invisible germs which eat up blood and cause itching feeling.

Scabies (kharuj) for that matter is believed to occur as a result of human blood becoming sweet, due to excess eating of sweets and hence attacked by germs which go on consuming blood and their movement in the body is believed to cause itching feeling. Thus according to Thakurs the PHC doctor's suggestion of using soap becomes irrational as they perceive the cause to be internal and not external. Thus the juice of neem (Azadrachta indica) is administered to kill the germs in the blood. Human body is perceived as a natural symbol when a patient gets scabies. During this context the concepts associated with disease etiology and cure are inter-linked with the Natural world.

The above given examples show how human body gets a divine,spiritual, cosmological, social and natural status depending on the community's notions of origin and cause of illness. Efforts are ritually made to meet the demands of the pathogenic agents in order to bring about an order and harmony in the relationship of man with the pathogenic agents.

***

CHAPTER - VI

NATURE AND ROLE OF ETHNOMEDICAL SPECIALISTS

As any highly developed society tends to have its specialized personnel, so does the folk society. If help is sought from medical practitioners, various types of specialists may be available, including herbalists, shamans, midwives, bonesetters and masseurs. A Therapist may specialize in only one type of skill or may combine several in the practice, while there is considerable material on distinction among the traditional therapists based on the variation in specialization (Nurge 1958 : Lieban 1962, Maclean 1969). The qualitative data collected on the practitioners of Thakurs has revealed that there are seven types of medical practitioners rendering health care services to their fellowmen since time immemorial. Each one has got a special role in treating and taking care of the sick in their community. These practitioners are as follows:

1. BHAGAT	-	A male socio-ritual curer
2. BHAGATIN	-	A female socio-ritual curer
3. VAIDU	-	Herbalist
4. HAD VAIDU	-	Bone Setter
5. MANTRIK	-	Aspecialized Herbalist expert in Scorpion stings & snake bites
6. SUINE	-	Mid-wife
7. POTDHARI	-	Assistant mid-Wife

1. Bhagat

A Bhagat is the principle medical specialist among all the other Thakur specialists. He is a professional socio-ritual curer, a diviner and an interpreter of supernatural phenomenon. A bhagat is one who is proficient in bhakti, which is a meaningful art of establishing contact with the supernatural beings and hence carried out by a bhagat because he is culturally assigned to serve his society members.

As stated by Sudhir Kakar (1982:89), that Bhagat may be compared to Shamans who generally specialize in script illness and generally salient characteristic of a Shamans is in their ability to go into voluntary and controlled trance, during their diagnostic or healing efforts.

A Thakur on the other hand describes the diagnostic rites and process of trance during the healing rites as a meaningful situation or event. They believe this action to be symbolic of entry of divine power into the bhagat's body which helps him to judge the origin and cause of illness. A bhagat gets power to diagnose and heal from "SUN" - the creator of universe and life.

It is very necessary for a Bhagat to continue to cure unless he gets a vision from the Sun God to give up his profession. If he stops, he is suspected to have devoted himself to sorcery. He must also practice his profession to fulfill his religious duty assigned to him by "SUN God". He does not work for money. A famous bhagat may pay a visit to another village, if called upon. A bhagat is always respected and given a higher status by the members of his society as an image of high moral and ethics. He is a mediator between God and his society. A bhagat plays dual roles as farmer and as a medical practitioner for his society. The office of a bhagat is socially transmitted from one generation to other in a family.

2. Bhagatin

A Bhagatin is a female Shaman. She holds the same status in her society as the bhagat does. A bhagatin gets the power of healing and diagnosing the cause of an illness from "Dantari" (Mother Earth) and the "Baya" (Planetary spirits/sisters of Mother of Earth). Her method of diagnosis also differs from the bhagat. She gets into a trance "Angat Vara Yeto", while the bhagat uses the metal pot technique.

A Bhagatin has destructive power, she can cast magico-religious spells on her enemies, where as a bhagat has protective powers and therefore he is superior and a more capable practitioner than a bhagatin. A bhagatin also has some knowledge of herbal medicine and prescribes it for mostly health problems of woman. She cures both male and female patients, while female patients prefer to go her first, in case she is not able to cure then they consult the bhagat.

Medical Functions Of Bhagats And Bhagatins

The medical functions of a bhagat and bhagatin are broadly classified by them are as follows:

A) Diagnosis of the origin and cause of illness

Shamanism is related to a system of beliefs about the causes and cures of diseases, with in a given cultural frame of reference. The healing performance of a shaman takes place in a group context, and the drama of diagnosing and healing is given a public recognition. The patient is surrounded by familiar people in a ceremonial or ritualistic situation to which he has become accustomed through witnessing curing rites for others.

Diagnosis of illness begins after setting the necessary objects of worship, cleaning rites of bhagats and Bhagatins, chanting prayers to "SUN" - in the case of bhagat and "Mother Earth" - in the case of bhagatin, laying the offering, music instruments (in this case drum - Dholki).The action of setting a stage of healing to start the diagnosis rite symbolically draws into operation on objective reality, by giving that situation or context a culturally recognized meaning.

The Diagnosis Rite

The methods, techniques or rituals of diagnosing illness differ from community to community. Among the Bhils of Dhule district, in the State of Maharashtra the Shaman (Badwa) uses prayer beads (abrus precatorius) to diagnose the origin and cause of illness. While the Koknas of Jawhar, Thane district use rice grains which are spread in a shifter to diagnose illness. (Tribhuwan Robin 1988 : 58).

There are two types of diagnostic rituals performed separately by the Bhagat and the Bhagatin to diagnose the cause of illness of their patients.

1. The metal pot technique (Tambya phirawane)
2. Getting into trance (Vara yene)

The metal pot technique (Tambya phirawane) is used by a Bhagat, while the Bhagatin gets into trance to trace the origin and cause of illness. The Bhagat also gets into trance at times to diagnose the cause of illness. Regarding what these two techniques are, how they are ritually performed, what objects are used and what 'ill' means to the Thakurs are highlighted in detail in the case studies of Bhagats and Bhagatins in this chapter. Thus, diagnosis is one of the most important aspect of the medical functions of a Bhagat and a Bhagatin.

Interpretations of the origin and cause of illness is followed by the diagnosis ritual. The diagnosis techniques help the bhagats and Bhagatins to trace the cause. Interpretation of the cause of illness is done on the basis of following pathogenic agents which can bring about illness.

Pathogenic Agents/Forces

1. Phirta Mela : The moving Planetary Spirits.

2. Zokyachya Devi	:	The Goddesses of Swing who dwell on the mountains.
3. Chokhy/Ratya Baya	:	The Spirits (Female) of the Devjati (upper caste)
4. Gandhicha Tap	:	Measles (Baya)
5. Kilyachya Devi	:	Goddesses of the Fort
6. Germany Baya	:	Spirits of the Britishers
7. Fodya Baya	:	Goddess of Smallpox
8. Vanachi Baju	:	Evil force of the forest
9. Pisha,Munja & Khais	:	Male Evil Spirits
10. Hadeli	:	Female Evil Spirit
11. Satvai	:	Mother Earth
12. Ilkat Mal Bhut	:	Evil Spirit of Wealth
13. Shel Bhut	:	Spirit of the goats
14. Kolha Bhut	:	Evil Spirit of the Fox
15. Waghya, Chedha, Khambya, Bhairi	:	Village Gods
16. Mariai	:	Goddess of the Mahar Caste
17. Bhavani	:	Goddess of the Mahar Caste
18. Malavarcha Chedha	:	The God of the Loft
19. Panch Mukhee Chedha	:	The five hooded Cobra
20. Gupit Bhut	:	Secret Evil Spirit
21. Dith Bhut	:	Spirit of the Evil eye
22. Mari Bhut	:	Evil Spirit of the Mahar Caste
23. Vir/Supali	:	Ancestral Spirits
24. Kuldev	:	Clan Gods

The above mentioned pathogenic agents are believed to cause illness. Depending on the cultural situations or context in which the illness might have occurred, the Bhagat or Bhagatin interpret one of the pathogenic agents responsible for causing illness.

Disease Treatment

The second most important function of a Bhagat and Bhagatin is treatment of disease using magico-religious and ritualistic healing techniques. There are again three types of treatments given by the Shamans :

1. Herbal Therapy

Which is purely administration of medicinal herbs or medical extracts of animals in a ritualistic fashion.

2. Magico - ritualistic treatment

Which involves the diagnosis rites, healing rites, the rites of offering coconuts, sacrifices, rituals of pleasing the pathogenic agents, driving out evil spirits, neutralizing evil effect and so on.

3. Combination of magico-ritualistic and Herbal/chemo therapy

Which involves both medication as well as ritualistic performance so as to give physical and psychological relief to the patient.

Medical Advice

One of the most important jobs of the Bhagats and Bhagatins is to render free medical advice to their patients on the following aspects :

1. The pathogenic agents that cause disease and the situation in which the diseases are caused.
2. How to prevent these pathogenic agents from causing illness.
3. Advice on dangerous areas such as, where the evil spirit, the Rakshas (Giants) and other pathogenic agents dwell.
4. The care that people must take and observe taboos of health.
5. Advice on maintaining good relationship with the pathogenic agents.
6. Advice on keeping certain holy objects or charmed objects to prevent illness.
7. Performing and presiding over healing rituals.
8. Offering coconuts and sacrifices and so on

3. Vaidu

A Vaidu (Herbalist) is one who has a vast knowledge of Herbal medicines and heals his patients only by giving herbal therapy. He prepares medicines from various plant parts such as root, shoot, bark, leaf, flower, seed, fruit etc. Besides administrating medicinal herbs he also uses animal extracts for treating his patients. He also advises his patients on diet.

It was observed that although a Vaidu deals with only Chemotherapy there is a lot of ritualistic behaviour associated with his profession which is common to that of a Bhagat. This ritualistic behaviour associated with collections, preparation and administration of medicines, the social taboos of his professions, the religious elements associated with his profession are all described in the case study form in this chapter.

4. Had Vaidu

A Had Vaidu (Bone Setter) is one who has a sound knowledge of the location of various nerves, veins, and bones in the human body. He heals fractures, swellings, sprains, joint pains, etc. using various herbal medicines.

He is an expert masseur, a bone setter and a skilled brandsman, As a masseur he uses various medicated oils such as Mauha Seed Oil (Bacia latifolia); Karanj Seed Oil (Pongamia pinnata); Monitor and Chicken fat oil and of course groundnut oil. He is a master bone setter among the Thakur medical practitioners. Branding is another form of therapy used by him. He heats iron rod and gently touches it on painful parts of thee body. The branding technique is popularly known as 'Chocha Dena'. Other details of Thakurs bone setters are presented in a case study form in this chapter.

5. Mantrik

A Mantrik is a specialized herbalist, who deals specifically with healing scorpion stings and snakebites, using Mantra techniques. He has a vast knowledge about the behaviour of different species of snakes and scorpions and hence give herbal cure to his patients, of course ritually accompanied by his Mantras which he chants to give his patient psychological relief initially.

Mantrik's office in a Thakur society is hereditary i.e. it is passed on from generation to generation. He undergoes a lengthy period of training and apprenticeship under the leadership and guidance of his Guru.

During his early phase of learning Mantras, a Mantrik is expected to get into the river right in the middle on a 'Poornima' (full Moon night) or 'Amosha' (No Moon night) to learn his Mantras. He takes 50 stones with him and each time he recites his Mantras he will throw a stone in the water. This he does for fifty times. He is expected to be totally naked while he is in water. This is a sought of assignment for him, which he does for a year or so especially during the summer and winter season for every fortnight.

Mantrik is so deeply specialized in curing snakebites and scorpion stings that he can handle almost any patient, however seriously he may be bitten.

Maruti Dalu Ughda a famous Mantrik of Sarai Wadi (hamlet) is known for curing scorpion and snakebitten patients. My informant Ramchandra Lobhie said, Maruti makes his patients face towards east. If the patient is bitten by a poisonous snake Dalu jumps in the well with a tumbler and goes right at the bottom of the well and get water from there. This water he splashes on his patient's face five times very hard. Then gives a herbal cure, while he is splashing water he chants Mantras taking the name of God Bhairi who is the source of healing power to a Mantrik. This act in most cases take away the fear of the patient even if he is not bitten by a poisonous snake.

Maruti was quite expert in curing his patients that he can exactly trace the snake which bit his patient, from the marks of the teeth.

A Mantrik also known a lot of preventive remedies for cultural etiologies as well as other natural causes of illness.

6. Suine (Midwife)

In almost all the Thakur hamlets deliveries take place at home, because of the cultural and ritualistic importance of the child birth ceremonies, which are carried out by Suine (a birth attendant).

The duties of a Suine are to give advice and medical aid to the expectant mother, to assist in delivering the baby and to treat any illnesses that might befall the new mother and infant. She has a vast knowledge of child birth techniques also the cultural behaviour expected during pregnancy and childbirth. She is also a masseur and knows the proper diet for the mother and child.

Although her knowledge of herbal medicine is not that extensive like the Vaidus and Bhagats, she does know some medicinal plants for ailments like urinary disorders, abortions, etc. Bhagubai Darwade a Suine of Bor Wadi knows a number of medicines and hence is a popular Suine of Kikwi village.

To become a Suine woman starts watching an accomplished Suine go about her duties. The office of a Suine is not exactly hereditary, but in most cases mothers tend to teach their daughters the skills of child birth. Most Suines teach their daughters-in-law the art of attending to a child birth and delivery.

A Suine always sees that a delivering mother faces the 'East' (a direction always associated with life). If a child is stillborn, mother's face is immediately turned to South (a direction always perceived by the Thakurs and associated with death). Placental waste (var) and the umbilical chord (nal) is buried on the western part of the house just adjacent to the cowdung plastered wall outside. A hole about 1 foot is dug to bury the umbilical chord to prevent it from being a tool of witchcraft.

At the same time the child and the mother bathe inside the house just opposite to the place of umbilical chord, for five days. A Suine gives bath to the child for twelve days. On the fifth day, which is a very important day because it is on this day the child's fortune is written by Satvai (Goddess of fortune) who comes in the form of a bird, rat, cat, dog, cow, etc. to visit the child.

On the fifth day at 8 o'clock in the evening the bathing place is worshipped, indirectly the Satvai is worshipped and food is kept for her to eat. This ceremony is headed by the Suine.

A Suine plays an important role in taking decisions, especially when it comes to repeated abortions and still births, which are attributed to sexual intercourse with evil spirits namely, Khais and Munja. Congenital deformities etc. are also attributed to breach of pregnancy taboos.

A severely deformed child is killed and buried, since he is believed to be a product of evil spirit and would be dangerous to the Thakur community. This decision of identifying the child as product of Khais or Munja is certainly taken by the Suine.

On the 12th day after a child is born it is put in the traditional swing (Jholi) and it is on this day the Suine is awarded a gift depending on the financial capacity of the donor. Mostly she gets a blouse piece, bangles and 5-10 Rs. for the 12 days service which she has rendered to the child and the mother.

7. Potdhari (Assistant Mid Wife)

The very word potdhari i.e. an helper who holds the stomach or an an assistant midwife. An assistant mid wife (Potdhari) helps the suine in delivering a child. Any midwife practices as a potdhari for 4-5 years till she becomes a perfectly trained mid-wife.

In case of emergency, that when a midwife is not available in the village the potdhari performs the delivery. She has a little knowledge of home remedies for minor ailments or health problems that befall the new child and mother. A potdhari gets Rs. 3-10 for her services rendered in delivering a child, depending on the socio-economic status of the family which the child is born. About other details of a potdhari (See case study in this chapter).

CASE NO 1
Medical Status - Bhagat
I. Personal Information

Name	:	Walku Hari Thorad
Sex	:	Male
Age	:	42 years
Marital Status	:	Married
Occupation	:	Farmer
Education	:	VII
Village Grampanchayat	:	Pathraj
Hamlet/Wadi	:	Nagyachiwadi
No. of years of Practice	:	20 years
Social Status	:	Bhagat

II. Various Steps Involved during the Apprenticeship period

Walku received training from his father who was also his Guru (teacher). Though Walku's father was his Guru the various steps involved were as rigorous as ever. Walku is of the opinion that to train to be a Bhagat is no ordinary task or joke. He describes the various phases through which the trainee has to pass (on the basis of his own experience).

A. Purification of one's Soul (Atma)

"The world, today is changing. Human beings are selfish, artificial and money minded. Their soul (atma) is striving for materialistic pleasures. Such an attitude has made the almighty 'Sun' very unhappy. Man no longer seeks the truth. So to become a Bhagat one must have a clean mind (mun), a clean soul (atma) and a clean body (pind), says Walku.

Thus one of the pre-requisites to becomes a Bhagat is to keep one's conscious clear, thereby purifying the body, mind and soul.

B. Becoming a true Devotee of 'Sun'

After cleansing one's body, mind and soul the next step is to become a true worshiper of the Sun God which means to observe the various taboos of the Sun God.

C. A Call from God

If an individual has sincerely fulfilled the above two requests he starts getting visions and dreams, the village God or the Sun God visits him and instructs him to take up the profession of a Bhagat.

D. The Training Period

The training is held during the period of Navratra (nine days before a festival called Dassera). During the nine nights Walku learned the chants, prayers, rites and words associated with the process of diagnosis and healing. During the first eight nights the student Bhagat has to stand in the river facing east and recite mantras (chants). This action is symbolic of the divine contact between the student Bhagat and the 'Sun' and 'Water' (water - brother of the Sun).

Walku was instructed to sit on a 'Shid' tree facing the east and recite mantras. This act symbolizes the integration of the human being with the divine being and the act of getting empowered. According to the Thakurs the Shid tree is the symbol of the Sun, it is male tree and symbolizes masculinity, indicating that the Bhagat must maintain his male identity and have no contact with any woman, other than his wife. The wood of Shid tree is not used as fire wood. It is known as the Guru

(Master of student).

E. Techniques of Diagnosis

During the first eight nights the teacher teaches the student the rites of diagnosis. A metal pot (tambya) is taken with some water in it. The student faces the east. Ash from the hearth is placed beneath and some ash is put in the pot. The student then rotates the tambya in a clockwise direction reciting the following mantras (chants).

Diagnosis Mantra (Chant) :

Rama, Ishwara, Parmatma Bhagwana
karta karta, kshirishticha palanwala,
Pashu, pakshi, kida, mungi, guj-guji
Manushya avtaar tujhyapasun
Nirman jhala ahey.
Khota bolaycha nahi, phasva phasvi karaychi nahi
Kay asel te agadi swachha manane bolayche

1. Phirta mela asel ka ?
2. Jhokycha devi asel ka ?
3. Chokya baya, Ratya baya asel ka ?
4. Gandhicha devi asel ka ?
5. Kilkacha devi asel ka ?
6. Germany baya asel ka ?
7. Phodya baya astil ka ?
8. Vavachi baju asel ka ?
9. Pisha, munja zombala ka ?
10. Hadeli, khais asel ka ?
11. Satvai ahey ka ?
12. Ilkat, mal bhut ahey ka ?
13. Shel bhut ahey ka ?
14. Kolha bhut ahey ka ?
15. Waghya, chedha, bhairi khambya-gaon dev ahey ka?
16. Mariai asel ka ?
17. Bhavani asel ka ?
18. Malavarcha chedda asel ka ?
19. Pach mukhi chedda asel ka ?
20. Gupit bhut asel ka ?
21. Mahari bhut asel ka ?
22. Kuldev astil ka ?
23. Vir, supali astil ka ?
24. Dhith bhut asel ka ?

Thus there are twenty four, pathogenic agents which are culturally recognized and may cause illness.

On translating the above chants the meaning is as follows :

Rama, Oh Lord, Thou art the creator or nature, animals, birds, insects, cows,

Human beings are your incarnations on earth.

They are created by you,

Whatever I diagnose is clean and true,

Nothing is fake or false.(The Bhagat then rotates the metal pot in a clockwise direction)

1. Is it the Baya (Band of planetary spirits)
2. Is it the Devis (Goddesses of the swing)
3. The Chokhya (vegetarian) and Ratya (non-vegetarian) goddesses.
4. Measles (Gandhi Tap)
5. Is it the Goddesses of the fort ?
6. Is it the Germany Baya (British authorities)
7. Is it the Fodya Baya (Goddesses of skin disease)
8. Is it the evil spirit from the jungle?
9. Is it pisha, Murya (male evil spirit)
10. Is it Hadeli (female evil spirit) or khais (male evil spirit)
11. Is it satvai ?
12. Is it the spirit of wealth ?
13. Is it the Shet Bhut ?
14. Is it the fox like evil spirit ?
15. Is it the village God ? (Waghya, Chedha, Khambya, Bhairi).
16. Is it mariai (the Goddess of Mahars)
17. Is it Goddess Bhavani ?
18. Is it Chedha of Wealth ?
19. Is it the five headed Chedha ?
20. Is it the secret evil spirit ?
21. Is it the spirit of evil eye ?
22. Is it the fighter spirit of Mahar ?
23. Is it Supali (female ancestral spirit) or Vir dev.
24. Is it the clan Gods ?

A student Bhagat is expected to know the above mantra by heart. It is believed that if one of the above pathogenic agents is the causative factor for the illness, the metal pot stands still when the name of the particular agent is chanted.

The student Bhagat is expected to learn this mantra for eight days and observe the following taboos strictly.

F. Taboos And Norms Of Shamanism

A number of rules and restrictions are imposed on the student Bhagat during the nine day training period and thereafter which have to be strictly adhered to

a. The trainee has to abstain from any type of non- vegetarian food for one year after his training.

b. During the nine-day training period he cannot leave or travel outside his village for he should be within the supervision of his village God.

c. He is not to sweep or make any use of the broom. This act is symbolic of cleansing away Bhakti (art of Bhagatism) out of the house.

d. He is to refrain from eating food which contains turmeric as long as he holds the post of a Shaman. The Thakurs associate turmeric with the female and categorize it as a woman. Hence a Bhagat who is empowered with the healing power from the Sun (Male God) cannot tolerate turmeric.

e. He is not supposed to eat food until the dead body of the person is buried. Death is a symbol of darkness and evil where as the Bhagat has light of the Sun God within him. Thus when death (darkness) occurs in the village it pollutes the food to be consumed by the Bhagat. After the disposal of the dead body the Bhagat's wife bring fresh water and prepares fresh food for the Bhagat.

f. While the Bhagat is eating his food and accidentally or on purpose the lamp is put off, the Bhagat should immediately stop eating his food. The putting off or extinguishing of the lamp symbolizes the interference of an evil force which is trying to pollute the Bhagat's food. When the lamp is extinguished, the evil force in the darkness pollutes the Bhagat's food. If the Bhagat consumes this evil/polluted food it will have an adverse effect on the food and on the pure light/power which is gift to him from the Sun.

g. The student Bhagat cannot cut vegetables or kill anything for a year. Restrictions such as not cutting vegetables and sweeping the house are culturally imposed so as to prevent the Bhagat from doing the woman's work. Killing is believed to be an evil act therefore a Bhagat does not kill.

h. The student Bhagat is not allowed to consume food prepared by a menstruating woman. Menstrual blood is symbolic of impurity and pollution. The hearth (chul) where the fire burns is believed to be incarnation of Holi (Goddess of Fire). The fire that burns in the hearth is a symbol of 'Sun' (Almighty). Thus a menstruating woman (carrying the pollutant menstrual blood) is not to face the holy fire and the divine Goddess (hearth). Anything that is good/pure (with reference to food) must not be touched by evil/impure (menstruating woman). If she cooks food she not only insults the 'Sun' and 'Holi' but also transfers her evilness to pollute the food she has cooked.

i. During the nine-day training period the student Bhagat should not indulge in sex. Loosing of semen is symbolic of loosing the shamanistic power in the Bhagat.

j. A Bhagat cannot eat food during the Grihan (solar eclipse). He eats and drinks water after the eclipse is over. Before preparing the food the chul (hearth) is smeared with cowdung and fresh food is cooked. It is believed that an evil force covers the sun blocking the life giving rays as a result of which the food and water becomes polluted. Those Bhagats who believe that they possess the light (power) of the Sun do not consume any food on the eclipse day.

k. While a Bhagat is eating and if he is called a 'Mang' or 'Mahar', he immediately stops eating as the caste groups 'Mang' and 'Mahar' are classified by the Thakurs as being lower in status and as the Rakshas (evil) Jati. A Bhagat is a special devotee of the Sun cannot be called such names as the utterance of such names pollute and have an evil effect on his food.

G. The Students Examination

The student Bhagat is subjected to a test by his guru on the ninth night to confirm whether he has mastered and to what extent has he mastered the techniques of diagnosis.

The guru makes the small heaps of rice and hides the following articles in them.

1. First heap	Supari (Areca catechu)
2. Second heap	Halad (Curcuma domestica) rhizome.
3. Third heap	Zendu (flower of Tagitus Species)
4. Fourth heap	Paisa (coin)
5. Fifth heap	Kharik (dried date)
6. Sixth heap	Badam (Almond)
7. Seventh heap	Kurud
8. Eighth heap	Kaulache phool
9. Ninth heap	Mogra
10. Tenth heap	Does not contain any article.

The student Bhagat sits outside his guru's house facing east with the metal pot containing water. Tha Bhagat (teacher) then instructs him to tell using diagnosis technique which article is placed in which heap. If the student Bhagat is unable to tell correctly the article hidden in the rice heal he fails the test and cannot become a Bhagat. Before the examination the student Bhagat has a bath, lights and offers an incense stick and a coconut to the Sun God facing the east.

On enquiring from Walku Bhagat why only ten heaps are taken and what is their significance in diagnosis ? Walku stated that the ten openings symbolizes the ten openings of the body (Daha Darwaze).

These openings are as follows : Eyes, Nose, Ears, Mouth, Central portion of the sternum (Atma/Soul), Naval opening, Vaginal/urethral opening, Wrist pulse, Pulse of the feet, and Anal opening (secret door).

Disease (Rog), evil or good forces enter the body through these openings and passes the soul (Atma). When the Atma of a person is controlled by a divine or evil being that individual becomes the part of the divine or evil world respectively. Thus the human body gets divine or evil status. Through the ritual healing process the disrupted order is reconstructed or order and harmony are brought back.

The articles in the ten heaps are associated with the ten openings of the body and are also symbolic of the ten planets in the cosmos. Walku said that every article has a colour which is associated with each planet respectively.

The colours of the articles are according to the Thakurs and are as follows :-

1. First Planet	Date (Blackish white)
2. Second Planet	Tagitus flower (Red/White)
3. Third Planet	Mogra (White)
4. Fourth Planet	Cucurma (Yellowish/White)
5. Fifth Planet	Almond (Creamish/White)
6. Sixth Planet	Arec nut (Brownish/White)
7. Seventh Planet	Paisa (Greyish/White)
8. Eighth Planet	Lin seed flower (Pinkish/White)
9. Ninth Planet	Wild flower (Kurud) (Pinkish/White)
10. Tenth Planet	No article/empty (White)

To the Thakurs, said Walku the human body is nothing but a representation of the whole cosmos ('Pinda Sarkha Khand'). The ten planets in the Universe have above said colours according to the Thakurs.

'Walku, why are the heaps made up of rice only?' To this question he replied that the Thakurs lived on rice as it is their only staple crop. They are nourished on rice and it is used in many rituals. Eg. after a person's death the soul migration ritual is performed during which ten balls of rice flour are made and put into the river. These ten rice flour balls represent the ten planets. The fifth ball represents the soul (jeev khada).

III. Atma (Soul) Fifth opening

The fifth opening in the body is associated with the fifth planet in the cosmos - Dantari. Dantari means mother Earth which among the planetary hierarchy is also ranked fifth by the Thakurs. Walku said that when an external force divine/evil in the nature causes illness, it takes control of the patient's atma (soul). When an evil force takes control of the patient's body the body becomes evil and it is at such a time that he as the Bhagat has to ritually purify the patients atma (soul) by driving away the spirit. Similarly if a divine entity causes illness then the patient's body becomes divine and the rituals performed are to appease the divine pathogenic agent. At such times the patient's body is worshipped.

'Walku, how do you co-relate atma with mother Earth?' Walku replied, 'Our body is made up of earth. The atma has elements like light, fire, water and air in it. All these are held together by the body (pind). The earth gives life and sustains life.

Thus, the entire set of rituals of a Bhagat are geared towards either purifying the atma by warding off or driving out the evil spirits and forces or to then please the atma in case a divine being visits the body thereby causing illness. The diseases such as measles, chicken pox, body sores etc. are perceived by the Thakur's as the visitation of Baya (Planetary Spirits) to the Earth (Soul).

IV. The Healing Rites Performed by a Shaman (Bhagat)

The outstanding characteristic feature of the Shaman's concept of illness is that the humans are integral parts of the ordered system, and, an illness is the result of some disharmony or disruption with reference to the natural, social, spiritual, ancestral, supernatural and the cosmic order. Shamanistic therapies via rituals lay emphasis on the restoration of harmony/balance between human relationships and the natural, social, spiritual, ancestral, supernatural and cosmological forces and agents.

The healing rites of Shamanism (in the Thakur Community) as classified/viewed by the Bhagats themselves are an order of culturally prescribed clinical rituals through which the patient must pass. The Bhagats have classified their healing rites into following categories :

Self Cleansing

The first and foremost step or stylized action in the ritual healing rites is the cleansing ritual. The Bhagat takes a bath or washes his hands and feet with water. Water is the symbol of purification and it is used because it is considered to be the brother of the Sun. It purifies the Bhagat who is now ready to enter divination.

Setting of the Healing Stage

The next step is to light an incense stick and this is placed at the door post of the Bhagat's house. The healing rites are always carried out in the Bhagat's house. Next, facing the East he bows to the Sun - the almighty. He then takes some ash from the hearth and applies it on the cowdung smeared floor. Fresh water is taken in a metal pot, which is placed on the spread ash. A pinch of ash is put into the water in the pot. Next, both he and his patient face east.

Diagram VI : 1. Demonstrates the manner in which various objects (used in the ritual) are arranged by a Bhagat.

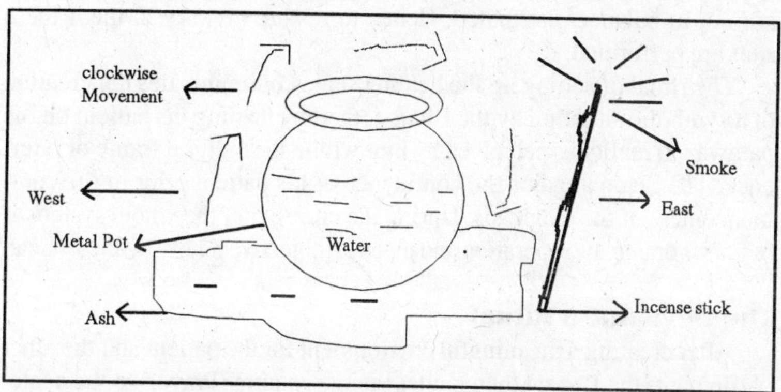

The action of facing east implies turning the patient's mind towards the supernatural, and creating a divine environment by setting the objects in a symbolic and meaningful manner, which is particular to the healing situation.

All the objects used for diagnosis have definite meanings and these are as follows :

a. The ash from the hearth (Surya Rakhad) symbolizes the body of the Sun.
b. The metal pot symbolizes the atma of the patients.
c. The ash placed below the pot symbolizes the body (pind) of the patient.
d. The smoke arising from the incense stick symbolizes the prayers sent by the Bhagat to the Sun God to heal his patient.
e. The light falling on the metal pot (Tambya) is symbolic of the healing power of the Sun.
f. Facing the east is calling the holy wind into the situation.

The objects are all arranged to invite (into the healing situation) the following elements -

a. Fire (Agni) - Through Surya Rakhad i.e.ash from the hearth whose source is the Sun.

b. Water (Pani) — Through purification, source is the Earth.
c. Light (Tej) — Healing power of the Sun.
d. Wind (Vara) — Facing East to receive the holy wind.
e. Earth (Atma) — The metal pot.

Walku Thorad (the Bhagat) explained that these five elements are very important in forming life. According to the Bhagat the atma is nothing but a combination of these elements. When illness occurs these elements are not in balance/distributed. Hence to restore divinity in them these rites are performed.

The ritual of setting up the healing stage communicates the creation of a symbolic situation by the Bhagat, thereby leading his patient on the pathway to reality as perceived by him within the cultural frame of reference. The Shaman gains the confidence of his patient prior to the commencement of the diagnosis. During the curing rite, the whole system of beliefs is drawn into operation and given an objective reality by the Bhagat.

The Devmantra Ritual

After creating a meaningful environment for the patient and the other participants the Bhagat then recites the Devmantra (Prayer) to the healer (Sun God). He faces the East while reciting the mantra and explained that the recitation of this mantra is done to obtain wisdom from the Sun God in order to diagnose the cause of illness.

Nadiche Mantra (Ritual of Diagnosis)

The ritual of diagnosis is popularly known as Nadiche Mantra. Nad means something has gone wrong or in other words it can be termed as disorder.

The Bhagat holds the lighted incense stick in his left hand and with his right hand spins the metal pot in anti-clock direction. While the metal pot is being spun he recites the causes. There is a standard list of pathogenic agents that are believed to cause illness, they are as follows -

1. The Phirastiya Baya

Planetary spirits in the form of locusts.

2. Jhokyachya Devi

Goddess of the swing residing in the mountains.

3. Chokhya Baya

Vegetarian Goddesses. Planetary spirits taking the form of upper vegetarian caste such as Brahmani Baya, Gujarani Baya, etc.

4. Ratya Baya

Planetary spirits taking the form of non-vegetarian castes such as Marathani, Kolani, Malani, Agarni Baya etc.

5. Gandhicha Tap/Measles

Interference of cosmic spirits.

6. Kilkahya Devi

Goddesses of the fort.

7. Germany Baya

Reference to harsh British rule.

8. Fodya Baya

Goddesses that cause small pox and chicken pox.

9. Vavachi Baju

Evil spirits from the jungle.

10. Pischa, Munja, Khais

Male evil spirits.

11. Hadeli

Female evil spirit.

12. Satvai

Wrath of mother earth, Goddess of life & fortune.

13. Ilkatmal Bhut

The spirit of the wealth.

14. Shel Bhut

Evil spirit of goat.

15. Kolha Bhut

Fox like evil spirit.

16. Waghya, Chedha, khambya, Bhairi

Village Gods.

17. Mariai
Goddess of Mahars.

18. Goddess Bhavani
Goddess of lower caste.

19. Chedha (Malcha)
God of wealth.

20. Panchamukhi Chedha
Chedha of five heads (referring to five hooded cobra).

21. Gupit Bhut
Unknown evil spirit.

22. Supali
Female ancestral spirit.

23. Virdev
Male ancestral spirit.

24. Drishti Bhut
Spirit of evil eye.

25. Mahari Bhut
Evil spirits of Mahar (lower) lower castes.

26. Kuldev
Clan Gods.

The above names of the pathogenic agents are recited sequentially and when the tambya (metal pot) stops spinning during recitation, the name being recited when the tambya stops is taken as the pathogenic agent which has caused the illness. The Bhagat also offers an explanation why the pathogenic agent has caused the illness.

Immediate therapeutic action is taken, which involves either cleansing the body (of the patient) driving out the spirit, satisfying the agent, asking pardon from the concerned agent.

Ibut Mantra - The Therapeutic Ritual

Ibut is the charmed ash which a Bhagat applies on the centre of the forehead between the brows of the patient. It is the symbol of the Sun's healing powers. This action is symbolic of fusing the divine force into the healing and which will aid in driving out or cleansing the evil force from the body. Walku was asked why the Ibut was applied on the forehead. He replied that the mother earth (satvai) visits the child on the fifth day after birth and writes the life span and fortune on the forehead. The "worms of life" (kidas) also reside there and are linked to all the systems of the body, including the soul. If the worms are disturbed or there is some dysfunction it directly reflects on the health. Hence in case of ill-health the Ibut is applied on the forehead as it is believed to possess the power to heal the kidas.

The Ibut mantra gives psychological relief to the patient. The Bhagat takes care of the physical ailments by administering medical plants and medicinal extracts from animals. There are rituals associated with collection, preparation and administration of potions, drugs and medical herbs.

Therapeutic Ritual Action

The entire set of actions of the healing ritual are geared towards the achievement of following aims.

1. Warding off/Neutralizing the Evil Effect

The ritual 'Drishti Phodne' i.e. destroying the evil effect or the agent (Drishti Bhut) responsible is a very common ritual in the healing process of the Thakur culture. Other rituals are performed to ward off or neutralize the evil effect (refer episode no : 18).

Driving Away Evil Spirits or Pathogenic Agents

The Thakurs believe that the evil spirits such as Pischa, Munja, Khais, Hadeli take control of the persons/patents soul (Atma) because of which he loses hs identity and is now an outsider in the Thakur community. The Bhagat starts by asking the name of the patient (actually he asks the evil spirit its name). Later on through out the ritual Bhagat addresses the patient by the name of the evil spirit.

The rituals are then performed to drive away the spirit and to meet his demands by offering it a cock or blood (for more details refer episode no : 16).

Satisfying The Demands of The Pathogenic Agent

It is believed certain pathogenic cause illness because their demands have not been fulfilled. For example if a person dies, and he was heavy drinker of liquor it is custom to offer liquor after his death so as to satisfy him. If this is not done then the spirit causes illness and its demands have to ritually met. (refer episode no : 23)

Worshipping or Pleasing The Pathogenic Agent

Thakurs believe as days are passing by, man is going away from God and forgets at times to perform divine duties such as offering a coconut or a sacrifice either to the village God or clan Gods. The Gods are displeased with human behaviour and pour down their wrath on mankind in the form of epidemics of measles, cholera, chicken pox etc. Thus the healing rituals are geared towards one goal i.e. to please the pathogenic agent.

Patching Up Relationships

The Thakurs believe that some illnesses are caused due to disruption of a man's relationship with his other fellowmen of his society or with the members of other tribes and caste groups. Witchcraft and sorcery are common examples of this category. Disruption of relationship could also be between man and the ancestral spirits or divine beings and so on.

Recreation of The Disrupted Cultural Order

Every culture has definite and set rules which govern human behaviour in different contexts or situations. There is definite pattern in which a house should be built and the rituals which are to be performed during and after completion of the house. If these rituals and rules are not followed then the owner is giving an open invitation to troubles and health hazards. (refer episode no. : 5).

Therapeutic Rituals Performed to Balance the Body Equilibrium

The members of the Thakur society believe that imbalance in the bodily constituents due to hot and cold elements cause illness. These elements may enter the body through food, air, medicines, exposure to hot/cold environment and so on. Rituals performed thus focus on balancing the body equilibrium and by giving to the patient a hot diet if the illness caused is due to a cold element and vice versa.

Actions of Excommunicating a Patient from the Social Circle

The Thakurs classify and practice three types of excommunication patterns as far a ill-health of a patient is concerned. Ex-communication of a patient is restricted to certain diseases and conditions of ill health. Three types of patterns of excommunication can be classified and are as follows.

a. Temporary Ex-communication

A menstruating woman is ex-communicated from the society including the family for a period of five days. During this period she is forbidden to cook , serve food or do any work. She is given food in separate dishes, her clothes are kept separate and she is not allowed to have any social interaction with any person. She does not attend nor take part in any ritual.

The Thakurs believe that menstrual blood is evil and pollutes the social atmosphere. It brings about diseases such as leprosy and venereal diseases. Consumption of food cooked by a menstruating woman leads to ill-health. She is not allowed to cook because she has to sit in front of the hearth (chulah) where the holy fire burns. She is temporarily ex-communicated for a period of five days, as contact with her is believed to bring misfortune. To be accepted back into the social circle of interaction, she has to undergo purification rites. She goes to the river washes the stained clothes and other clothes, has a bath. After the bath she bows down facing east to the Sun. When she comes back home she lights an incense stick and is now ready to interact with her family and members of her community. Thus she is accepted back into the social circle. (refer illness episode no. : 29).

Permanent Excommunication

Leprosy patients are excommunicated from the Thakur society. The Thakurs believe, leprosy is caused (in case of males) due to sexual intercourse with a menstruating woman. In the case of women lepers, cause of the disease/deformity is explained as if she must have cooked food and consumed it during her menstrual periods or she must have consumed food prepared by another menstruating woman.

Leprosy is associated with deformity and disorder of the human body. What does not have a form and order is evil. According to the Thakur culture the human body is related to the cosmos. Any deformity in the human body implies disruption between the body and the cosmic forces. Since this relation cannot be patched up the patient is excommunicated. (refer episode no. : 12)

Excommunication of the Soul

Diseases such as albinism and congenital deformities are held in great contempt. Child born with above disease is believed to be the offspring of the evil spirits Munja or Khais. These spirits are believed to have mated with the mother without the knowledge of her husband. Thus letting a child afflicted by either of these grow up in the Thakur society is an open invitation to the evil spirits. Hence such evil (child with the disease) cannot be a part of good (Thakur Society) and has to be done away with. So the suine (midwife) kills these children either by choking the neck of the child or placing a basket smeared with cowdung on the child so that it dies of suffocation.

The burial of such a child is done in a different and interesting manner. The child is buried with its dorsal side facing the Sun. This action is symbolic of ex-communicating the soul of the albinos or the congenitally deformed child from the good Thakur society.

Rituals or Methods Associated with Collection of Medicinal Herbs

Herbs and animal sources of medicine are ritually collected. Walku does not allow his shadows to fall on the source of medicines, as the shadow blocks the life giving rays of the Sun and the healing power that is being continuously transmitted to medicinal plants through the light. Shadow (darkness) is a symbol of death in this context.

Rituals or Methods Associated with Preparation of Herbs

Walku does not store prepared medicine. According to the Thakur, plants are living and they possess a soul in their roots. If a prepared medicine is stored then its freshness disappears and it will be dead and therefore be ineffective.

Walku prepares the medicine on the spot. He faces east during preparation as this is the direction of life.

Rituals Associated with Administration of Herbs

While administration of medicine a Bhagat sees to it that he faces the east. This action is symbolic of praying to the creator of life "Sun" to make the medicine effective and restore good health to the patient.

CASE NO. 2
MEDICAL STATUS - BHAGATIN
1. Personal Information

Name	: Mathura Agivale
Sex	: Female
Age	: 40 years
Marital Status	: Married
Occupation	: Housewife
Education	: Nil

Village Grampanchayat	: Pathraj
Hamlet/Wadi	: Nagyachiwadi
No. of years of Practice	: 5 years
Social Status	: Bhagatin (female shaman)

2. Apprenticeship

There is no specific and definite period or time for training to be a Bhagatin. To be one, thewoman should be sincere, honest, have a pure soul (swachha atma), be an ardent devotee of mother earth and should be willing to serve humanity willingly and unselfishly. Thus unlike other practitioners the Bhagatin has no period of apprenticeship at all.

3. Beginning of Career

Mathura fulfilled all the requirements and also possessed all the required qualities. She was then visited by mother Earth (Dantari) and her sisters (Baya) in a vision and was instructed to take up the profession of a Bhagatin and serve mankind. She told her vision to some women and then announced to the khot (village head). Every one was happy to hear the news and soon everyone in the village had heard the news. On every Tuesday Mathura would get into a trance (Angat vara yene). She would be possessed by planetary spirits, Baya, believed to be sisters of mother Earth. Initially her getting into a trance was a publicly witnessed phenomenon. Soon people became aware that she was a divine medium who could solve their health problems.

4. Diagnosis

There is a vast difference in the techniques adopted by a Bhagat (male shaman) and a Bhagatin (female shaman). A Bhagat uses a tambya (metal pot) and a Bhagatin gets into a trance to identify the cause of the illness.

A Bhagatin gets into a trance while a drum (dholki) is being played. She lets her hair loose and rotates her head in an anti-clockwise direction. The dholki is played because the Bhagatin is possessed by female spirits (Baya). The dholki symbolizes the female gender. The moving in an anti-clockwise manner is symbolic of the divine powers present in Mathura and she assumes a divine status and is able to diagnose the cause of the illness. Mathura was asked how and which part of your body is occupied by the spirits, She replied 'vara yeto' which means through the wind the planetary spirits get into the body and enter either through the nostrils ot mouth and take complete control of the atma, hence the bodily movements are controlled by the Baya. Mathura was asked if she was aware of what she spoke during the diagnosis rite. She replied that it was not she who speaks but the Baya and she speaks on their behalf.

How long does the state of trance last Mathura ? she answered, "it depends upon the severity of the patients illness. If the patient iis possessed by an evil spirit it takes a long time to drive out the evil spirit and to fulfill his (spirit's) demands such as offering blood, coconut, driving at out using a whip or holding the hair and slapping the patient". Mathura, do you chant prayers during diagnosis?. "No, I only light an incense stick, the smoke gets into the air. This is my prayer to the Baya to visit me and help me diagnose the illness". "Do you have certain days of getting into a trance ?". "Yes, the Thakur Bhagatins get into a trance usually on Tuesdays as it is the day of Baya (Bayancha var). Most of my patient visit me on Tuesdays".

"What happens if a patient is possessed by evil spirit and visits you on any other day ?". Mathura replied that she gets into a trance, she prays to mother Earth and lights an incense stick as a call to the Baya. My son when he is there plays the dholki, the sound of which is a symbol of the Bhagatins cry/desire to call the Baya and help herin the diagnosis of the illness".

Thus the setting of the diagnosis scene is very important for the Baya to visit Mathura.

1. She first takes a wash or bath - This symbolizing her purification with water (holy) 2. Lighting the incense stick - This symbolizes that the smoke merges with the cosmos and reaches the Baya as a form of the Bhagatin's prayer to call for help.
3. Prayer to mother Earth - This symbolizes that the mother Earth who is superior than the Baya instructs them to help the Bhagatin.
4. Playing the drum (Dholki) - The sound of the dholki symbolizes the call of the Bhagatin to the Baya to get into her body and take control of the soul.
5. Lighting a Lamp - A lamp is lit in a plate. Other articles of worship such as coconut, kunku (pink powder), halad (turmeric powder) etc are also placed. The flame of the lamp symbolizes the presence of the Sun God. Thus setting the diagnostic articles before getting into a trance plays a very important and meaning role for the patient and the practitioner.

5. Therapy

Mathura is consulted mostly by patients who have psychological problems such as possession of evil spirits, sorcery, witchcrafts, evil eye, wrath of Gods and Goddesses etc. Mathura diagnoses by getting into a trance. The therapy used by her is the 'Ibut therapy" - applying the charmed ash on the forehead of the patient. On enquiring why the charmed ash is applied only on the forehead. Mathura replied the ill-health of the patient is determined by the degree of disturbance caused to the soul (atma). The only way to reach the divine power of the atma is to remove the evil effect and to remove the evil effect charmed ash is applied on the forehead which is believed to be the point of fortune. The mother Earth writes the fortune of the patient on this point and when the atma leaves the body it goes out through the eyes, nose or mouth. Thus ill health is believed to be a warning of the patient's death and hence the charmed ash (divine touch) is applied on the forehead.

Other than "Ibut therapy" the Bhagatin also uses techniques such as whipping the patient who is possessed by evil spirits, recites prayers commanding the evil force to leave the patient and so on.

6. Medical Knowledge

Mathura's knowledge about medicinal herbs and medicinal extracts from animals and natural sources is very limited as compared to other practitioners. However she knows a lot of home remedies to cure common ailments such as cold, cough, fever etc. She also follows the same rituals connected with collecting, preparing and administrating herbal medicines as done by the Bhagat.

7. Taboos

A Bhagatin refrains from eating food prepared by a menstruating woman nor does she cook food while she is menstruating. Menstrual blood is believed to be evil and a social pollutant. Any menstruating woman interacting with her family members and others is believed to pollute the atmosphere. Mathura does not get into a trance while she is menstruating as she is aware of the "Baya's aversion" for menstrual blood.

8. Method of Giving Up the Profession

When a Bhagatin becomes too old or physically unable to perform her duties she is again visited by the mother Earth or Baya in a vision and asked to discontinue.

9. Thanksgiving

The Thakur Bhagatins do not take any money for the services they render. As per wish of the patient she is a given a bottle of liquor, a feast or a coconut or a cock/hn or a blouse piece.

10. Divine Links

The Bhagatin gets the divine power to heal and diagnose the illness from the Baya and mother Earth. Thus there is great involvement of the religious element in detecting and curing illness.

CASE NO. 3

MEDICAL STATUS - Had Vaidu

1. Personal Information

A. Name	:Hema Raovji Shingva
B. Sex	: Male
C. Age	:85 years
D. Marital Status	: Married
E. Occupation	: Farmer
F. Education	: Nil
G. Village Grampanchayat	: Shillar village
H. Hamlet/Wadi	: Shilarwadi
I. No. of years of practice	: 70 years
J. Social Status	: Had-vaidu

2. Procedure of Medical Apprenticeship

Hema's family are traditional bone setters. The knowledge has been passed down from father to son since generations. Hema being the eldest in the family was taught by his father the art of bone-setting. The period of apprenticeship for Hema was almost 30 years until the death of his father. His training included thorough knowledge of anatomy, physiology, techniques of bone-setting, massaging, study of medicinal plants and more important location of various nerves and branding points on the body. He also learnt the cultural taboos of his profession, the rites of collection, preparation and administration of herbs and medicines.

3. Beginning of Career

Hema Raovji Shingva started his career as a bone setter when he was 30 years old and was doing his apprenticeship under his father. Hema's father had a vision in which he was instructed by the 'Sun God' (God of life) that Hema should carry on with the family tradition and thus serve his fellowmen. This vision was publicly announced. Hema was taken by his father to the village God where he (Hema) took an oath that he will abide by the norms, rules and observe the taboos of the profession and that he will use his medical knowledge only for healing and never to harm anyone. He then offered a coconut.

Hema began his career by giving massages to his father's patients who came with the complaints of swellings. He then shifted to branding patients with hot iron rod. The bone setters and their patients believe that the branding therapy i.e. placing hot iron rod on severely painful points on the body is very helpful in relieving pain. From branding he then slowly turned his attention to the practice of the technique of blood letting. Initially the technique of blood letting was monitored by his father as there is a lot of risk involved in its practice.

Hema next focused on the art of setting bones. Initially he was helped by his father till he had mastered the art. He was quick to learn the administration doses of plant medicine. He also did not face much problem in identifying medicinal herbs used in his profession. The tribals seem to be good students of Systematic and Economic Botany.

4. Reasons for Taking Up the Profession

On enquiring from Hema why did he choose this particular profession, he replied that (Sun God) 'Parmatma' had assigned this duty of serving sick and the suffering to his family and added that God would definitely reward them (his family) for serving his people. He would reward them in heaven (Swarg).

5. Divine Links With the Profession

Bone setting is always fused with mysticism. Religious elements are always part of this mechanical therapy. Rites related to collection, preparation and administration of medicines are always followed and observed. Hema believes that he gets the power to heal from the Sun God. Before touching a patient Hema asks for help from the Sun God and to maintain his healing power he offers a coconut every Thursday to the village God and abides by the norms of his profession.

6. Taboos Associated with the Professiona. Unless and until a lamp is lit Hema does not eat his dinner

It is believed that with the setting of the Sun the light goes out and darkness prevails, but when a lamp is lit it symbolizes the presence of the Sun and that the Sun God is with him. The lighting of the lamp is thus symbolic of the Sun and its light (Tej) and that it is present with the practitioner. The presence of light is symbolic to divinity and purity. Darkness is evil, it spoils the food and water which the practitioner has to eat. Thus the food is polluted. If the bone-setter consumes food in the darkness, the light of the Sun (Tej) present within him is put off and he is then unable to heal his patients.

b. He Does not consume food prepared by menstruating woman

Menstrual blood symbolizes impurity and social pollution. If a menstruating woman touches the practitioner's food, she pollutes it as the blood symbolizes evil. When it flows out her interaction with others spreads evil and hence she is avoided in the menstruating period. If the practitioner consumes the polluted, the healing light (Tej) within him is put off. The Tej is no longer present in his soul (Atma).

c. If a woman delivers in Hema's house, he does not eat food touched, cooked or served by her

The Thakur's believe that the effect of the evil menstrual blood within the body of the woman lasts for twelve days after delivery. They believe the menstrual blood which did not flow out for the nine months and nine days of pregnancy is present in her body.

d. While eating his food, if a lamp is put off Hema stops eating

As soon as the light is put off darkness prevails and takes control of the situation and pollutes the food. If he consumes this food the healing light within his atma may be put off.

e. If death occurs in the village, Hema does not eat till the body is buried

Death is evil according to Hema and his profession. It spreads darkness over the village. The medical practitioners therefore abstain from eating as death pollutes their food. If this food is consumed it may cause hindrance in their profession. After the burial of the dead body, Hema has a bath and eats food prepared from freshly drawn well water.

f. On a Solar Eclipse Hema fasts

Solar eclipse (Surya Grihan) according to the Thakurs is a bad omen. They believe that the Sun God is blocked by evil forces 'Spirits of Mangs and Mahars' (caste groups). Due to this blockage the life rays of the Sun do not reach the earth. Whatever light comes to the earth is evil. The darkness (evil effect) pollutes the food. Hence all medical practitioners fast. After the eclipse is over fresh water (Navin pani) is used to prepare fresh food.

g. Hema abstains from eating food in a wedding

Turmeric is used to cook food at the weddings. Turmeric (halad) according to the Thakurs is symbolic of a woman and is associated with a married woman. A medical practitioner does not consume this food to avoid contact with a woman.

h. He does not chase a dog away while eating

It is believed that the Sun God takes the form of a dog to test the practitioners faith. If the practitioner offers food to the dog then he is a true devotee of the Sun God.

i. On the day of the Solar eclipse he takes a lighted incense stick and rotates it in an anticlock direction over all the medicinal plants he uses for medicinal purposes

During a solar eclipse darkness prevails because evil forces have blocked the light of the Sun. It is feared that the medicinal plants in his house may lose their power. Thus the Thakur culture has designed ways and means to retain it. The burning incense stick symbolizes the Sun and its life giving rays. On enquiring from Hema why this ritual is performed, he replied the this ritual is performed so that the plants may be peaceful and get the rays of the sun through the incense stick. The smoke from the incense stick neutralizes the evil effect of the Solar eclipse (Grihan).

7. Healing Rituals

a. Rituals or methods ot diagnosis

Hema Shingva uses two methods for diagnosis -
i. Observation and/or
ii. Enquiry

i. Observation

He observes the swellings, fractures and touches various parts of the body and the nerves to gather information about the seriousness of the case.

ii. Enquiry

Hema enquires from the patient a detailed history of the accident.

b. Rituals or methods associated with the collection of Herbs

Herbs and animal sources of medicine are ritually collected. Hema does not allow his shadow to fall on the sources of medicines as the shadow blocks the life giving rays of the Sun and the healing power that is being continuously transmitted to the medicinal plants through the light. Shadow (darkness) is a symbol of death in this context.

c. Rituals or methods associated with the preparation of medicines

Hema does not store prepared medicines. According to the Thakur's plants are living and they have soul (atma) in their roots. If the medicine is prepared and stored its freshness disappears and it is dead and will be ineffective.

Hema prepares the medicine in the presence of the patient/his relatives. He faces east during the preparation as the east is the direction of life. This action symbolizes the transmission of healing power of the Sun God (creator of life) into the medicine. Hema chants the name of the Sun God. If the relatives of the patient are present they also time to time chant the name of the Sun God. The patient present gets not only physical relief after consuming the medicine but also psychological relief as he is present during the divine situation of preparing the medicine.

d. Rituals or methods associated with administration of medicines

Both, the practitioner and the patient face the east while the medicine is being administered. During administration the practitioner chants mantras (prayer) asking/requesting God to heal the patient by making the medicine effective (Bhagvana Hya davyala Gun Yeude).

e. Therapeutic measures employed

The bone setter makes use of five different therapeutic measures.

1. Massaging

The bone setter is an expert at healing swellings/complaints of body ache using massage techniques. He makes use of different types of oil. The most popular being oil of Pongamia Pinnata (oil prepared from tha fat of monitor - a reptile). He also uses groundnut oil. He also recommends herbal applications for swelling and body aches.

2. Branding or 'Chocha Dene'

This technique is often used in cases of severe pain. An iron rod is heated and applied to the points of the body where there is severe pain. More than one point may be branded at a time. Problems like severe stomach ache, joint pains, arthritis etc. are treated using this treatment.

3. Blood letting

Thakurs believe that diseases such as migraine, head ache are a result of accumulation of spoilt blood in the affected part of the forehead. This spoilt blood should be let out. Hence the practitioner recommends that a cut be made on the forehead to let out the spoilt blood or the petiole of the Mango leaf is thrust hard into the nostril of the affected half to let out the blood, or a corrosive fluid of semicarpus anacardium (Bibva) seed is applied on the affected part of the forehead to remove the spoilt blood.

4. Bone setting

First Hema sets the bone with his hands using techniques taught to him. After setting the bone, bamboo sticks are used to support the dislocated or fractured bone which are tied with cloth. For setting the bone he usually recommends external application. One of his commonly used application is the latex of the 'Mahua' tree (Madhuca Indica) which is applied on the fracture after setting it. On the latex Nagli seeds (Eleucine Coracana) which are semi-ground are applied to give a cooling effect to the site. The Thakur's believe that the sticky nature of the latex joins the bone.

5. Hot Medication Therapy

Hema also employs and prescribes hot medication therapy to his patients. These include application of hot water bath, hot herbal packs to the swelling.

8. Thanksgiving Rituals or Practices

As a token of appreciation Hema's patients after getting cured give him a coconut. This he ritually offers to the village God as a token of appreciation for His help and success in curing the patient. Hema never accepts cash as it is a taboo to make his profession an income earning means. But appreciation in kind is welcome. He accepts liquor or a feast given to him.

9. Method of Retiring From the Profession

Bone setting as a profession is practiced till the bone setter has strength to handle his patients. He is instructed by the Sun God through visions and dreams to give up the profession. This is then announced publicly. Before giving up the profession the bone setter sees to it that a younger practitioner is ready. In Hema's case his three sons are trained bone setters.

10. Symbols and Meanings Associated with the Profession

The 'Sun God' is the symbol of healing. All the healing rites associated with bone setting revolve round the sun. The Sun is the centre in the ritual healing associated with bone setting. Thus, this profession is not only mechanical but is fused with divine aspects and is treated as incomplete without the combination of the two.

Every action involved in healing has a symbolic and meaningful connotation. The action of instructing the bone setter through visions and dreams to take up the practice and continue it till old age shows his relation with the divine force 'Sun', uplifts his image in his society. The Thakur culture has historically designed norms which fuse with divine elements thereby imposing certain responsibilities (Status and role) that a person must shoulder to maintain the cultural system. In this case norms imposed on medical practitioners fused with divine elements compel him to render health services through their profession.

Facing 'east' (direction of life) while collecting, preparing and administrating the medicine is symbolic to directly inviting the healing power of the Sun to combine with the medicine. The cultural taboos imposed on a medical practitioner have been historically designed to ensure his continual service to mankind.

The Thakur society has also designed ways and means to give thanks to the practitioner. Cash is not accepted by the bone setter (cultural/professional taboo). This practice ensures that if the bone setter becomes popular he does not misuse his curing ability. Hence in kind liquor, clothes or feast is given to the bone setter.

CASE NO 4
MEDICAL STATUS - MANTRIK
1. Personal Information

A. Name	: Hasu Rama Padir
B. Sex	: Male
C. Age	: 48 years
D. Marital Status	: Married
E. Occupation	: Farmer
F. Education	: Nil
G. Village Grampanchayat	: Nalde
H. Hamlet/Wadi	: Nalde Wadi
I. No. of years of practice	: 30 years
J. Social Status	: Mantrik

2. Procedure of Medical Apprenticeship

A Mantrik's office in a Thakur Society is hereditary, i.e. it is passed on from one generation to another. Hasu had to undergo a lengthy period of training and apprenticeship under the able leadership and guidance of his Guru (teacher). Hasu's father Mr. Rama was his teacher. There are a number of phases which Hasu had to pass to become a Mantrik. These steps as described by Hasu are as follows.

a. The Preparatory Phase

One of the most important criteria for becoming a Mantrik is purification of one's atma (soul). The Thakurs believe that Medical Practitioners are mediators between God (Sun) and Man. Thus for a medical practitioner it is necessary he cleanses himself to be a devotee of God Sun.

b. A Call From God

When an individual who wants to become a Mantrik becomes a true devotee of Sun and makes up his mind to abide by the rules and regulations that are laid on him by the progression of Mantrik. Such true devotees receive a call from Sun God to take up this profession. Many a times its through dreams and vision these devotees are instructed by the almighty (Sun) to take up the profession.

C. Training Period

As a preliminary part of the training the Mantrik student is taught Mantras (chants) to reduce and/or neutralize the poisonous effect of scorpions. The various herbs that are used for scorpion stings and snake bites, the ritual healing associated curing cases of scorpions and snake bites, are also part of the training.

The major part of the training is during the Navratra (nine days before a festival call Dasera). During these nine nights a Mantrik learns chants, prayers, rites and words associated with the process of diagnosis and healing. A student Mantrik goes to the river in the night at 1 am., he gets into the water with 50 stones (small ones). he faces the east (the direction of life). Each time he recites a mantra he throws one stone in the water. He repeats his mantras for 50 times. Getting into a river water means getting a divine feel. The Thakurs believe that water is the brother of the Sun. Facing the east is symbolic of inviting the Sun's power in the body of the Mantrik. He enters naked in the river for it is believed that there is no other thing such as clothes on his body to block the power of the Sun and water. While he is doing this no woman is supposed to be around. It is believed that the skill of Mantrik is associated with masculinity and therefore there should not be any feminine intervention.

After the nine days of training in rituals and Mantras a Mantrik student is taken by his Guru (teacher) to the village God. A coconut is offered by the student. This act is symbolic of the ordination of the student and his dedication to work as a Mantrik to serve his people, that he will not misuse his knowledge to harm anyone.

3. Taboos and Norms of a Mantrik

a. A Mantrik is not to sweep his house or make any use of broom in the house. This act is symbolic of chasing away his skill out of the house.

b. He refrains from eating food which contains turmeric as long as he holds the post of a Mantrik. The Thakurs associate turmeric with female and categorize it as a woman. This taboo reminds him that he cannot fiddle with more than one woman (his wife)

c. He is not supposed to eat food until the dead body of the person is buried. Death is a symbol of darkness and evil where as the Mantrik has light of the Sun God within him. Thus when death (darkness) occurs in the village it pollutes the food to be consumed by the Mantrik. After the disposal of the dead body the Mantrik's wife brings fresh water and prepares fresh food for the Mantrik. He cleans himself with fresh water by taking a bath then has his meal. Death in this context is a symbol of (evil darkness) that pollutes the food. Water is a symbol of cleansing.

d. While a Mantrik is eating his food and accidentally or on purpose the lamp is put off, the Mantrik stops eating his food. The putting off or extinguishing of the lamp symbolizes the interference of an evil force which is trying to pollute the Mantrik's food. If the Mantrik consumes the food (evil) polluted by the darkness it will have an adverse effect on the good and pure light/power which is a gift to him from the Sun.

e. A Mantrik is not allowed to consume food prepared by a menstruating woman. Menstrual blood is symbolic of impurity and pollution. The hearth (chul) where fireburns is believed to be an incarnation of Holi (Goddess of Fire). The fire that burns in the hearth is a symbol of the Sun. (All mighty).

f. He does not kill a snake. A snake is believed to be a God, namely chedhoba/Bhari. It is worshipped by the Thakurs so that the actual snake does not bite them. A Mantrik recites chants in which he pleads to the Gods namely chedhoba and Bhari to heal the patient and to remove his poison from his body.

g. While a Mantrik is eating if he is called a "Mang" or "Mahar", he immediately stops eating as the caste groups "Mang" and "Mahar" are classified by the Thakurs as being lower in status and as the Rakshas (evil) jati. On solar eclipses the Thakurs believe the spirits of Mang and Mahar block the Sun with darkness. A Mantrik who is a special devotee of the Sun cannot be called such names as the utterances of such names have an effect on his food.

4. Beginning of the Career

Hasu began his career as a Mantrik when he was 18 years old. In his initial period of practice he always consulted his father regarding the healing of his patients. As the years passed by he became an expert. He has now mastered all the techniques of ritual healing taught to him by his father.

5. Reasons for taking up the profession

Hasu classifies two reasons for taking up this profession.

i. The office of Mantrik has been their family tradition, with an aim to serve the humanity with an unselfish motive.

ii. He had a call from God through vision to take up this profession.

6. Divine Links With The Profession

The healing profession of a Mantrik is not restricted to giving only medicinal herbs to cure scorpions stings and snake bites. The fact that he is is called a "Mantrik" means a "Chanter" who heals his patients during chants in a ritualistic fashion. Besides administering herbs a Mantrik brings into play the entire belief system during the healing processed.

Secondly his profession is very much linked with divine and mystical elements. He gets the healing power from the Sun. He performs certain rituals to maintain his healing power. He refrains himself from breaking any taboos that have been historically imposed on his profession through culturally set norms.

7. Healing Rituals

A. Rituals or Methods of Diagnosis

There are three methods used by a Mantrik to note the severity or complexity of his patient's story by a scorpion or bitten by a snake.

a. Observation - Of the colour of the bitten portion of the body.

b. Type or pattern of the sting or bite to note which species of scorpion and snake has bitten.

c. The temperature of the body of his patient, i.e. to what extent it is hot/cold.

B. Rituals or methods associated with collecting medicinal herbs

Mantrik like the other medicinal practitioners also follow culturally prescribed norm of collecting medicinal herbs. They do not let their shadow fall on the plant. Shadow is symbol of darkness which blocks the light and the power of life that comes from the east in the plant. Shadow interrupt this power.

C. Rituals or methods associated with preparation of medicines

A mantrik always faces the east while preparing his medicines, he symbolically invites the healing and life giving power of the Sun to combine or fuse with his medicine so that it heals his patient faster.

D. Rituals or methods associated with administration of medicines.

Both the mantrik and his patient they face the east while the medicine is being administered. This action symbolizes the request of both mantrik and his patient to the Sun for a quick recovery, through his life giving and healing power.

8. Therapeutic Measures Employed

Mantriks use a number of therapeutic measures to heal their patient and they are as follows.

a. Medicinal Herbs

Use of medicinal herbs to cure patients of scorpions stings and snake bites is a very common feature of a Mantrik's treatment.

b. Blood Letting

At times the Mantrik cuts the part which is bitten by a snake and allows the blood to flow. This action is associated with removal of poison.

c. Sucking the poison

The bitten part is sucked by a Mantrik and spat out. Mantrik who is a devotee of the Sun has power to suck the poison that is in the patient's body. The Thakurs believe that the poison of a snake turns the human blood blue. Because the poison takes control of the atma and hence the blood in all the parts of the body turns blue. Sucking the poison means cleansing the patient's atma of the blue effect, which makes it dysfunction.

d. Healing through chants

Mantriks also use chants to cure cases of scorpion stings. The chant is a prayer requesting the scorpion to reduce its "Aag" (pain). This chant is popularly known as "vinchu utarnyache mantra".

e. The ritual of "pani marne"

An interesting ritual is performed by a mantrik to ward off the poisonous effect that gathers on the atma (the fifth opening). He takes his patient to a well. He has a metal pot (tambya) with him. He faces towards the east and jumps in the well and fills the tambya with fresh water from below and then come up. He then makes his patient face the east and splashes the holy water on his face five times.

The tambya is a symbol of the patient's atma which is affected with poison. Water from the well's bottom is considered to be fresh since pure water that comes out of the spring is believed to be brother of the Sun God, it is holy. In this situation water symbolizes a cleansing agent that purifies or cleanses the poisonous effect. Why five times splashing is done because the human atma is situated on the fifth place in the order of the ten body openings. Why facing the east is because along with the holy water a mantrik also invites Sun's life giving healing power to cleanse the poisonous effect.

It is a shared cultural belief that a person's atma is situated in the fifth position in the order of the bodily openings. This ritual aims at removing the poisonous effect which exists on the patient's atma. This scene is also co-related with the fifth position of Earth in the cosmos. Life is associated with earth.

f. Healing by initiating Vomiting

In case of snake bite which is not delayed for a long time, the Mantrik administer herbs or medicines to initiate vomiting in the patient. Thc logic here is that some thing comes in (poison) and it has to some how go out, thus when a patient vomits it is believed that the poison also is vomited out.

g. Combinational Therapy

Very often herbal therapy is favoured with mystical elements by the Mantriks to treat their patients. He not only chants mantras requesting the snake and/or scorpion to reduce the pain but also gives medicinal herbs to cure the patient. Thus chants take care of the fear and anxiety part of the patient giving him psychological relief and medicine gives him physical relief.

9. Thanks Giving Rituals or Practices

As a token of appreciation Hasu's patients after getting cured give him a coconut. This he ritually offers to the village God as a token of appreciation for his help and success and curing the patient. Hasu never accepts cash as it is a taboo to make his profession an income earning means. But appreciation in kind is welcome. He accepts liquor or feast. The Thakur culture has designed this norm in such a way that the divine forces control a mantrik not to accept cash.

10. Method of Giving Up The Profession

The profession of a mantrik is practiced till the mantrik has strength to handle his patients, to jump into the well to perform the 'pani marne' ritual. before giving up his profession a mantrik sees to it that he trains his eldest son. If he does not have a son he trains his brother's son or a true devotee of Sun.

11. Symbols and Meanings Associated With The Profession

Every action, word, chant, object, relationship, gesture and utterance used in healing process by mantrik has a symbolic and meaningful connotation. These include the norms imposed on a mantrik means a lot to him and his people. The norms are symbolic of marking the mantrik as a special person from the others, giving him a higher status. Most of the activities such as not sweeping the house, not consuming the food prepared by a menstruating woman, not consuming turmeric and so on reflect his manly higher status which is dominant in his society. In fact all male medical practitioners are devotees of 'Sun' (male) God, while the female practitioners such as bhagatin, suine and potdhari are devotees of (mother earth) female Goddess. Normative behaviour hence reflects the dominance and superiority of males over females in the Thakur society.

CASE No 5

MEDICAL STATUS - Vaidu

1. Personal Information

A. Name	: Palu Kamlu Lobhie
B. Sex	: Male
C. Age	: 50 years
D. Marital Status	: Married
E. Occupation	: Farmer & Daily wage labourer
F. Education	: Nil
G. Village Grampanchayat	: Pathraj
H. Hamlet/Wadi	: Lobhyachi Wadi
I. No. of years of practice	: 38 years
J. Social Status	: Vaidu (herbalist)

2. Procedure of Medical Apprenticeship

Palu was given a comprehensive training under the guidance of his father, since Palu's childhood. His major subjects were identification of medicinal plants and their collection, administration, preparations and all the rituals and norms associated with the profession of a vaidu. Palu initially saw his father work and slowly followed his foot steps to be trained for ten years until his father expired.

3. Beginning of Career

At the age of 12 years Palu began treating his patients on minor complaints such as stomach ache, head ache, cuts, wounds etc. He would consult his father before treating a patient. He practiced with his father for ten years till he became an expert.

4. Reasons for Taking Up the Profession

The Vaidu profession has been the family tradition of Palu's family. The eldest son of every generation takes up the charge. Palu's grandfather (Changu) passed on his knowledge to (Kamlu) then (Palu) and now Palu's son (Bhau) is under apprenticeship. Secondly the profession is considered to be an assignment from God.

5. Divine Links with the Profession

The vaidus believe that they are appointed by God almighty (Sun) to serve humanity. It is the Sun God who gives them the healing powers to heal the people. Vaidus offer the Sun a coconut every Sunday. They believe that plants which contain medicines are often mixed with "Tej" (light) of Sun.

6. Taboos Associated with the Profession

A. The vaidus fast on solar eclipse, they do not eat nor drink. They believe that the 'Sun God'who gives them the power of healing and who is a life giver and sustaineris blocked by an evil force and therefore the life giving Sun raysare blockedand hence the food and water becomes polluted due to this shadowed effect. If evil food is consumed their body may be polluted and even they may be a subject to death.

B. Palu does not consume "turmeric" because in the Thakur classification turmeric is associated with a female. Brides are applied turmeric. It is believed if the Vaidu takes turmeric he automatically becomes dishonest to his wife and goes for another wife. The consumption of turmeric is therefore a taboo as it is linked with female cult.

7. Healing Rituals

A. Rituals or Methods of Diagnosis

A detailed enquiry of the type of sickness or suffering is made by the vaidu from his patients. At the time Nadi (pulse) is also checked. Colour of eyes and skin is checked. In case of fever the patients body is felt to check for the temperature. The vaidu also enquires from the patients what type of food was consumed by the patients during illness.

B. Rituals or Methods Associated with Collecting Medicinal Herbs

Palu observes certain rituals and religions norms to collect plants. he collects his plants on Sunday because its the day of the 'Sun' and Tuesday because its the day of his village God Bariri. While collecting a medicinal plant he does not allow his shadow to fall on the plant for it is believed that the shadow blocks the Sun life giving rays and therefore the medicine becomes ineffective.

C. Rituals or Methods Associated With Preparation of Medicines

Medicines as per medical norms areprepared facing the east (the holy direction) from where rises the almighty (Sun). It is believed that the life giving power is combined with the medicines.

D. Rituals or Methods Associated With Administration of Medicines

If medicines are to be administered the vaidu makes his patient face the east and then makes him take the medicines. Facing east (the direction of life) symbolizes the patient's urge to ask the 'Sun' pardon for his wrong doings and requesting the Sun to cure him.

8. Therapeutic Measures Employed

Depending on the type of illness and Palu's judgment about its origin and cause he employs the following types and therapies.

a. Herbal Therapy -

He uses medicines prepared from the various bodily parts of the plants to cure diseases of his patient.

b. Branding Technique -

Palu uses a hot iron rod to brand the severely painful parts of the patient's body.

c. Massage -

For swelling and sprains he prescribes or himself massages.

d. Fumigation -

In case of tooth decay Palu prescribes fumigation of smoke of solanum xantho carpum fruits.

e. Blood letting -

In case of migraine head ache the affected part is punctured with corrosive fluid of semicarpus anacardium. There is yet another method to let the blood out, that is by pushing a mango leaf petiole hard into the nostril of the affected side.

9. Thanksgiving Rituals or Practices

Palu accepts gifts such as chicken, liquor or a feast or a coconut from his patients. If given a coconut he offers it to the village God "Bhairi". Gifts given to Palu are mostly in king for taking cash does not fit into his frame work of being a socially devoted and dedicated vaidu.

10. Method of Giving up the Profession

Palu says that the vaidus give up their profession when the village God or Sun instructs them to stop their profession. When a person's body starts degenerating there by loosing its vital power in old age or when a person starts loosing his teeth.

11. Symbols and Meanings Assocaited with the Profession

The effectiveness of cure or treatment with whatever therapies which are employed by Palu are because of the healing power or the light (Tej) of Sun which is there in him. The herbal or chemo-therapy is linked with number of social, cosmological, natural, spiritual and supernatural symbols and meanings. The various actions of the vaidu profession are an inter-play of these symbols which are brought into play and represent the cultural whole. Each action is interrelated to another concept or sphere of social life. Every object, material and action has some meaning behind it.

CASE No. 6
MEDICAL STATUS - Suine
1. Personal Information

Name	: Rakhma Chahu Padir
Sex	: Female
Age	: 55 years
Marital Status	: Married
Occupation	: House-wife
Education	: Nil
Village Grampanchayat	: Kotimba

Hamlet/Wadi : Kotimba
No. of Years of Practice : 35 years, attended approximately 900, deliveries.
Social Status : Suine

2. Procedure of Medical Apprenticeship

Rakhma's mother was a midwife. She often heard her mother talking about deliveries and the advice she gave to expectant mothers. She was aware of the rituals performed after delivery etc. Thus from the beginning she was exposed to such an atmosphere. Rakhma later got married into a family where her mother-in-law happened to be a midwife. Rakhma worked with her mother-in-law as a potdhari (assistant midwife) for five to six years and was trained to serve as a midwife.

3. Beginning of a Career

Rakhma began her career as a midwife at a young age of 20 years. She began to practice as a midwife after serving with her mother-in-law as a potdhari. Before she undertook her first delivery all by herself she had a vision in which Satvai "mother earth instructed Rakhma to be a "punjarin" (midwife).

4. Reasons for Taking Up the Profession

There are two reasons why Rakhma took up this profession.

a. After her mother-in-law was a midwife and this tradition had to be carried on.
b. She had a vision in which Satvai instructed her to take up this profession.

5. Divine Links with the Profession

Rakhma gets the power to conduct her deliveries successfully from mother earth. She performs certain rituals which are necessary to keep up her status as a midwife. She observes certain divine restrictions during delivery such as making the delivering woman face west performing the 'Panchvi Pujan' ritual in which offerings are given to the mother Earth on the fifth day of delivery.

6. Taboos Associated with the Profession

1. A Suine is not allowed to participate in the healing ritual namely 'Jagran of the Baya'. The Baya are the planetary spirits, barren and believed to be sisters of mother Earth. The Suine is not allowed to participate because she performs the menial jobs like cleaning women's menstrual blood and delivering children.

2. The Suine does not offer a coconut. She is only allowed to light an incense stick. The coconut is a symbol of masculinity and the water in it symbolizes the sperms.

3. She is prohibited from cutting a cock or a goat for sacrifice. Killing is a symbolic of manliness and hence all sacrifices are offered only be males.

4. She is not allowed to attend the ritual of 'Mothur-Med' as this ritual is performed only be male members.

7. Rituals performed by a Midwife/Suine

a. Ritual of Delivering a Child

The midwife lights an incense stick to the village God after bathing. She prays for good luck and success in performing the delivery.

She carries some ash of the incense stick (Ibut) and applies it on the forehead of the expectant mother. This action symbolizes that the almighty God will help the mother to delivery safely. This action strengthens the belief of the mother that the delivery will be safe and normal.

In case the delivery is delayed, the Suine goes and worships a Rui (Calotropis gigantia) plant and pleads with her to deliver the child safely and quickly. In this context the Rui plant (for the Thakurs) is a symbol of mother Earth. This plant is also given importance on other important occasions like marriage etc. It is believed that the Rui plant has the ability to make a bond or to bind. Hence a man who gets married for the fourth time, first weds the Rui plant and this symbolizes that now he cannot break away from the fourth wife.

The latex of the Rui plant never dries up and is symbolic of the mother milk. The plant grows where there is water and is used to cure other ailments like guinea worms, asthma, abortion and delayed deliveries. The Thakur's therefore look upon this plant as a mother. Therefore the Suine worships the plant. In case of delayed delivery the root of the plant is placed at the nape of the woman's neck. Root of plantain or some mud of an anthill may also be placed at the nape.

In case of prolonged delay in the delivery, charmed ash from the Bhagat (Shaman) is brought and applied on the forehead of the parturient woman. Another measure is to wet a part if the husbands loin cloth in a little water and give the water to the woman to drink. These actions symbolize the moral support from the almighty as well as the husband.

2. Ritual of Cleansing the Mother

After delivery the midwife takes care that both the mother and the child are well cleaned. After delivery she presses the mother's stomach to remove the evil menstruating blood and clean the mother with water (holy). The water is considered to be the brother of the Sun God and is used in most rituals and acts as a neutralizing agent which neutralizes the effect of evil.

3. Squeezing the Breast Milk

The Thakurs do not allow the mother to feed the new born for five days. They believe that the child must not be given this milk as it is cheesy or thick in nature and causes digestive complications in the child like diarrhoea or dysentery in the child. Hence the milk is squeezed out on a cloth and is poured and the cloth is washed in the river, to prevent the milk from becoming an object of witchcraft or sorcery to harm either the mother or the child. On enquiring why does the milk become thick, the answer was that the menstrual blood of the woman, the spermatic effect of the husbands sperms and the faeces of the child make the milk thick.

4. The Burial of the Umbilical Chord

The fertility of the woman, her sexual behaviour, her feminine nature etc. are linked to the mother Earth by the Thakurs. The midwife takes a palas life, places it on the umbilical chord in the center with some rice, gulal (red powder), a coin and a wick. The leaf is then buried (along with the things placed on it) on the outside of the western wall of the house. A temporary bathing place is made for the mother and child to bathe. Thus, the used bathe water is allowed to flow over the buried palas leaf as the water helps the chord to decay and perish. Thus the chord is prevented from becoming an object of withcraft and/or sorcery.

5. Turning Over the Palas Leaf

A Thakur woman who does not wish to bear more children buries the placenta of the child in an inverted position. This means that the concerned family must stop having children. The same things mentioned above are placed on the dorsal surface of the leaf, the leaf is then inverted, now the ventral side faces up and it is then buried. This symbolizes the mother Earth's desire or the wish for the family to stop producing children. This ritual expresses or symbolizes a cultural check on population growth.

6. Bathing Ritual

Symbolism plays an important role in bathing ritual. The umbilical chord is buried outside the west wall of the house. A temporary bathing place is constructed on the inner side of the west wall and both the mother and the child are given bath for five days by the Suine. The bath water is allowed to flow on the buried umbilical chord (Outside the west wall). Thus ensures that the umbilical chord gets decayed and perishes and thus does not become an object of witchcraft or sorcery.

During the bath the woman faces west as mother Earth resides in the opposite direction i.e. the east. Also during the delivery the woman faces west so that the mother earth first sees the child on delivery.

7. The Ritual of Panchvi Pujan

On the fifth day after the birth of the child, the elaborate ceremony of Panchvi Pujan is held. This ritual is performed between 12 to 1 pm in the noon when the Sun is right on the head. The house is cleaned, clothes are washed, the house is smeared with cowdung. Above five feet away from the temporary bathing place of the mother and the child a circular pattern with cowdung is made. The following objects are placed on this cowdung pattern- Rice grains, Date (1), Almond (1), Betel nut (1), Rhizome of Turmeric (1), Nada, Incense stick, Kumkum, Gulal, andCalotropis leaves(5).

These objects are offerings made to the mother Earth. If the newborn is a boy then a coconut is offered and if it is a girl then dry copra is offered. The coconut with water is symbolic of sperm and the copra which is half symbolizes the womb of the woman which receives the sperms.

On the west wall inside the house five circular patterns are drawn by the punjarin (midwife). She uses the following powders and the order is adhered - 1. Kunku - pink powder, 2. Gulal - red powder, 3. Halad - yellow powder, 4. Shendur - Orange powder, and 5. Abir - black powder.

The five patterns form a square which represents Satvai. THe punjarin worships Satvai and presents the offering depending on the sex of the child and makes an obeisance to the deity. The child placed in a Topli (basket) with the head pointing east is presented to the deity. A nada or string is tied to the child's wrist and sacred ash is applied to its forehead. The mother then bows down and worships Satvai.

It is believed that on the same day in the evening/night Satvai comes in the form of a rat, dog, cow or any other creature and writes the fortune on the forehead of the child. Satvai comes in at 12 o'clock midnight. She also writes the life span of the child. The Thakur's say for the above explanation (Satvai Kapalavar Aakshar lihite).

The entire ritual of Panchvi Pujan brings into account the importance of mother Earth (Satvai) as the mother of all life present on the Earth. She gives life (birth) to every creature on earth. Mother Earth is given a motherly status in this ritual. The basket in which the child is placed for five days is symbolic of the womb of mother Earth where life is nurtured. She exercises control over the child for five days and hands the child over to the Thakurs on the day of Panchvi Pujan.

8. The Ritual of Warding off the Evil Spirit

The Thakurs believe that both, the new born and the mother are likely to becomes the victims of 'evil eye' (Drishti). The people who cast evil eye are the barren women (wanjuti), witch (Bhutali), sorcerer (Bhutala) members of the tribe, members of the Kathkari tribe, members of the lower caste groups viz, Mangs, Mahars, Chamars etc.

Rituals for warding off evil eye and evil forces are different for the new born and the mother. On the fifth day, the Suine applies sacred ash on the mother's forehead and ties a coloured string and a piece of orris root around her neck. Both the sacred ash and the root are charmed by the Bhagat and hence ward off evil effect. Another measure adopted is the mother should carry a sickle when going out for defecation. Iron absorbs evil and the sharpness of the sickle is symbolic of a means to destroy evil.

To ward off evil eye affect among children and mothers, five chillies, a piece of broom stick and some salt is taken and ritually rotated over the patient five times. These articles are then thrown into the fire. The crackling noise that is produced is symbolic of destruction of evil effect. The hotness of the chillies has the ability to absorb evil and irritate it till it is destroyed in the fire. To prevent children from becoming victims of the evil eye, the Thakurs make a special chain of black and yellow beads and tie it around the child's neck to ward off evil.

9. Rituals of Collecting Herbs

All the medicinal herbs collected by the Suine for administration are collected in a ritualistic fashion. The Suine always faces east during collection, she does not allow her shadow to fall on the plant as the shadow symbolizes darkness and block life giving power from the rays of the Sun. If the shadow falls it is symbolic of the plant loosing its medicinal value.

10. Rituals of Preparation

Even while preparing the medicinal decoction and powder, the Suine faces east as the healing power, life giving power of the almighty Sun God comes from the eastern direction. This rite is performed to combine the divine elements (healing power of the Sun) with the natural elements (Medicinal plants) and this makes the medicine very effective.

11. Rituals of Administration

While administering the medicine the Suine is particular that both, she and the patient face East. This action is symbolic of praying to the creator of life to restore the patient's life.

12. Functions of a Suine

The duties of a Suine center around the mother and the new born. She also gives dietary advice to the expectant mothers, she delivers children and treats illness that may befall the new born and/or the mother. She also performs the ritual of Panchvi Pujan. She has a vast knowledge of child birth techniques and cultural behaviour associated with pregnancy and child birth.

She does not have extensive knowledge of herbal medicines, but she is well aware of the medicinal remedies for urinary and menstrual disorders, abortion and other gynaec problems. Most Suines pass on the art of child delivery and their knowledge to their daughters-in-law as observed in the Thakur community.

13. Some Medicines Given By the Suine

Plant	Part Used	Sickness and method of administration
1. Piper nigrum	Seed	7-8 seeds of pepper and 2 stalks of synzium aromaticum,2 pinches of tea leaves with 1/2 spoon of sugar are powdered and mixed in a cup of water are taken as a remedy to accelerate delayed deliveries.
2. Riccinus	Root	Riccinus root is placed at the communus nape of a woman to speed up the delivery.
3. Calotropis	Root	The same as above. Gigantia
4. Musa Paradisica	Root	The same as above.
5. Butea Mono-	Flower	Flowers of Butea monosperma sperma are heated and placed on the abdomen of a woman suffer ing from kidney stones.
6. Calotropis	Root	The root is ground and soaked Gigantia in coconut water for a period of twelve hours and is then taken as a remedy for abortion.

14. Thanksgiving Ritual/Ceremony

The midwife literally slogs for twelve days after assisting the mother in the delivery, she washes their clothes, gives both of them a bath, performs rituals for a period of twelve days. She is paid Rs. 5/- by the Thakurs and is given a coconut.

Among the Mavchi tribe the Havakis (midwives) are paid Rs. 40/- to 50/- per delivery (Tribhuwan Robin and others, 1992). The Thakur Suine therefore prefers to attend to the deliveries of the Maratha caste people as they give her Rs. 25/- or a blouse or a sari and food for her twelve days labour. She is also given grains by the Marathas.

CASE NO. 7
MEDICAL STATUS - Potdhari
1. Personal Information

A. Name	: Anni Balu Pingale
B. Sex	: Female
C. Age	: 50 years
D. Marital Status	: Widow
E. Occupation	: Farming
F. Education	: Illiterate
G. Village Grampanchayat	: Pathraj
H. Hamlet/Wadi	: Lobhyachiwadi
I. No. of years of practice	: 10 years and has managed 50 deliveries
J. Social Status	: Potdhari

2. Procedure of Medical Apprenticeship

Anni's husband expired ten years ago, since then she has been practicing as a Potdhari (assistant midwife). She has been trained by the midwife of Lobhyachiwadi. Her training included learning to give medical advice to expectant mothers, assisting in deliveries performing rituals, learning the taboos of midwife profession.

3. Beginning of the Career

Anni began her career as a Potdhari at the age of forty. The word 'Potdhari' literally means to hold the stomach. Anni was taught the art of holding the pregnant woman's foetus and pushing it as she delivers. Initially she had to take advice from the midwife, but with ten years of experience behind her. she can even manage deliveries.

4. Reason/s For Taking Up the Profession

After the death of her husband, Anni had a vision in which God Bhairi - village God instructed Anni to take up the profession. Mother Earth also called upon her and asked her to serve the people through this profession.

5. Divine Links with the Profession

Anni is a sincere devotee of 'Dantari' (mother Earth) who she believes gives her the courage and strength to handle deliveries. Anni applies Ibut (charmed dust from the Earth) on her forehead facing the west. This action is symbolic of fusing herself with the divine power. While delivering the child she faces East (Sun) and while assisting in the delivery she faces west (Earth).

6. Taboos Associated with the Profession

A Potdhari does not have much status compared to the other medical practitioners. She comes last in the hierarchy of medical practitioners i.e. she ranks seventh. She is not allowed to participate in healing rituals. She is not allowed to offer coconut for it contains water and it is symbolic of masculinity. The water is symbolic of sperms. She is not allowed to offer a sacrifice Killing or cutting an animal is associated with manliness and bravery and hence she in excluded from the rite.

7. Potdhari and Ritual Performance

A potdhari does not play any role in performing major rituals of maternal and child health. Her major job is to assist the midwife (Suine) in delivering the child, massaging the woman. However, rituals concerned with warding off the evil eye are performed by the potdhari. Rituals such as this can be performed by any other woman and hence the potdhari does not have any ritual/s to perform which are specific to only her profession. Compared to the midwife, a potdhari does not perform any specific ritual, and enjoys no reputed status.

8. Medical Knowledge

Compared to the midwife and other medical practitioner, a potdhari does not possess any knowledge of medicinal herbs and other potions administered. She is however aware of the home remedies concerned with common ailments such as cough, colds, fever, cuts, wounds, etc. After practicing as a potdhari for atleast five to ten years she becomes an expert student of medicinal plants used to cure diseases which may effect the new mother and the new born.

9. Thanksgiving Rituals and Ceremonies

Among the Thakurs the potdhari is given Rs. 1.25np. as a token for assisting the midwife, by the family members of the pregnant woman. She is also offered a meal along with the midwife. If the potdhari is called to assist the midwife while carrying out the delivery of a woman belonging to the Maratha caste she is given Rs. 5/- as her fee for the labour put in. The midwife and the potdhari function as a team but the midwife in no way gives away monetary aid to the potdhari for her help. The potdhari's fee is paid by the family.

§§§

CHAPTER VII

RITUAL HEALING

Therapy in ethnomedicine is a vast subject, it includes both magico-religious and mechanical and chemical procedures (Lieban 1973:1044).

Lauglin (1963) has made the point that the success of human species is in no small measure due to the ability to cope up with medical problems, and an assessment of indigenous medical systems, including those of non-literate societies, shows an impassive array of practices that demonstrate therapeutic knowledge, including trephining, bone setting, removal of ovaries, obstetrics including caesarean section, laprotomy, Unulectomy, comparative anatomy, autopsy, cautery, inoculation baths, poultices, inhalation, laxatives, enemas, ointments and cupping (Ackernecht 1942, Simons 1955, Laughlin 1963, Haurd 1969).

The pharmacopoeia of ethno-medicine is copious and includes such proven drugs as quinine, opium, coca, cinchona, copaiba, curare, chaulmoorga oil, ephedrine and rauwolfia (Lieban 1973:1045). Quisumbing (1951) lists more than eight hundred known medicinal plants in the Philippines alone, including flora efficacious in the treatment of a number of maladies, such as asthma, diarrhoea, malaria, diabetes and kidney ailments to mention only a few.

Literature on disease and treatment in primitive medicine, has pointed out that most data on treatment, in general ethnographic techniques used, a list of disease in which they are applied, and of statements as to the possible objective effect that such measures have. It is obvious that such descriptions are valuable as they, omit just the points needed for our special (anthropological) inquiry. What are the ideas underlying these therapeutic acts, and under what circumstances (with or without ritual) are they performed? (Turner 1967:299).

Since Ackernecht (1946) wrote, there have been several praiseworthy attempts to answer his queries, directly or by implication, but by and large there have been few systematic discussions of the relationship between the treatment of practices of a specific tribal society. Thus merely documenting medicinal herbs and describing therapeutic techniques from an emic perspective does not give an in-depth analysis of a community's medical culture.

An anthropologist's job is to document and understand ethnomedical phenomena as defined and understood by the natives from an emic perspective. Ethnomedical studies must unravel the deeper meanings and symbolic normative forms of beliefs regarding health and disease. The question which a researcher must constantly ask himself while collecting data is 'Why the natives behave the way they do? And what cultural symbols and meanings shape their illness and treatment experiences.

Foster G.M. (1983:21) has pointed out that 'The therapies found in every society stem largely from prevailing causality beliefs, which form the rationale for treatment. What ever source of power, the primary role of Shaman, priest, witch finder or a medicine man is to identify the deity, ghost, or other agent that has caused illness, and then determine how to placate or overcome it. Until the causal agent has been discovered, therapy is believed to have little effect.

The entire drama of ritual healing begins with the tracing the origin and cause of illness and to identify what has gone wrong, where, how and why? This job of tracing the pathogenic agents is done by medical specialists and often elderly members of a community. Once the cause is traced the second phase is to heal or get rid of it. The entire process of healing in ethno-medical accounts is popularly known as 'ethno-medical therapy' or 'ritual healing'. This chapter aims to reveal the entire set of ritualistic actions, gestures, utterances, rituals, objects, colours, substances, chants, prayers, songs etc. and their meanings and symbolic forms as viewed by the Thakurs and to show how these ideas prevade wider realms of belief and action. Before getting into the data of ritual healing it is necessary to understand what a ritual is and how healing processes become ritualistic.

What is a ritual?

The term 'ritual' though seems to be a simple matter, few terms in the study of religion have been explained in more confusing ways. For example, Edmund Leach (1968:524) a cultural anthropologist after noting the general disagreement among the anthropological theorists, suggests that the term 'ritual' should be applied to all the cultural sets of behaviour, that is the symbolic dimension of human behaviour as such regardless of its explicit religious, social or other content.

According to David Lotz (1987:405), a ritual is referred to as those conscious and voluntary repetitions and stylized bodily actions, that are centred on cosmic structures or sacred presence, he includes verbal behaviour such as chants, songs, and prayers in the category of bodily actions. Kartz and Kirkland (1988:1179) are of theview that 'Rituals are stylized, repetitive, arbitary and exaggerated forms of behaviour'.

Turner (1967) uses the term ritual to 'prescribe formal behaviour for occasions not given over to technological routine, having reference to beliefs in mystical (non-empirical) beings or power'.

Rituals are thus a set of stylized bodily actions (which may include iconic symbols such as acts, objects, words, gestures, prayers, songs, chants and other things) performed in a culturally defined place, situation or context by certain actor/s only, encompassing basic rules to accomplish given tasks or goals in any social sphere with in a given cultural frame of reference.

A number of social scientists interested in socio-cultural functions of rituals in different spheres of life have pointed out varied functions of rituals which are as follows -

1. Rituals encourage cohesion (Gluckman 1970).
2. Rituals facilitate transition (Van Gennep 1960).
3. Rituals define conceptual categories (Mary Douglas 1966).
4. Enhance individual and group autonomy (Kartz P. 1981).
5. Help resolve social conflicts (Gluckman 1970; Turner 1967).
6. Endow culturally important cosmological conceptions and values with persuasive emotive force, thus unifying individual participants into a genuine community (Geertz and Turner).
7. Ritual actions express and communicate shared socio- cultural meanings which are symbolically transacted through the medium of ritual action (Munn 1973).
8. They reveal the knowledge of meanings of symbols involved in them (Hongiman 1959).
9. They are modes of symbolic communication (Firth 1973).

From the theoretical understanding it is observed that rituals are set of culturally governed symbolic activities, which gain meaning with in a given context, situation or culturally defined place and that these rituals reveal socio-cultural concepts of the natives and are performed to accomplish tasks or goals in any social sphere.

Ritual Healing

The process of ritual healing has been conceptually defined as the culturally designed clinically meaningful reality of health behaviour through which a sick person passes to get cured, wherein participant actors such as elderly members of the family and village, ethno-medical specialists and others follow cultural specific ritualized forms of therapies including herbal, mechanical and magico-ritual to cure the patient depending on the community's notion of the origin and cause illness, thereby abiding with all medical and socio-cultural norms of healing situations (Tribhuwan Robin 1993).

It includes the culturally prescribed symbolic andnormative forms of behaviour and stylized bodily actions, gestures, utterances, trance states, chants, prayers, words and use of certain holy objects by the healers to diagnose the origin and cause of illness and then to employ the necessary therapies in order to restore the health of the patient.

Healing ritual actions express and communicate shared socio-cultural meanings which are symbolically transacted through the medium of ritual action (Munn 1973:589). Rituals reveal the natives' knowledge of meanings and symbols involved in them. (Hongiman 1959:506).

Forms of Healing Rituals

Lieban Richard (1973:1044) has pointed out three types of ethnomedical therapies or healing procedures which include chemotherapy, mechanical and magico-religious therapeutic procedures. Besides employing these therapies depending on the perception of the origin and cause of illness of the patients, indigenous healers use certain chants, prayers, use of patterned sounds, movements, colours, shapes, odors etc. as therapeutic techniques (Roseman 1988:811-818). Roseman further goes to state that, healing performance presents a moment of articulation between two domains of knowledge and action : musical composition, performance and effect on the one hand; indigenous cosmology, illness etiology and the pathogenicity of emotions on the other hand.

Laughlin (1963) states that in many cultures medical practices are often fused with religious practices. Glick (1967) states that even when mechanical or chemical therapy is employed, magico-religious elements may also be an essential part of the prescription, or the treatment may be regarded as incomplete without the attention of mystical factors involved in the etiology of the illness.

Shiloh (1961) describes indigenous Middle Eastern medical beliefs that attribute a burn or a fall from a high place, such as a house top or a tree, to an evil spirit or evil eye. In such cases the bruised or torn flesh is dressed with curative preparations and bandaged, and broken bones are set, but concurrent with such straight forward treatment there will be a search for the evil spirit or evil eye responsible for the accident.

Herbalist surgeons in Ethiopia employ pragmatic means to treat illness, including an elaborate pharmacopoeia but mysticism is often mixed with materia medica, the name of a curative plant may not be said aloud, for instance, because this would enable the spirit causing disease to defend itself against the therapy. (Messing, 1968). In the Philippine's, healers may prescribe a simple decoction of certain plants for illness but the leaves will have been picked from the east side of the plant, because that is the direction in which the sun rises, and the healer may have learned the prescription itself from a spiritual benefactor who conveyed it to him in a dream or vision (Lieban, 1967).

The above studies point out that therapeutic techniques are not merely administration of medicinal herbs and warding off pathogenic agents it is much more than that. There is a lot of symbolism and mysticism involved in ritual healing behaviour and hence therapeutic procedures are fused with ritualized forms of behaviour in order to accomplish a task or a goal that is reflected in the disease etiology other than only healing the patient. Healing rituals hence express and communicate the knowledge of medical symbols and their inter relationship in the light of the cultural system. In this chapter, the interplay of symbolism, ritualized behaviour and therapy of the Thakur ethno-medicine is examined with reference theories of ritual healing and the theory of culture by David Schneider. The data collected on ritual healing of the Thakur medicine has shown following forms of healing rituals which are associated with herbal, mechanical and magico-religious therapies.

A. Rituals Assocaited with Herbal (Chemo) Therapy

Plants, animals, vegetables and minerals with known medicinal properties are found in every eco-climatic regions, from rain forests to deserts. They provide the basic ingredients not only for traditional medicines, but also for climatic derivatives for modern allopathic medicine (Tribhuwan Robin and Peters Pretti 1992:20). The healing properties in plants, vegetables, animals and minerals if viewed at from an etic (scientific) point of view are due to virtues of vitamins, alkaloids, mineral salts, hormones and so on. Contrary to the etic (botanical) approach of studying chemo or herbal therapy, there is a emic (anthropological) approach which defines things are perceived by the natives. The anthropological approach unravels the conceptual and symbolic aspects of herbal or chemo therapy while botanical approach restricts itself to taxonomy, morphology and pharmacology of the medicinal plants.

All the Thakur medical practitioners including Bhagats, Bhagatins, Had vaidus, vaidus, Mantriks, Suines and potdharis follow a culturally accepted pattern of administering medicinal herbs. These ritualized forms of normative behaviour are meaningful and express cosmological and body symbolism conceptions.

i. Rituals or Methods Associated with Collection of Herbs

All the medical practitioners observe certain taboos while performing the ritual of collecting medicinal herbs. They see to it that their shadow does not fall on the plant and face east while collecting it. They believe that the shadow (symbol of death in this context) blocks the life giving rays or healing power of the Sun (the life giver) that is being continuously transmitted to the medicinal plants through the light. Thus the falling of the shadow symbolizes the blockage of healing power from the Sun to the plant as a result of which that plant becomes ineffective.

Before collecting the plant the practitioners utter a prayer to the 'Sun' and also to the plant requesting for its efficacy and quick relief to their patients. Secondly they also believe in treatment with freshly plucked plants. If a plant part is plucked and its medicine is administered after a long time it does not have life and is not effective. The rationale here is that life (fresh plant charmed with divine power) treats an unhealthy body and removes evil from the body.

Medicinal plants collected and administered on Sundays and Saturdays give quick relief. It is believed that 'Sunday' - is the day of Sun God and 'Saturday' - the day of Maruti - the monkey God of medicine. Tuesdays are also considered to be auspicious as it is the day of planetary spirits - Baya (Sisters of Mother Earth).

FLOW CHART VII : 1. DEPICTING SYMBOLIC ASPECTS THAT THE ETHNO-MEDICAL SPECIALISTS ASSOCIATE WITH THE RITUALS OF COLLECTING HERBS

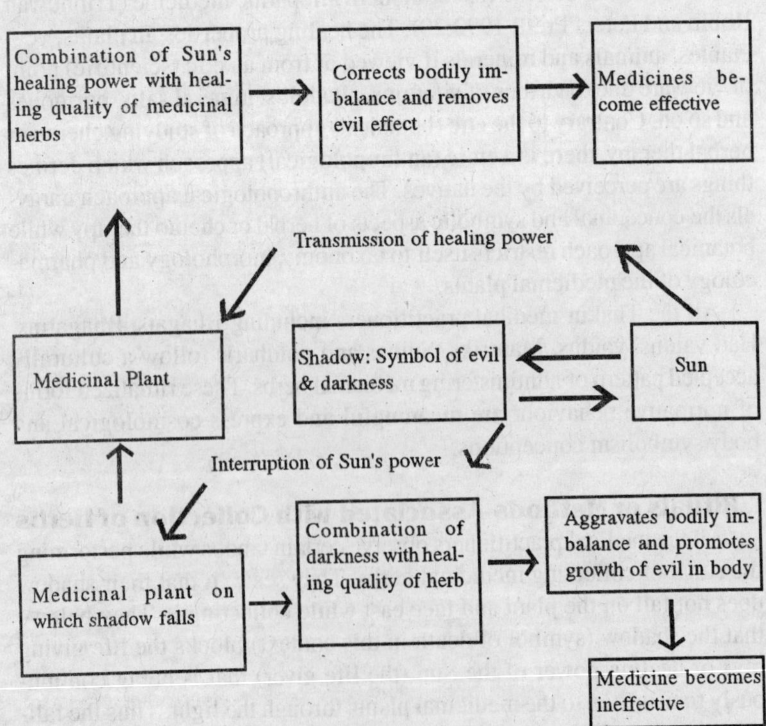

ii. Rituals Or Methods Assocaitde With Preparation Of Medicines

Preparation of medicines also has a lot of meaningful behaviour associated with it. All seven types of medical specialists including Bhagats, Bhagatins, bone setters, herbalists, Mantriks, Suines and potdharis prepare their medicines facing east (the holy direction). They believe that the healing power of Sun should combine with the medicine so as to make it very effective. Whether it is day or night the Thakurs follow strictly the above rule while preparing the medicines. A prayer is also recited while preparing medicines so as to invite the healing power and that it should be kept trapped in the medicine.

iii. Rituals Or Methods Associated with Administration Of Medicines.

Before the medicine is administered all the medical practitioners first face the east and pray to the 'Sun' - the life giver to make the medicine more effective. It is only after this short ritualized behaviour that he/she administers medicine. He then makes the patient also to face east while taking the medicine.

The Thakur symbolism of collection, preparations, administration of medicinal herbs thus highlights 'Sun' - the life giver and healer as the central symbol. Sun's rays have life giving and healing power and when blocked by 'shadow' - darkness/evil, prevents the healing/divine power from combining with the medicinal plants and hence that herb on which the practitioner's shadow falls is believed to be ineffective.

Secondly, the concept that fresh plants should be collected, prepared and administered holds true for the Thakurs. They believe that if a medicinal herb is collected and kept for long time it dies and hence its Ras (essence) looses its medicinal value. Life (fresh medicinal plant) corrects illness (intermediatary stage between life and death). It is therefore very necessary that fresh medicinal plants are administered.

A significant element in an ethnomedical specialist's ability to ritually collect, prepare and administer herbal medicines is to create a symbolic and meaningful situation through culturally recognized normative actions and behaviour, wherein healing entities and forces are called upon to empower the naturally available medicine. Hence the medicinal herb gets a special divine status due to entry of healing power. Medical specialists contribute towards creating a culturally recognized clinical and meaningful reality by setting a stage of healing and drawing the necessary powers and forces to act on the ill-health of the patient and also to remove/fight evil forces the cause illness.

Intrinsic Qualities Of Medicines

Most data by ethnographers on primitive medicines has highlighted documentation of medicinal plants, the parts used and the method of administration. Such descriptions are no doubt valuable as they are, but omit just the points needed for our social enquiry. What are the ideas underlying these therapeutic acts and under what circumstances (with or without ritual) they are performed ? What concepts do the natives hold as far as the intrinsic qualities of the medicines are concerned. Turner Victor (1567 : 343) has pointed out the concepts regarding the intrinsic qualities of medicinal plants used by Ndembu. For instance Cremaspora trifolia is used as a remedy for male sterility and the reason why it is used states the rationale of the natives, "A white medicine, makes semen white". Similarly Afzelia quanzensis, administered as a remedy for stomach disease is taken because "its bitterness kills disease".

The researcher has made maximum efforts to focus on collecting anthropological data on medicines used by the Thakurs than giving it a botanical touch. The charts given below highlight the plant and animal. Sources of medicines used to cure diseases and their rationale for using these medicines.

TABLE VII : 1
MEDICINAL HERBS

S.No.	Botanical Name Local Name	Disease or Disorder	Reason for use Plant part used
1.	Semicarpus anacardium Biba	Migraine	Seed fluid being corrosive helps to rupture forehead Seed skin to let out the spoilt blood.
2.	Solanum xanthocarpum Ran Wange	Tooth decay	Fruits put on charcoal and smoke inhaled through the Fruit mouth. Fruit smoke irrita- tes the worms in the deca-yed tooth & worms are spat out.
3.	Tridax procubens Pala Leaves	Cuts	Leaf extract applied on Dagdi fresh cuts/bruises. Clots blood and cools the cut.
4.	Azadrachta indica Neem Leaves	Scabies	Leaf extract mixed with water is taken orally to kill the worms in the blood. Bitterness kills the disease.
5.	Calotropis gigantea Rui Latex	Abortion	Root paste mixed with coc-onut water kept over night & taken early in the morning. Latex is hot in natu-re & ruptures foetus of 1-3 months.

6.	Dioscorea bulbifora Dudhkand Corm	Breast milk defficiency	Raw corm is eaten to prod- uce breast milk.
7.	Pongamia pinnata Pivli rui Latex	sore-eyes	Latex is applied in eyes to remove heat & redness as latex is believed to be cold in nature.
8.	Carrisaa carandis Karvanda Root	Snake bite	Root chewed & extract swa- llowed to induce vomiting in or der to throw out poi- son.
9.	Vitex negundo Nirgudi Leaves	Swelling	Leaves heated in a pan and tied on the swollen part to disperse the blood clot and relax muscles.
10.	Calotropis procera Pandhari Rui Leaf	Boils	A leaf is tied on the boil. Latex is believed to be hot in nature and hence ruptures the boils.
11.	Musa paradisica Keli Root	Delayed Delivery	Root is put under the neck of a woman to accelerate the process of delivery.
12.	Ficus glomerata Umber Sap	Chicken pox	Filtered latex from roots which symbolizes sperms of Moon is given orally to patient, who symbolizes female spirits of planets.
13.	Ficus glomerata Umber Latex	Fractures	Latex mixed with Ragi pas- te is applied on fractures &tied with bamboo sticks. Latex is be- lieved to join bones.
14.	Plumeria rubra Chapha	To induce sterility	Paste of flowers mixed with 1/2 cup of milk is Flower given to fertile woman to induce sterility. They be- lieve this tree does not bear fruits and hence the woman will not bear a child.
15.	Holarrhena-antidys- entrica Kuda	Diarrhoea	Two spoons of bark powder mixed with water taken twice a day. Bark powder cools digestive system.
16.	Terminellia chebula Hirda Fruit	Cough	Fruits chewed 2-3 times a day to clean phelgm.
17.	Capsicum fruiticens Mirchi Fruit	Evil-eye	Five chillies are ritually revolved around patient to absorb evil-effect & put in fire to be de

			stroyed.
18.	Bauhinia racemosa Shid Leaf	Arthrities	Tobacco wrapped in shid leaf is smoked to transfer heat to painful parts of joints and to remove the cold air present in there.
19.	Tectona grandis Sagwan Leaves	Wounds	Ash of tectona leaves is mixed in chicken fat oil & applied on wounds. It is believed to kill the germs.
20.	Butea frandosa Palas Flowers	Kidney stone	Flowers heated and tied on the belly of a patient su- ffering from kidney stone. This remedy dis solves the stone naturally.

The Thakurs classify the intrinsic qualities of plants into two major categories.

1. Natural Qualities :-

They believe that medicinal plants have certain intrinsic qualities such as hot, cold, bitter, healing, sweet, sour, pungent and so on which are responsible for healing diseases. For example ailments such as Arthritis, cough, cold are believed to be caused due to entry of cold air/water in the body. This imbalance is then corrected by administering medicinal plants having hot qualities or hot diet is recommended. Another instance where scabies is believed to be caused due to growth of worms in the blood. To correct this imbalance "bitter juice" of Neem (Azadrachta indica) is taken to kill the worms. There are many instances, but I am reporting only few here.

2. Supernatural Qualities :-

Certain plants are interpreted in the Thakur culture and are believed to have supernatural powers to cleanse impurity and ward off evil or evil effect. For example chillies are used to ward off evil-eye effect. Chilly in this situation symbolizes fire (hotness) which destroys the evil effect casted on the patient.

Besides the use of different medicinal herbs to treat diseases the Thakurs also use medicines prepared from the different bodily parts of the animals. The kathkari tribe makes maximum use of medical extracts from animal sources (Tribhuwan Robin & others 1993). The chart given below explains the Thakur conception of the intrinsic qualities of animal sources of medicines.

TABLE VII : 2
ANIMAL SOURCES OF MEDICINE

S.No.	Animal Local Name	Disease or Disorder	Reason for use Part used
1.	Mongoose Mungus Skin	Spirit Possession	The skin of Mongoose tied in a cloth and is worn on the arm to ward off evil spirit.Mongoose has destr-uctive powers.
2.	Mongoose Mungus Hair	Asthma	The hair of mongoose are burnt. Its ash is mixed with Jaggery syrup and taken twice a day as a remedy for Asthma.Hair has a heal ing quality to heal lungs.
3.	Cat Manjar Teeth	Rat bite	Powder of cats teeth mixed with pongamia pinnata seed oil is applied on wounds caused by rat bites. They believe rat's poison is absorbed by cat's teeth powder.
4.	Tortoise Kasav Blood	Asthma	A tea spoon of freshly extracted blood of tortoise is taken as a remedy for Asthma. Blood is be lieved to be hot in nature.
5.	Hen Kombdi Anus	Burns/wounds	Oil extracted from the anus of hen is applied on burns and wounds. It has a cool-ing and healing effect acc -ording to Thakurs.
6.	Hen (alive) Kombdi	Snake Bite	A live Hen's anus is placed on the part bitten Anus by snake to pull out the poison.
7.	Bat Vatwaghul Entire body	Asthma	Fatty precipitate prepared from bat's body is taken for asthma. It clears out the cold in the lungs.
8.	Monitor Ghorpad Fat	Joint pain	Oil extracted from Monitor fat is used for massaging joint pains. The heat in the oil removes cold ness in the joints.
9.	Goat Bakri Milk	Sore-eyes	4 - 5 drops of Goat's milk is put in the eyes. It is believed to give be lieved to give cooling effect and cleanses eyes.
10.	Cow	Chicken pox	Cow's urine is holy and is used to

	Guy Urine		purify a patient suffering from chicken pox. It is applied exter-nally.
11.	Fox Kolha Skin	Facial Paralysis	A cap made out of fox skin is worn by a paralysis patient. Face gets its original form. Skin is hot and corrects the imbalance of air in the face.
12.	Tortoise Kasav Head	Piles	Tortoise head is placed on the affected part.Its head which goes in and comes out of the shell is compa- red to the tip of anus.
13.	Wild dove Parva Meat	Asthma	Wild dove's meat is consu- med as a remedy for Asthma Asthma is believed to be caused due to presence of cold air in lungs. Meat is hot in nature and helps to remove this air.
14.	Deer Becker Horn	Swellings & Sprains	Horn paste mixed with alum is applied on swellings.It disperses the clotted blood in the swellings.
15.	Peacock More Claws	Ear ache	Oil extracted from peacock claws through filtration technique is used to cure ear ache.
16.	Cow Guy Dung	Evil-eye	Cow dung is used to ritua- lly absorb evil-eye effect
17.	Wild Boar Ran Dukkar Tooth	Evil spirits	Tooth of a wild boar is always kept to ward off evil spirits.

Mechanical Therapies

Mechanical therapies include bone setting, massaging, blood letting, attending delayed deliveries, removing guinea worms, abortions, removing unwanted substances from the body etc. The table given below explains the Thakur perception of mechanically employed therapeutic actions and concepts associated with it.

TABLE VII : 3
CONCEPTS OF MECHANICAL THERAPIES

S No.	Disease Local Name	Concepts of Therapeutic Actions
1.	Migraine	Migraine is believed to be caused due to accumula

	Arshi	tion of spoilt blood in the forehead.To remove the spoilt blood the petiole of mango leaf is thrust heard into the nostril of the affected side and let the blood flow out. Thakurs also use the seed fluid of semi car pus anacardium to let the blood out.
2.	Guinea Worms Naru	A small stick piece is used to roll the guinea worm out of the body.
3.	Bleeding Rakta Vahane	To prevent bleeding, cold water is quickly applied to a cut.
4.	Scorpion sting Inchu chavne	A Mantrik sucks out the poison using his mouth. In case the patient is frightened the Mantrik fetches water in a metal pot and splashes it five times on the face of the patient ritually by using healing chants.
5.	Cobra bite	The anus of a hen is placed on the Nag chavne poison. Then a medicinal herb is given.
6.	Cholostrom milk Naska dudh	Cholostrom milk is considered to be spoilt, since it is thick in nature it can not be digested by the child. Child gets loose motions. Therefore, cholostrom milk is squeezed out for 3-5 days. They believe that it becomes thick because of the spermatic effect and the presence of menstrual blood which is converted into cholostrom milk during the period of nine months of pregnancy.
7.	Abortion Garbha padne	Fresh twig of calotropis gigantia tied to a string is inserted into the uterus to abort a child. The latex of calotropis is believed to be hot in nature and ruptures the foetus.
8.	Prolonged wounds Zakham	Prolonged wounds are believed to be results of intrusion of millets, bone, or some objects using witch craft techniques. These objects are removed by the Bhagat (Shaman), by cutting the wound open to trace the object causing suffering to his patient.
9.	Delayed delivery Lambavaleli Koni	Deliveries are delayed because the midwife or the family concerned have deviated from the divine norms of 'Satvai' (Goddess of fertility - mother earth) In such case mud (earth) is charmed and put on the forehead of the delivering woman.
10.	Swellings Suj	Swelling according to Thakurs are results of blood clotting in a part- icular place.To disperse, this blood massage techniques using medicated oils are employed.
11.	Arthritis	Arthritis is believed to be caused due to presence

	Vat	of cold air in a painful joint. To remove this cold air an iron rod is heated and gently touched on the painful part. This technique of branding is popularly known as 'Chocha dene'.
12.	Evil eye Drishti Lagne	The effect of evileye is mechanically and magically removed using five chillies and salt by revolving it five times around the patient to absorb evil effect and then putting it in fire to be destroyed.
13.	Albinism Munjache por	An albino is believed to be an off-spring of a white male evil spirit namely 'Munja'. Whatever is product of evil must not exist in good (human society). Therefore the albino children are killed by choking their neck and buried in an inverted fashion to be sent to the world of evil spirits.
14.	Congenital Deformities Knaisache por	Congenitally deformed children are also considered to be off-springs of another male evil spirit namely 'Khais' which are also killed and bur ied to be sent to the world of evil spirits. If it grows in human societies it may cause harm to Thakurs.
15.	Menstrual blood of a new mother Koni baicha Veetal	Menstrual blood does not come out for nine months during pregnancy After delivery the woman's belly is pressed to remove the blood. Menstrual blood is believed to be evil and can cause health prob lems to the mother such as thickening of breast milk etc. It is hence removed out of the body.

Ritual Healing

Ritual healing has been defined as 'those culturally prescribed normative therapeutic actions and/or ritualized forms of behaviour of ethnomedical specialists, patient, family and/or village elders and other participants, historically designed in order to compromise with the pathogenic agents (social, natural, spiritual, supernatural, ancestral and cosmological) so as to reorder or bring about harmony of the disrupted cultural disorder, there by restoring the health of the patient.

Healing rituals or therapeutic actions are performed depending on the community's notion of the origin and cause of illness. Thus what is diagnosed to have been caused spiritually is treated spiritually by Shamans. Presentations of disease etiology is a pre-requisite to creating a symbolic stage or situation to proceed with the concerned healing ritual. The Shamans have a standard list of pathogenic agents who cause illness (ref case study of Bhagat in Chapter VI).

Classification of Healing Rituals

All the seven types of medical practitioners and the elderly people classify three categories of healing rituals and these are as follows -

1. Ritual of Inviting Healing Forces : Dev Mantra

The ritual of Inviting Healing forces (Dev Mantra) includes setting up of a divine stage, the cleansing of the Shaman (Bhagat/Bhagatin) by bathing or having a wash, lighting an incense stick, bringing holy objects like metal pot, ash, water etc. and after having set the stage reciting a prayer to Lord 'Sun' to send his healing power into the Bhagat and in to the healing objects and give the Bhagat the ability to diagnose, the healing, origin and cause of illness. The 'Dev mantra ritual' differs from practitioner to practitioner. For instance, the Bhagat and Bhagatin (Shamans) perform complex rituals wherein the degree of ritualized and symbolic forms of actions are greater than those used by mid-wives, bone setters, herbalists etc. who only recite prayer to ask either 'Sun', mother earth or village god to help them treat their patient successfully.This is a stage where physical objects and social situations, or contexts get a meaningful reality.

2. Ritual of Diagnosis : Nadiche Mantra

The diagnosis ritual is performed to identify pathogenic agents responsible for causing illness or bringing about misfortune. Bhagats (male Shamans) use metal pot, filled with water. A pinch of ash is added in it. The metal pot is then spun on some ash in a clockwise movement chanting the diagnosis rite (nadiche mántra : refer Bhagat's case study in Chapter VI) in order to trace the originator of illness. The Bhagat faces east (holy direction) while the rite is being performed. He utters the names of 24 major pathogenic agents, out of which one of them could have caused the illness. The spinning metal pot stands still at the name of pathogenic agent which has caused the illness.

Meanings of Diagnosis rite

The meaning of these actions and objects used in a diagnostic rite are as follows -

1. Metal Pot - symbolizes the patient's 'soul' (atma) which is believed to be possessed by good or evil forces.
2. Pouring water - in the pot symbolizes integrating 'water' (holy element) with the troubled atma or soul.
3. Putting ash - Ash symbolizes "Sun's body" (fire element).
4. Bhagat facing the east - East is believed to be a holy direction, because 'Sun' the creator of life and healer comes up from there. The Bhagat gets knowledge and wisdom to diagnose the cause from east.
4. Reciting the names of 24 major pathogenic agents which could be

natural, cosmological, social, spiritual, supernatural and ancestral is itself a proof that illness is an expression of disharmony or disruption of man's relationship with the above said pathogenic agents.

5. Anticlock movement of metal pot - Anticlockwise movement is believed to be auspicious because that is the movement of the cosmological, spiritual, supernatural and natural forces. The movement of blood, water, air, heat and light in the body is believed to be anticlockwise. Sound health is symbolic of anticlockwise movement of body substances and element. Clockwise is symbolic of ill-health. The clockwise movement of metal pot symbolizes illness of the patient, some thing goes wrong, the metal pot is spun in a wrong way (clockwise) and not the right way (anticlockwise).
6. The entire set of actions performed by the Bhagat during the diagnosis rite are meaningful and cross cut into other domains of Thakur culture.

In case of a Bhagatin (female Shaman), while she is in trance, during the diagnosis rite she leaves her hair open and moves her head in clockwise manner. This movement again symbolizes the cultural disorder, that some thing has gone wrong some where. This wrong is expressed through the illness of a patient. She gets the power from planetary spirits (Baya - sisters of mother Earth) and also from mother earth (Dantari). Diagnosis rite hence aims to uncover the distorted or disrupted cultural order which is patched up through the ritual healing.

3. Therapeutic Ritual : Ibut Mantra

After having traced the origin and cause of illness the members of theThakur family and/or community prepare themselves to compromise with pathogenic agents, appease them, satisfy them, praise them, ask pardon for deviant behaviour or administer medicine to the patient. The therapeutic ritual or Ibut Mantra, comprises of other sub-rituals that are culturally prescribed and vary depending on the perceived origin and cause of illness.

a. Rituals of appeasing

Diseases such as chicken pox, measles, body sores, boils etc. are believed to be caused due to visitation of the 'Baya' (sister of mother earth - planetary spirits). They dwell in the body of the patient for 7-14 days. Baya are not evil spirits. They are good spirits and visit human beings to check their behaviour in case of deviance. They enter the human body in the form of hot air which burns blood and ruptures skin as a result of which body sores are formed. In such situations the 'Baya' are appeased, worshipped and praised by setting up a 'Ghat' and are requested to leave the patient. Appeasing the Baya is not a responsibility of the patient or his family members but the entire village. During the visitation of Baya a patient's body gets a divine status and he/she is well cared for.

b. Rituals of Compromise

Certain diseases in a particular cultural context are believed to have been caused by certain pathogenic agents who demand offerings from patients. The midwives often said that deliveries of some woman get delayed because of intervention of 'Munja' (evil spirit). He delays the delivery. In such case themidwife enquires from him his demands. He is then promised a cock sacrifice or a coconut. Sometimes mother earth delays the delivery. She is also promised a coconut. Some times children fall sick as a result of wrath of ancestral spirits. If the souls of grandparents are not given food on pitra Amosha they bring about misfortune and illness. To treat the patient the Bhagat first compromises with ancestral spirits (Virdev and Supali) (refer episode no 23).

c. Rituals of warding off pathogenic agents and/or evil effect

Both male and female Shamans perform the rituals of warding off evil pathogenic agents and evil effect cast through evil eye. When a patient is possessed with an evil spirit the Bhagat ritually whips the evil spirit out or commands him with authority to leave the patient. (refer episode no 15). Similarly a Bhagatin while she is in a trance she very tightly holds the hair of the patient possessed with the evil spirit and slaps him and commands the spirit to leave the patient.

Certain rituals are performed by the Thakurs at home to ward off evil effect. Five chillies are spun in a clockwise movement over a patient who becomes a victim of evil eye. These chillies along with some salt are thrown in the fire. Chillies absorb evil and this evil (effect of evil eye) is destroyed by fire in the hearth. (Refer episode no. :18).

There is also a very common belief among the Thakurs that witches and/or sorcerers (Bhutali and Bhutala) introduce certain objects into the body of their enemies due to envy or jealousy. The Bhagats ritually diagnose and then remove these objects from the body of their patients.

Rituals of Killing Pathogenic Agents :

Albinos and congenitally deformed children are believed to be the off springs of munja and khais (Male evil spirits). These children are killed by the midwives and buried in the sun. The logic behind this behaviour is what is produced by a evil spirit must go back to the world of spirits and cannot grow in the human society. It is therefore killed, by choking its neck or by covering it with a basket smeared with cowdung using suffocation method. (Refer episode no. : 1).

e. Rituals Of Purification :

Menstrual blood is believed to be a pollutant, evil, impure and hot in nature. It causes disease if a man or a woman comes in contact with a menstruating woman. Thus for five days a menstruating woman is socially discarded from her social system. She does not cook nor work nor interact with anyone not even with her husband. Food cooked by her if consumed causes leprosy. On the fifth day she goes to the river, cleanses herself by taking a bath. She washes her clothes. She then turns to the east bows down to the sun. Before interacting with anyone in the house she lights an incense stick. Menstruation according to the Thakurs is illness of impurity and calls for purification after its scheduled period.

f. Rituals of Collecting, Preparing and Administering Medicinal Herbs :

Patients with only physical problems such as cuts, wounds, fractures, stomach ache, diarrhoea etc are treated by using medicinal herbs or medicines extracted from animals. Even the collection, preparation and administration of medicines is ritualized because of the essence of meanings associated with this behaviour. (Refer Case studies of medical practitioners in Chapter VI).

4. Rituals of Prevention :

The belief that both good and evil forces cause illness, is part of medical system of Thakurs. These pathogenic agents could be natural, social, spiritual, supernatural, cosmological and ancestral. The Thakur society is a very insecure society - politically and economically with no social support from the other social groups. There has been too much exploitation from the 'Devjatis' - the upper caste (who help the Thakur in times of trouble but in return extract maximum). It is because of this feeling of insecurity perhaps the Thakurs take their problems at a spiritual level to be solved.

They classify over 24 pathogenic agents that cause illness due to various reasons such as failure to perform a divine duty or rite,a taboo and so on. Thakurs are aware that they must not deviate from the culturally accepted norms of behaviour. Thus many rituals of prevention are performed. For instance a goat is sacrificed by every Thakur village once a year to the village God (gaondev) to protect their health. A lime with five chillies is hung on the door post to ward off evil effect. The clan God, ancestral spirits, cosmic entities and other deities are appeased from time to time so as to avoid their wrath. Burial of the umbilical chord is yet another example of preventive ritual. It is buried so that it does not become a magical device to harm the child or mother.

5. Rituals of Thanksgiving :

The entire process of ritual healing ends with a smali ritual of thanking the originator or curer of illness. The originator of the cause is either given a coconut, a sacrifice or grains in appreciation for freeing the patient from illness. The curers (ethnomedical practitioners) are either offered a feast along with a drink and sometimes clothes. Midwives and potdharis are paid in cash.

Role Of Numbers In Healing :

Symbolism of certain numbers is an important phenomena observed in Thakur ritual healing. No's 5, 10 and 7 are often recited or referred to or used in ritual healing. All the above said numbers have symbolic function in ritual healing.

Number **'ten'** in some situations refers to the ten cosmic planets, or ten bodily openings (Daha darwaje), or ten small heaps of rice during the training period of a student shaman. Number ten is also used in death ritual, when ten rice flour balls are prepared and left into the river to merge with the cosmos. These ten rice balls symbolize the ten spirits that dwell in the human body. Thus number ten is associated with health differently in different contexts. For instance when the 'Baya' (planetary spirits) visit human body (by causing chicken pox) they enter through the ten doors of the body (Ref page 31).

Number Five :-

Number five is the most important number in the ritual healing because the Thakurs classify hierachially the bodily openings into ten, and the fifth one is the 'Soul' (atma). In the cosmic hierarchy mother earth is positioned at fifth place. Atma is a symbol of life. Whenever illness occurs the 'Atma' or 'soul' gets disturbed. Hence rituals of diagnosis, cater to warding off the good or evil spirit which takes charge of the Atma.

The metal pot (tambya) is a symbol of the patient's atma which is spun by Bhagat, (all five directions i.e. North, South, East and West and sky) to detect the pathogenic agents that cause illness. Then therapeutic actions are performed ritually to drive away, or appease the evil or good effect in the atma. For example when a person is possessed with evil spirit a Bhagat whips the patient five times. Five because 'atma' or 'soul' is situated on the fifth place in the bodily opening hierarchy. It is only when the fifth whip is struck the evil spirit leaves the patient's atma.

Similarly when a person is bitten by snake a mantrik ritually removes the poison from the 'atma' (soul) by splashing water fetched from the well in a metal pot, on the face of the patient five times. Water here symbolizes purifier which cleanses poison from the 'soul' (atma). If a patient's is tried by splashing water only trice or four times the therapy will never work. Because both Mantrik and patient share the same belief that 'atma' is situated on the fifth position in bodily hierarchy and needs to be cleansed. There are other instances of number five in health beliefs of Thakurs. Water in this context becomes a symbol of purification.

On the fifth day after the birth of a child a ritual of 'panchvi punjan' is performed by the midwife. This is performed in order to offer the child to Mother earth (Satvai - Goddess of fertility and fortune). Mother earth takes the form of an animal, bird or insect to visit the child and write his/her fortune and life span on the forehead. Again there is use of number five to perform this ritual.

Another instance where number five is used is in warding off evil eye. Women of the Thakur tribe take five chillies revolve it five times around a patient in clockwise manner to absorb the evil effect into the chillies and throw it in the fire to be destroyed. The reference of five in this context again is symbolic of the 'atma' - soul that unseen force which is attacked by evil effect. Chillies in this context become a symbol of absorption of evil effect. Fire becomes a symbol of destruction. Thus when we analyze the objects and actions of this ritual it is symbolic of following explanation according to Thakurs.

A. 5 chillies - symbolic a medium of absorption of evil effect. B. 5 times revolving chillies around patient - symbolizes the action of absorbing evil effect from patient's atma onto the chillies . The atma is situated on the fifth place.C. Action of throwing the chillies in fire - symbolizes transferring of evil effect which is absorbed in chillies into the fire.

D. Fire - is a symbol of destruction of evil effect in this context.

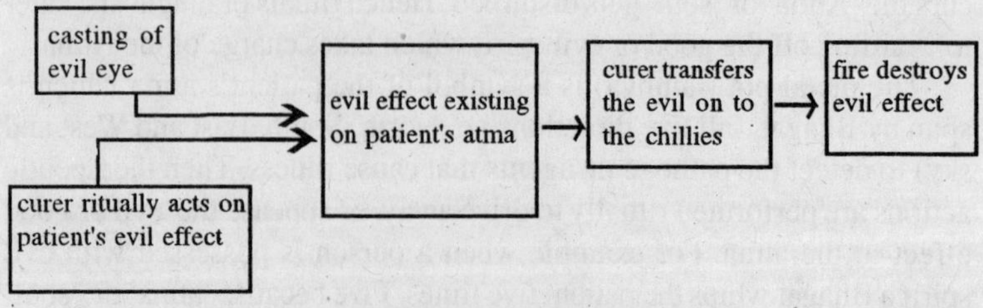

Similarly a ritual popularly known as ritual of 'pani ghalne' - meaning to pour water is performed on the fifth day during a patient's illness who is suffering from chicken pox. Chicken pox is believed to be caused by the female planetary spirits (Baya). These female spirits are virgins. Their sister mother earth (Dantari) has a husband. Baya do not have. They express their desire to have sex with the moon. On the fifth day watery sap is collected over night from the root of Ficus glomerata and is given to the patient on the fifth day. The tree is worshipped before cutting its roots for sap. It is believed that the Baya are satisfied. On making the Thakurs analyze this ritual's meaning. They explained it as follows.

a. Chicken pox patient - is a symbol of virgin 'Baya' - female planetary spirits.
b. Ficus glomerata - is a symbol of moon.
c. Watery sap which is white in colour - symbolizes the semen of moon.
d. Administration of watery sap to patient - symbolizes the sexual intercourse of moon with Baya.
c. Assimilation of the watery sap by patient - symbolizes the sexual satisfaction of Baya.
f. Administration of watery sap on fifth day - symbolizes satisfying the Baya which dwell in patient's atma (5th position).
g. Pani ghalne ritual - pani - refers to moon's semen and ghalne refers to put into.

The ritual of pani ghalne is in itself an expression of the relationship of cosmic entities (in this case the moon and Baya). The sexual frustration which arouses in the female planetary spirits (Baya) is symbolically brought into play at the social level where Ficus glomerata tree (male tree) symbolizes the moon, while the patient's body symbolizes the 'Baya'. Drinking of the root sap by the patient is symbolic of releasing the semen of the moon in order to satisfy the Baya.

Role of "Panch Amrut" - Fluids of purification

During the 'Jagran' ceremony - i.e. while singing songs of praise to appease the Baya (planetary spirits) to leave the patient. Any person who enters the house where 'Jagran' ceremony is being performed, the owner of the house sprinkles 'Panch Amrut' - a solution comprising of five fluids namely milk, honey, cows urine, coconut milk and water. These five fluids purify the atma (Soul) of the participant before he participates in the ritual. Again the use of number five, because atma is situated on the fifth place in the hierarchy of body openings.

Turner (1967:50) has emphasized the polysemic nature of the ritual symbols, with different meanings of the same symbol becoming paramount in different contexts. This polysemy is an obvious quality of symbols used in the healing rituals of the Thakurs. For instance, 'water' in one context such as this is a symbol of purification where as else where it becomes a symbol of 'absorption' of evil effect and in some other context it becomes a 'divine' symbol where in Thakurs associate water as the brother of 'Sun' - creator.

Contrary to Victor Turners views on polysemy of symbols, the Thakur ritual symbols also show that within a given context many symbol have same meaning. FOr instance, 'Panch Amrut' - combination of honey, milk, water, coconut milk and cow's urine all of them are symbolic of purification. There isyet another phenomena observed about symbols in Thakur ritual healing is that a symbol in a given context means many things. For instance 'Albino child' which is believed to be off spring of 'Munja' - male evil spirit is killed by the Suine. The Thakurs attribute many meanings to albinism -

ALBINISM
- Off Spring of evil spirits
- Symbolizes body deformity
- Symbol of evil world
- Sexual harassment of male evil spirits of other castes and tribes

Five Cosmic Entities and Human Body

Thakurs classify five cosmic entities in the order of divine beings in their hierarchy of Gods and Goddesses -

1. Sun } As the source of light, heat and fire for
2. Moon } sustenance of body and soul.
3. Water - from clouds and earth which contribute to form blood, breast milk, semen etc.
4. Wind - from the cosmos helps in physiological process of the body.
5. Earth - gives food and water for bodily growth.

The Thakurs believe that imbalance in the bodily heat, light, fire, wind, water etc. causes illness. Body should be able to balance the exact proportion of the above elements. Any changes occurring in atmosphere according to Thakurs has an effect on the human body. For instance during the solar eclipse most Thakurs especially medical practitioners, pregnant women and adults fast. They do not eat food on solar eclipse, because sun is blocked by a 'Black evil entity' and therefore cannot emit life giving light, fire or heat to life on earth. The effect of darkness pollutes food and water on earth and therefore food is not consumed.

Thus the cosmic entities namely, sun, moon, wind, water, earth and Baya are closely associated with human body and health. Their reference in ritual healing is very frequent, I would stress that their discussion is central theme of ritual healing, because these forces or entities are often referred or associated with preventive, promotive, curative, and even destructive aspects of health are concerned.

Role of No. Seven

Number seven has been referred to as an auspicious or very lucky number in the Bible. Its reference is associated in Genesis Chapter to creation of Universe in 7 days. God, the father rested on 7th day and sanctified it. In revelation chapter, No. 7 has been referred in many instances. Number 786 is believed to be very lucky by Muslims.

Contrary to the Christian belief, Thakurs consider the number seven to be an unauspicious one. It is a symbol of evil, trouble, ill-health, danger and so on. Thakur sorcerers and witches take a cloth and make 7 knots and magically transfer evil power in it. It is believed if any person crosses it he or she falls sick. Misfortune or trouble is termed by the Thakurs as 'Sade sati'. Illness caused due to wrath of Satvai (Mother Earth) is termed as 'sati' - meaning seven. Medical specialists revealed that the sorcerers and witches always use No. 7 while performing rituals of destruction. For example, a Bhagat said that a sorcerer takes a lime and pricks seven thorns thereby hurting his opponent. The lime in this context symbolizes the soul of the victim, and the seven thorns the hurting spells. This ritual is known Muth marne. Thus No. 5, 7, 10 are meaningful and play an important role in order to fulfill the purpose or aim of the ritual.

Purpose of ritual healing

The basic purpose in performing healing rituals is to restore a patient's health. In doing so a number of goals as mentioned below are achieved through ritual healing. Symbolism of the purpose/goal of ritual healing lies in disease etiology.

The analysis of Thakur ritual healing shows following classification of the purposes or goal involved in performing healing rites.

1. Diagnosis or identification of the originator of illness.
2. To resolve social, religious, political, cosmological, ancestral, spiritual etc. conflict at spirit level.
3. To appease Gods, Goddesses, supernatural forces, ancestral spirits etc. in order that they lessen a patient's trouble or prevent their wrath from falling on a village.
4. Rituals of healing are performed to ward off
   a. evil spirits
   b. evil effect

c. evil eye
d. spirits of evil animals eg. fox
e. to remove evil objects from the body

5. To purify pollutant bodies, eg. menstruating women, women who are victims of sexual intercourse with evil spirits.
6. To balance the lost bodily equilibrium.
7. To satisfy and fulfill the demands of pathogenic agents.
8. To compromise with pathogenic agents both good andevil regarding social deviance or wrong doings.
9. In order to meet basic needs such as buying clothes, ornaments, eating good food during the state of ill health.
10. Ritual healing also calls for social gatherings to sing praises to the life givers.
11. To reconstruct the disrupted harmony or relationship and order with social, natural, spiritual, cosmological, ancestral and supernatural entities and forces.
12. To prevent misfortunes, troubles and sickness by performing rites of prevention.
13. Finally to tune one's health with the cosmos.
14. To absorb and neutralize the evil effect through symbols (objects, actions, chants etc.) having power of absorption.

As regards to the various stages or procedures through which a sick person passes during the process of ritual healing is highlighted in the second section of this chapter - 'Ethnomedical pathway - a Conceptual model'.

Ethnomedical Pathway : A Conceptual Model

The Model

The major structural components of any ethnomedical system are : disease classification, etiological categories, ethnomedical specialists, their nature and role, forms of therapies and preventive measures (Lieban 1973:1043-47; Foster G.M. 1981:18-21; Fabrega 1977:201-28).

The above mentioned structural components are symbolically and meaningfully inter-related within their own cultural frame of reference. These structural components are evident in a rationalized sequential mode of treating a patient, depending on the community's notions of the origin and cure of illness.

A patient thus passes through the various phases of culturally constructed clinically meaningful reality, in order to get cured. Participant actors such as family heads, village elders, relatives and medical specialists thereby play situational role in the healing process in order to restore

FLOW CHART VII : 3 ETHNOMEDICAL PATHWAY : A CONCEPTUAL MODEL

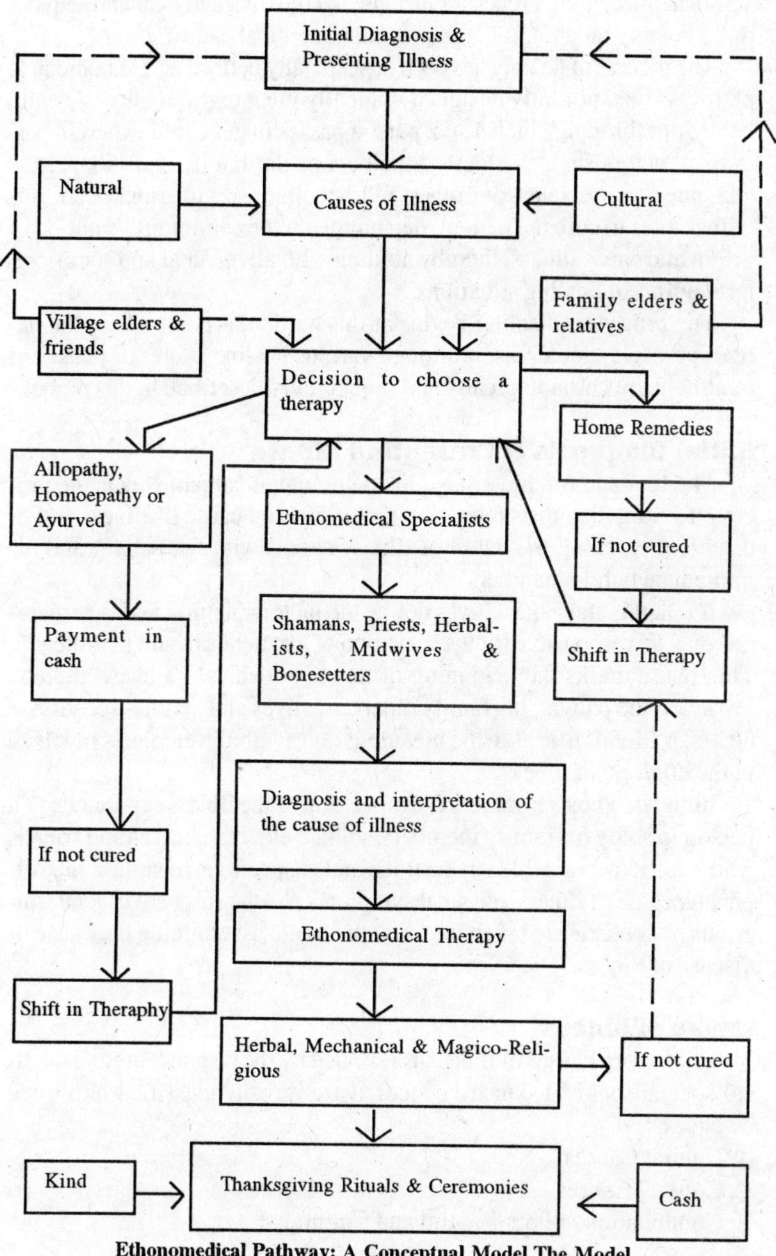

Ethonomedical Pathway: A Conceptual Model The Model

the health of the patient.

It is in this regard the model throws light on the various processes of healing attended upon the sick person. It highlights as to how participant actors in the healing process contribute to construct a logical and sequential clinically meaningful reality or Ethnomedical pathway.

The process of healing has been conceptually defined as 'Ethnomedical pathway' i.e. culturally designed clinically meaningful reality of health behaviour through which a sick person passes to get cured, wherein participant actors such as elderly members of the family and village, the ethnomedical specialists and others follow culture-specific ritualized forms of therapies to cure the patient, depending on the community's notion of origin and cause illness, thereby abiding with all medical and socio-cultural norms of healing situations.

The process of healing begins at this particular point where the natives perceive that a person through various healing stages or phases of treatment are chronologically and sequentially described in this model.

Initial Diagnosis & Presenting Illness

The first and foremost stage in an ethnomedical pathway is the process if initial diagnosis regarding the origin and cause of illness and/or disease. Searching the cause of illness begins with the patient and his immediate family members.

It is at this stage the natives define the factors (natural and supernatural) that are responsible for the transition of a patient's health to ill-health. This phase marks the beginning of an ethnomedical pathway, thereby involving the patient, his family elders, relatives and at times the village elders or friends to search the meanings and symbolic elements involved in the etiology of illness.

Initial diagnosis involves an explanation of the illness experience of a person to study his family members, village elders, relatives and friends who contribute valuable suggestions and suspections regarding the origin and cause of illness, physical symptoms and the suspected social situations or contexts are taken into account while ascertaining the cause of disease of illness.

Cause of Illness

Etiology or causes of illness as revealed by the respondents and medical specialists of Thakur tribe studied are broadly classified into three categories :

1. Natural Causes
2. Cultural Causes
3. Combination of both Natural and Cultural

1. Natural Cause

Of diseases are the influence of environmental factors such as heat, cold, diet, wind, accidents, etc. which upset the bodily humours and equilibriums. The excess and/or less influence of the above mentioned environmental factors affect the human health. Thus ailments such as cold, cough, arthritis are attributed to have been caused by excess influence of cold substance or winds by the Thakurs and the Kathkaris. In such case the therapies always comprise of hot foods and/or medicinal herbs.

What is perceived to have been caused due to cold substances or cold environmental factors is treated with hot foods and remedies or therapeutic procedures. So is the case with what is perceived to have caused due to hot substances or hot environmental factors is treated with cold foods and remedies of therapeutic procedures.

The data showed that minor ailments such as cold, cough, head-ache, migraine, asthma, cuts, wounds, sprains, fractures, burns, dysentery, diarrhoea, scabies, fever etc. may be categorized as having been caused due to environmental factors.

2. Cultural Causes of the illness

May be defined as those causes perceived or attributed to the intervention of culturally recognized supernatural, spiritual and magical pathogenic agents. Foster G.M. 1983:19, has pointed out that 'in ethnomedical accounts causes of illness are commonly described as magical or supernatural in contrast to natural.'

Thus illness caused by angry deities, ghosts, ancestors, witches, sorcerers, etc. falls into the second category, while those caused due to upset in the body humours and consequently loss of body equilibriums fall into the first category (Natural causes).

The cultural causes of illness and disease as Thakur tribe studied are classified as follows :

1. Sexual intercourse with menstruating women
2. Disruption of human relationship with cosmic entities and forces
3. Possession of evil spirits
4. Sexual intercourse with spirits
5. Evil Eye
6. Witchcraft and sorcery
7. Breach of taboo or failure to perform divine duties
8. Disruption of human relationship with ancestral spirits
9. Deviance from culturally set norms and order of house construction or design
10. Breach of social pollution taboos.
11. Disruption of the relationship of Thakurs with other tribes and caste groups.

12. Disruption of man's relationship with flora and fauna.
13. Disruption of man's relationship with his deities.

Beliefs, understandings, perceptions and comprehension regarding the origin and cause of illness and the supernatural agents such as deities, ancestral spirits, ghosts, etc. that cause illness however show inter-cultural variation.

For instance the Thakurs believe that there are three types of evil spirits that exist namely, Khais, Munja and Hadeli which cause illness. (Chaphekar 1960:89), while Warlis believe that Pisha (an evil spirit moving in the jungle) is responsible for causing illness (Tribhuwan Robin 1988:30).

3. Combination of Cultural and Natural elements in the origin and cause of illness

Besides natural and supernatural categories of the causes of illness, there is yet another category which combines both natural and supernatural elements in the origin and cause illness. Hence therapies employed by the medical practitioners or family elders (in case of home remedies) is often a combination of two therapies.

Therapeutic procedures or medical practices are often fused with magico-religious activities. Thus even when mechanical or chemical therapy is employed, magico-religious elements may also be essential part of the prescription, or the treatment may be regarded as incomplete without the attention of mystical factors involved in the etiology of the illness (Glick 1967; Lieban 1967; Messing 1968; Lieban 1973).

Illness experiences which have the combination of the natural and supernatural elements in the origin and cause of illness are treated in combined therapeutic fashion. Thus Budhya Katwara, aged 26, a member of the Thakur tribe, resident of Thakur wadi, kashele village, Karjat Tehsil, Raigad District got right arm fractured. He was immediately rushed to a local bone setter of Nalde wadi. The bone setter gave herbal as well as mechanical therapy to Budhya and set his fractured bone.

That evening Budhya had high fever. He did not havehis dinner. The fever was there for three-four days. Kamli, his mother then consulted a Bhagatin from Kotimba village. When she got into a trance and diagnosed the Budhya was possessed by an evil spirit. She interpreted that Budhya was cutting wood of a Banyan tree on which dwells the Khais (a male evil spirit).

The day he got fractured was an 'Amosha' evening (new moon evening) during which the evil spirits are active. She gave Kamli the holy ash and instructed her to put it on Budhya's forehead and after having done this a black coloured cock was given to the evil spirit in order to leave Budhya. Thus natural and cultural causes in this case were combined.

Decision To Choose Therapy

Therapy in ethnomedicine ranges from home remedies to herbal, mechanical and magico-religious provided by the medical specialists. Besides culturally recognized therapeutic procedures and practices, there are other forms of therapies such as homeopathy, allopathy, ayurvedic and so on, which are also employed during the course of treatment especially when there is a shift from one therapy to another. When herbal therapy is found to ineffective the patient may shift to allopathy, homeopathy or magico-religious or any other form of therapy to get cured. So is the case with other therapies which are employed initially may later be ineffective.

Once the processes which involves classifying the origin and cause of illness and identifying the pathogenic agents and forces associated with it. The natives then decide on choosing a therapist, a home remedy and any other form of therapy which may include allopathy, homeopathy, ayurved and so on.

The decision makers who decide to choose a therapy often take into consideration factors such as what type of disease it is ? The pathogenic agents and forces associated with it ? The situations and contexts in which the disease occurred ? The seriousness of the disease ? The symptoms associated with it ? The suspected suggestions or advice lent by people regarding the origin and cause of illness.

Having thought upon these questions related to the disease, the natives then decide to choose either a home remedy, a specialized therapy provided by the ethnomedical specialists or straight away decide to go for allopathic, homeopathic or ayurvedic treatment.

Nature and Role of Ethnomedical Specialists

When illness or disease occurs, it is either ignored or treated at home using home remedies or referred to a medical specialist. If the treatment is to be sought, a variety of ethnomedical specialists may be available using herbalists, shamans, diviners, bone setters, priests, masseurs and midwives.

Therapists may be either specialized in one type of skill or may combine several in one (Lieban 1962 b). All these medical specialists are looked upon with great respect by the members of their community. The ethnomedical specialists play a dual role in their societies i.e., as practitioners as well as farmers, artisans, or whatever economic activities they

Table VII : 4

A CROSS CULTURAL VIEW OF ETHNOMEDICAL SPECIALISTS

S.No.	Tribe	Specialist	His/Her function	Method of Diagnosing Illness	Therapy Employed
1.	The	Bhagat (Shaman) Divining Identity Interpretation of super-natural phenomena Performing healing rituals and employing magico-religious therapy Protective functions of warding off evil effects, Spirits and evil forces. Performing thanksgiving ceremony and offering sacrifices on behalf of the patients.	Diagnosing & Interpreting the cause of illness.	A Thakur Bhagat uses a Metal pot (tumbler) containing water and a pinch of ash from the earth. Facing the divine east direction, he spins the tumbler slowly in an anti-clock manner chanting mantras to diagnose the exact cause of illness.	Magico-religious & at times combination with Herbal

Table VII : 4 {Cont.}

2.	Wa	Bhagat (Shaman)	Same as above	The Bhagats of Warli tribe use a grain shifter in which small heaps of rice grains are made to diagnose a patient's illness.	Magico-religious & Herbal
3.	Ka	Bhagat (Shaman)	Same as above	An iron sickle (koyta) is used by the kathkari Bhagat to diagnose a patient's illness by sticking a metal coin to this sickle during the diagnosis ritual.	Magico-religious & Herbal
4.	Bh	Badwa (Shaman)	Same as above	Among the Bhils the Shamans who are popularly known as Badwas use Abrus precaterius seeds & jowar grain to diagnose illness by spreading a cloth on the floor and making heaps of these seeds.	Magico-religious & herbal
5.	Th Ka Wa	Bhagatin (Female Shaman)	Same as above	The Bhagatins get into trance to diagnose and interpret the cause of illness.	Magico-religious
6.	Bh	Badvi (female Bhil Shaman)	Same as above	Same as above	Same as above
7.	Th	Vaidu	Tha vaidu collects,	Checking the pulse,	Herbal

Table VII : 4 {Cont.}

	Ka Wa	(herbalist)	prepares and administers herbal medicines for his patients and gives them dietary advice.	feeling body temperature observing the body colour asking patient questions about illness.	therapy
8.	Th Ka Wa	Had-vaidu (Bone-setter)	Setting bones, massaging swellings & sprains, the Bone setter are also specia-lized in Branding bodily areas of severe pains with hot iron rod. They also use medicinal herbs.	Feeling, massaging and observing.	Medicinal and Herbal
9.	Th Ka Wa	Suine (Mid-wife)	Give medicinal advice to the expectant mother. To attend deliveries, recommend diet for the child and mother. Bathing the new born. Performing birth rituals such as burying the umbilical chord etc. Administer herbal medicine for gynecological problems.	Palpitating and feeling	Mechanical therapy
10.	Bh	Hovarin (Mid-wife)	Same as above	Same as above	Same as above
11.	Th Ka	Potdhari (Assistant midwife)	To assist the Suine in and in her absence manage deliveries.	Palpitation or feeling	Mechanical

Table VII : 4 {Cont.}

12.	Th	Mantrik (Scorpion sting and snake bite curer)	A mantrik uses both a ritualistic style and herbal therapy to cure scorpion stings and snake bites.	Checking the depth of the sting and mark of the snake bite. Know the intensity of their poison.	Herbal and magico-ritualistic

Note

*** Th = Thakurs**
*** Ka = Kathkaris**
*** Wa = Warlis**
*** Bh = Bhils**

are involved in.

Qualification for folk medical roles vary considerably. In some cases, formal training is required for the practitioners (Metzger & Williams 1963) in others a long apprenticeship may be customary. A post of a medical practitioner is hereditary, that is medical knowledge restricts to particular clan or family in the community.

Every therapist has a specific role and function to play in the healing process. Thus a shaman according to Micheal Harner (1973:IX) is a man or woman who has direct contact with the spiritual world through a trance state and has one or more spirits at his/her command to carry out his/her bidding for good or to cure persons affected by other spirits or simply acting in their own violations.

A priest on the other hand is a religious functionary whose supernatural authority is bestowed upon him by a cult or organization. In contrast to a shaman, he derives his powers directly from the supernatural sources (Hoebel, 1958:657).

In most societies the priest also play an important role in healing patients by performing healing rites.

Bone setters provide treatment for mechanical injuries such as sprains, broken bones, massaging, and using branding techniques (Kurian J.C. & Tribhuwan Robin 1990:255). The bone setters have a sound knowledge about position of bones, nerves, veins, and arteries in the human body.

Mary Schutlur (1979:22) refers to a mid-wife as one who is always a female and is necessarily not a diviner. Her duties are to give advice and medical aid to expectant mothers, to assist in deliveries and to treat illness that may befall the new mother and child. To fulfill her duties a midwife prescribes a few herbal medicines, knows massage techniques and recommends proper diet for the mother and child.

A herbalist is one who necessarily does not use magico-religious elements in herbal therapy. He also advises his patients on diet to be taken during the ill-health.

Not every society may be having all these different types of medical practitioners may be specialized in more than one area of therapy. Thus, many Bhagats (shamans) combine magico-religious as well as herbal therapy as they are specialized in both types of therapies.

Table VII :

4 in this chapter shows the different types of medical specialists of four tribes namely the Thakurs, Kathkaris, Bhils and Warlis highlighting their medical function, the type od diagnostic methods used and the therapeutic procedures employed by them. This table is prepared on the basis of an empirical study conducted on four medical system (Tribhuwan Robin

& Gambhir R.D. 1990).

Diagnosis & Interpretation of the Cause

The data in the Thakur medical system has shown that there is a culturally recognized and set pattern or standard of diagnosing illness which is unique in every culture.

Diagnosing and interpretation of the cause and origin of illness is a very important phase on the ethnomedical pathway wherein medical practitioners consulted, confirm the actual cause of illness after consulting the divine entities by performing diagnostic rituals and/or by getting into a trance.

Methods of diagnosing illness differ from culture to culture. Table VII : 4 given in this chapter highlights the different methods of diagnosis found in the four tribal medical systems of Maharashtra based on an empirical and comparative study conducted on the Thakurs, Kathkaris, Warlis and Bhils (Tribhuwan Robin & Gambhir R.D. 1990).

Therapy

Therapy in ethnomedicine is a vast subject. It includes magico-religious, chemical and mechanical procedures (Lieban 1973:1044). Therapies found in every society stem largely from prevailing causality beliefs, which from the rationale for treatment. Thus depending on the community;s notions of origin and cause of illness therapy takes its meaningful course towards the medical specialist concerned.

Illness believed to have natural causes are handled in non-magical and non-religious fashions. Thus excessive cold may be extracted from the body by warm baths, use of 'warm' herbs or by 'hot' poultices. Similarly excessive heat may be removed from the body with 'cold' herbs, cold leaves applied to the temples or diet which is believed to have cold qualities.

Illness believed to have caused as a result of supernatural or magical intervention is treated by shamans, diviners or priests who are believed to be interpreters of supernatural phenomena. The simple logic is that what comes spiritually has to be healed spiritually and takes its own course towards spiritual healers to get cured finally.

Many a times, even when mechanical or chemical therapies are employed, magico-religious elements may also be an essential part of the prescription, or the treatment is incomplete without the attention of mystical factors involved in the etiology of illness (Glick 1967). In such situations medical practitioners administer fashion to their patients to make the treatment meaningful.

The data has revealed that during the course of treatment patients tend to shift from one therapy to another depending on the suggestions and suspections contributed by the elderly members of the family and village. Thus what may be initially attributed to have caused naturally tends to be interpreted to have caused as a result of supernatural or magical intervention.

Shift in Ethnomedical Therapy

In his study the Magic Healing Techniques Among The Baluhis of Central India, Stephen Fuchs (1964:122-24) has stated that 'Baluhis are aware of the fact that certain diseases have natural causes and so they first look for natural remedies to cure them by resorting to household medicine, when these medicines fail to cure an illness, friends and relatives send their advises that certain deity or spirit has been offended and has sent the illness in revenge. Hence a Janka (herbalist-cum-diviner) Badwa (shaman) is consulted.

This trend of shifting from one therapy to another during the illness progression has been observed as a common trend in all the four ethnomedical systems studied. What may ne initially thought or perceived to have caused naturally is interpreted and attributed to have supernaturally caused in the course of ethnomedical pathway.

We have classified and discussed the following criteria factors or situations which promotes the shifting from one to another therapy during the course of an ethnomedical pathway :

1. The prolonged duration of the disease.
2. Cultural events, situations, actions, circumstances, places etc. in which the disease might have occurred.
3. The degree of severe pains caused due to the disease or health program.
4. Suggestions and advice contributed by the elderly members of the family and village regarding the suspected origin and cause of the illness.

Given below are the four illness episodes from the Thakur, Kathkaris, Warlis and Bhil tribes respectively supporting the above mentioned four factors.

1. The prolonged nature of the disease :

Illness episode No. 1 :

Babu Pandurang Pawar aged 45, a member of Kathkari tribe, resident of Kathkari Wadi, Kashele Village, Karjat Tehsil, Raigarh, got his little right hand finger cut while catching crabs. Babu applied a medicinal herb and tied his finger with a piece of cloth.

A week later his finger became still worse. Babu used to cry in pain. Having found that household medicine was not effective, he consulted a vaidu (herbalist). The herbalist treated Babu for a week, but his medicine also did not work. By now, it was already two weeks that Babu was suffering from this wound.

Babu's old father Pandurang, instructed Babu to consult the Bhagat from Kaute Wadi. The Bhagat (Shaman) diagnosed Babu;s health problem ritually and interpreted that Babu has become a victim of witchcraft. A witch has filled a dog's bone piece into Babu's little finger. She was suspected to be from Babu's community. The Bhagat gave Babu some holy ash and instructed him to apply it on his forehead once a day after his bath. Babu did this for another week. Even this did not work.

He narrated his experience to the village school headmaster, who met Babu in the village fish market. The headmaster suggested and convinced Babu to go to the PHC Doctor and take allopathic treatment. Babu then went to the PHC Doctor and took treatment for ten days and got his wound on the little finger of the right hand healed.

Thus the prolonged nature and duration of the disease at times forces a patient to shift from one therapy to another, till it finally gets cured. During this period the patient and his family members are willing to change and consult as many therapists available.

Illness Episode 2 :

Kashinath Nama Dhole, aged 37, a member of the Thakur tribe, resident of Khande Wadi, Pathraj village, Karjat Tehsil, Raigarh district, lost his father in the month of June, 1988. A week later his son Palu - a twelve year old boy fell sick. He had fever during this period. Kashinath Palu felt that after giving a herbal decoction Palu would feel better.

Palu was treated with herbal decoction for 5-6 days but he did not get well. In the initial stages, Kashinath was of a view that Palu's fever was as a result of playing in the rains. When Kashinath's father's brother suggested the Palu would have been afflicted by some supernatural power. Kashinath decided to take him to the Bhagat.

According to Kashinath's paternal uncle, Palu was affected by the warth of ancestral spirits. Kashinath consulted the Bhagat. Thus, Ambo Thorad, the Bhagat from Khondewadi was consulted. He used the metal pot diagnosis technique and ritually interpreted that the cause of Palu's illness was due to the 'warth of the ancestral spirits' i.e. the soul of Kashinath's father.

Ambo Bhagat (shaman) said that the soul was not offered liquor and bidis while performing the death rite and hence the soul is troubling Palu. The shaman also instructed that the concerned spirit (Vir) must be given liquor and bidis as well as offered a cock.

The situation in which Palu's illness occurred was right after the death of his grandfather (a cultural event). Hence the origin and cause stemmed from the concept of 'wrath of ancestral spirits'.

Most illness origin and cause is interpreted to be associated with cultural events, inauspicious occasions, movement of cosmic objects, evil places etc. For instance, it was observed that all the four tribes, namely, Thakurs, Kathkaris, Bhils and Warlis believe that evil spirits disturb or trouble human beings and cause illness during the new moon (Amosha) and full moon (Poornima) nights.

3. The degree of severe pains caused due to disease or health problems.

Illness Episode 3 :

Narayana Padu Dore, aged 35, a member of the Thakur tribe, resident of Thakur wadi, Kashele village, Karjat Tehsil, Raigarh District, suffered from kidney stone problem during the summer of the year 1989. His stomach bulged up since he was not able to pass urine because of the kidney stone problem. He would cry in pain.

During 2-3 days of severe pain, Narayana would constantly complain about the pain and behave as if someone was hurting him. His father and mother were relied worried. One of his uncle's suggested that Narayana should be taken to a Bhagat (shaman).

Narayana was taken to his father-in-law, who was a Bhagat himself, who diagnosed the origin and cause of Narayan's illness and interpreted that a Kathkari woman was filled nachni (Millet) in Narayana's belly. Her evil spells were hurting him and hence he was crying in pain. Thus the cause of Narayana's illness was attributed to the severe pains caused by witch-craft spells.

Finally suggestion contributed by the elderly members of the family and village to choose therapies depending on the then suspected notion of the origin and cause of illness.

Illness Episode 4 :

Rama Valvi, aged 42, member of the Bhil tribe, resident of Mundalwad village, Akrani Taluk, Dhule District, was bringing his cattle home in the eve of May 1988. As he was approaching his village, he saw a dog walking quietly towards the hillside. He picked up a big stone and hit it very hard. The dog ran about 50 to 60 yards away and looked back at Rama.

Rama returned home, had his dinner and was relaxing in front of his house. He started feeling cold and after some time he was shivering. After an hour he had fever. His master told him to take rest. It was during the midnight hours when Rama had high fever. He started crying and shouting. His uncles who were next door came to enquire as to what happened to Rama. After a short discussion one of his uncle's suggested to Rama's father that he might have been possessed by an evil spirit as he is behaving like a mad person. Rama's father then went to summon the Budwa (shaman).

Soon after the arrival of the Budwa, Rama started still more roughly. The Budwa diagnosed and interpreted that Rama had been possessed by an evil spirit. Rama had disturbed the spirit which was in the form of a dog, on its way to the hillside. The evil spirit was hot with a stone by Rama and therefore it took control of Rama's body.

The Budwa then performed certain rituals then whipped the evil spirit out of Rama. One week later on, on the new moon night, Rama's father offered a coconut and two hens to this spirit.

Thanks Giving Rituals and Ceremonies

Therapeutic procedures are often followed by thanks giving rituals and ceremonies. Every society has certain ways and means of expressing gratefulness to the originators or the causative pathogenic agents and also to the curers (medical practitioners) for restoring the health of a patient.

The medical specialists are given gifts or payments in kind and recently in cash. At times a bottle of locally prepared liquor and a meat feast serves the purpose of practitioners who refuse to take cash or gifts in kind. On the other hand, angry deities, ghosts, spirits etc. are offered sacrifices of goats or fowls. It is at this point the ethnomedical pathway completes its course.

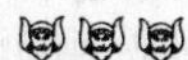

CHAPTER VIII

SUMMARY AND CONCLUSION

Since the last couple of decades, considerable literature is available, both by medical and social scientists, on biological and socio-cultural aspects of health and disease. Almost every anthropologist since the end of 15th century has included too often in passing some or the other reference to medicine or disease in his/her monograph.

Anthropological interest in medicine stems from the fact that health and disease though scientifically understood as biological in nature are related to people's belief system. The theoretical concern of Anthropology in medicine is made explicit by Lieban (1073:1034) by stating that,"Medical Anthropology encompasses the study of medical phenomena as they are influenced by social and cultural phenomena and social and cultural phenomena as they illuminated by their medical aspects.

Health is an aspect of culture. Henry Siergist, the medical historian stated that every culture has developed a system of medicine and thus medical history is but one aspect of the history of culture, as all aspects of culture are integrated.

Throughout the ages man has been devising ways and means to take care of the sick in the community. (Newell 1975 : 55). Every culture has developed its own beliefs and practices regarding health and disease. It is to such beliefs and practices related to health and disease which are products of indigenous cultural developments and not explicitly derived from the conceptual framework of modern medicine, the term, "Ethnomedicine" is applied (Hughes 1968 : 99).

Studies on ethnomedical accounts have highlighted tribal illness concepts, body symbolism, nature and role of ethnomedical specialists, various forms of therapies, ritual healing, ethnophysiology, preventive medicine, witchcraft and sorcery and so on. (Foster GM 1976, 1983; Fabreya 1977; Hughes 1968; Douglas 1970, 1975; Lieban 1973; Turner; Nitcher & Nitcher 1981; Young Allan 1982; Kleinman 1980; Hahn & Kleinman 1983).

Next to Africa, India has a considerable size of tribal population. In comparison to the numerous studies carried out on African and Latin American tribes in the field of ethnomedicine. two cultural Anthropologists (Marriot 1955, Carstairs 1955) were among the first to carry out formal social science studies on health and medicine in India in rural settings. Other who surveyed the Indian Health scenario in rural India include Opler (1963); Hasan (1967); Djurefedth and Lindberg (1975); Bhatnagar (1978) Zurbeig (1984) and Khare (1963) who conducted a study of folk medicines in north Indian villages.

Morbidity studies related to beliefs and practices of the people were conducted in India by Bharara (1951) on small pox, Dhillan Karim (1961) on Malaria, D.B. Banerjee (1961) on T.B., Mutatkar R.K. (1979) and Pathan B.R. (1986) on leprosy. Besides these studies Kakar (1976), Shukla (1980), Joshi Vibha (1986), Singh I.P. (1988), Chaudhary (1986), Kurian J.C. and Bhanu B.V. (1980) also carried out social science studies related to health and disease in Indian Settings.

Most of the above quoted studies have been carried out in rural settings and predominantly by medical sociologists. There are very few studies conducted on ethnomedicine in India by Anthropologists, on Indian tribes. Reference to disease and medicine is of course given in the monographs written on Indian Tribes. But a full Health Monograph highlighting symbolic and meaningful aspects of medicine has not been published to date. This study has made an attempt to unravel the symbolic and meaningful aspects of ethnomedicine of the Thakurs as a symbolic system not in its own right but as a representation of the cultural whole.

Beliefs form among every people, a system of symbols and meanings (Schneider 1976:20). This system can be seen as a group of sets of propositions and perceptions of people regarding the world, which on further examination, reveal themselves to be ordered in their relationships to one another.

An attempt has been made in this study to show how medical symbols (acts, words, objects, ideas, relationships, colours, songs, chants etc) stand for,suggest and reveal cultural realities other than themselves. That the domain of ethnomedicine is not confined to a single area of social life but represents not only the Thakur culture but also is a part of the greater social system (The Hindu Caste (Jati) system). The Dev and Davan jati system according to the Thakurs is a social system of all the caste and tribal communities which are divided into two groups namely the Devjatis (God like social groups) and the Davan jatis (the giant, Rakshas) like social groups. The study also points out how structured and ordered is the relationship of Thakurs with the natural, supernatural, social ancestral, spiritual and cosmological forces and entities. That disruption or disturbance of this relationship signals ill-health, misfortune or death.

The natural, cosmological, spiritual, supernatural, social and ancestral world of the Thakurs is symbolically and meaningfully ordered. Following the theoretical understanding og (Lec 1950, Hallowell 1955, Schneider 1969, 1976, Turner 1967, 1972 and Mary Douglas 1970, 1975) this study has made an attempt to show that any domain of social life (which includes ethnomedicine as well) is built on a frame work of implicit meanings. That these meanings are not confined to a single area of social life but the same pervade the whole social system. That the state of ill-health is an expression of cultural disorder and through ritual healing disrupted order is recreated (Camaroff 1981, Carpa 1991, Munn 1973).

The introductory chapter presents in a systematic manner the significance of studying symbolic aspects of ethnomedicine, its areas including the lacunae. This chapter also presents the main focus of the present study, its significance, definitions, concepts and aims and objectives. It also deals with the theoretical overview of ethnomedicine.

The chapter on methodology presents the research population for the study, the research tools and techniques of data collection and the processing and analysis of data. The chapter on ethnography of the Thakurs briefly highlights the life style of the target population with special emphasis on their Maternal and Child Health Care Beliefs and Practices.

The findings of the research including the discussions and interpretation have been presented in five chapters namely Illness Ideology, Body Symbolism, Ethnomedical Specialists, Ritual Healing and Summary and Conclusions.

The chapter on Illness Ideology gives comprehensive details,of what the Thakurs perceive to be the origin and cause of illness. The various contexts and situations wherein disease is defined as illness and more significantly how illness etiology reflects the Thakur conception of cultural disorder and/or disharmony of man with social, spiritual, cosmological, natural and supernatural entities/forces. Besides this a detailed account of the manner in which cultural meanings shape illness experience is presented in the form of 50 illness episodes.

Body symbolism chapter throws light on the Thakur concept of body physiology and more importantly on the various symbols and symbolic forms expressed through the body during the state of ill-health. The study also pointed out how human body during the process of ritual healing gets a natural, social, spiritual and supernatural status.

The chapter on ethnomedical specialists gives a comprehensive picture of the nature and role of seven types of medical practitioners in the form of indepth case studies. It covers the symbolic aspects of apprenticeship, taboos associated, rituals associated with collection, preparation and administration of drugs, diagnosis, healing and thanksgiving rituals and their meanings and other therapeutic actions.

Ritual healing, chapter focuses on the Thakur's concepts regarding intrinsic (healing) qualities of medicine used by them. The entire set of actions, objects, songs, words, chants, gestures and uttrances etc. in a ritual healing contexts are explored so as to understand their meaning as perceived by the natives. Besides this a conceptual model has been evolved which aptly describes the entire process of culturally designed clinically meaningful reality through which a sick person passes. Finally the last chapter gives a brief summary of the thesis and highlights various conclusions drawn from the findings.

The definition of Health from an outsider's perspective as 'a state of complete physical, mental and social well being and not merely absence of disease or infirmity', differs very much from an insiders perspective. What constitutes a state of sound health varies to a great deal from culture to culture.

The state of sound health as understood by the Thakurs is explained as follows :

1. The state of sound health is one in which an individual's body, mind and soul (pind, mun and atma) maintains form and order as perceived by the Thakurs in their cultural frame of reference.

2. A state of sound health is one in which there is a harmonious co-ordination between the mind, body and soul.

3. That the body, mind and soul are pure and not filled with evil or taken charge of by evil spirits, pathogenic agents and natural harmful pathogens.

4. That the cosmic elements such as light, air, heat, water, earth which control the body physiology are in a balanced conditionor proportionate form in the body.

5. A state of sound health is a state in which man as a social animal maintains a clear and perfect relationship with his tribesmen, with other caste groups and tribes, with his deities, the ancestral spirits, with cosmic forces and agents etc.

6. A healthy person is one :

a. who has an ability to with stand extreme cold and hot conditions.
b. a person who has the ability to work and walk for long time in the sun.
c. who has an ability to digest monitor's meat, Dioscorea (corm), and Nachni porridge (Eleucine coracana) with raw milk.
d. a person who lives for longer time is considered to be healthy.

e. a person is physically fit, because he exersices. (Mehenat Karne).
f. a person who is able to walk long distance.
g. a healthy person's body is not deformed.
h. a healthy person is one who has red blood. More the blood in the body more the strength. Black blood is a sign of old age. Yellow, green, dark red, white discharge is a sign of ill-health.
i. a healthy person is one who can resist and fight disease without taking medicine. Healthy person is not lazy, nor does he sleep during the day time.

Human beings (Manev) according to the Thakurs is a microcosm of the Universe, 'Khand Sarkha pind' - meaning human body is a reflection of the Universe. Their explanation for this statement is that the human body has ten bodily openings (Daha Darwaze) namely eyes, nose, ears, mouth, soul (atma), pulse wrist, naval opening, urethal/vaginal opening, pulse of the feet and the anal opening (Gupta darwaza), symbolize the ten planets (Nav graha and a Gupta darwaza). They believe that these ten bodily openings resemble the ten planets of the cosmos. The soul or atma which is on the fifth position in the bodily opening hierarchy resembles with the earth, which is also on the fifth position in the planet hierarchy.

Human body, exists because of Sun, Moon, Stars, Earth, Air, water, light, Heat (fire), Natural environment, Planets, Clouds etc. In fact the entire body physiology is controlled by the cosmic elements and their movements. For instance the Thakurs believe that air in the body contributes to the smooth functioning of blood circulation, digestion of food, excretion of waste matter and so on. Water taken in the body along with the blood in turn produces breast milk, semen, vaginal fluid etc. Water also helps in digestion, excretion of waste matter etc. Heat (fire) in the stomach boils food and converts it down into liquid form which later is turned into blood (strength). The light present in the eyes helps a man to see. Besides this, cosmic elements control other bodily systems.

Soul (atma) according to the Thakurs is composed of wind, fire, light and water. It dwells in the cage of ribs in the body (earth). Atma (soul) is composed of cosmic elements. Mother Earth (Dantari) which is on the fifth position in the planetary hierarchy resembles the soul (Atma) which is on the fifth position in the bodily opening hierarchy.

A human body without atma (soul) is a dead body. because atma is composed of the major elements of the cosmos namely fire, light, water and air and that the human body cannot survive without it. Atma is therefore associated with life. Infact all these life giving elements namely water, air, light, fire, earth (mud) and vegetation (food) are available for man on earth. When man ploughs the earth, plants seeds, waters it, plants use produced because they get earth, air, water, light and heat available on the earth. That means the Earth and Sun which are the sources of life giving elements are immediately linked with existence of living human body (life). Sun, earth, plants, air, light, water etc therefore are very closely linked with health. Hence Illness Ideology, Body Symbolism and Ritual Healing concepts of the Thakurs express these cosmic entities/forces as control or dominant symbols.

When a person dies, on tenth day in case of married males, ninth day in case of married females and seventh day in case of bachelors and spinsters, a rite of soul migration is performed. Thakurs prepare ten rice flour balls which are ritually worshipped by a Brahman (priest) and thrown into the river. These ten rice flour balls symbolize the ten spirits of the body openings and atma (soul) - which in this ritual is termed as 'Jeev Khada', also is included in these ten spirits. The throwing of these rice flour balls symbolizes the leaving or migration of the ten spirits into the cosmos. Thakurs call it this way - 'pind khandala milto' - meaning body merges with the cosmos.

Disproportionate ratio of the cosmic elements in the body means ill-health. Absence of cosmic elements in the body means death. For instance, entry of excess cold or heat in the body makes the blood too hot or cold and leads to imbalance of the body humours. In case excess cold air enters the body a person is likely to get arthritis or joint pain. Such cases are treated with hot remedies, i.e. branding techniques, an iron rod is heated and touched on painful points. If an ailment is believed to have been caused due to entry of excess heat in the body, it is treated with cold remedies or diet.

Maintenance of correct proportion of cosmic elements in human body becomes very important as far as sound health is concerned. Atma (soul) which is the seat of life is believed to be attacked by spiritual, cosmological, ancestral, social, supernatural and natural forces or entities. According to the Thakurs when a person is possessed by evil spirit, it means that the patient's atma (soul) is taken charge of by the evil spirit. Hence socially, the patient looses his social status and gets a spiritual status. When the shaman beats the spirit ritually to please the pathogenic agent to leave the patient rituals of compromise are performed. Depending on the community's origin and cause of illness and the entry of social, spiritual, cosmological, supernatural and ancestral pathogenic agents. Human body simultaneously gets social, spiritual, cosmological, supernatural, ancestral or natural status.

MODEL VIII : 1. The State of Ill-health : A Conceptual Model

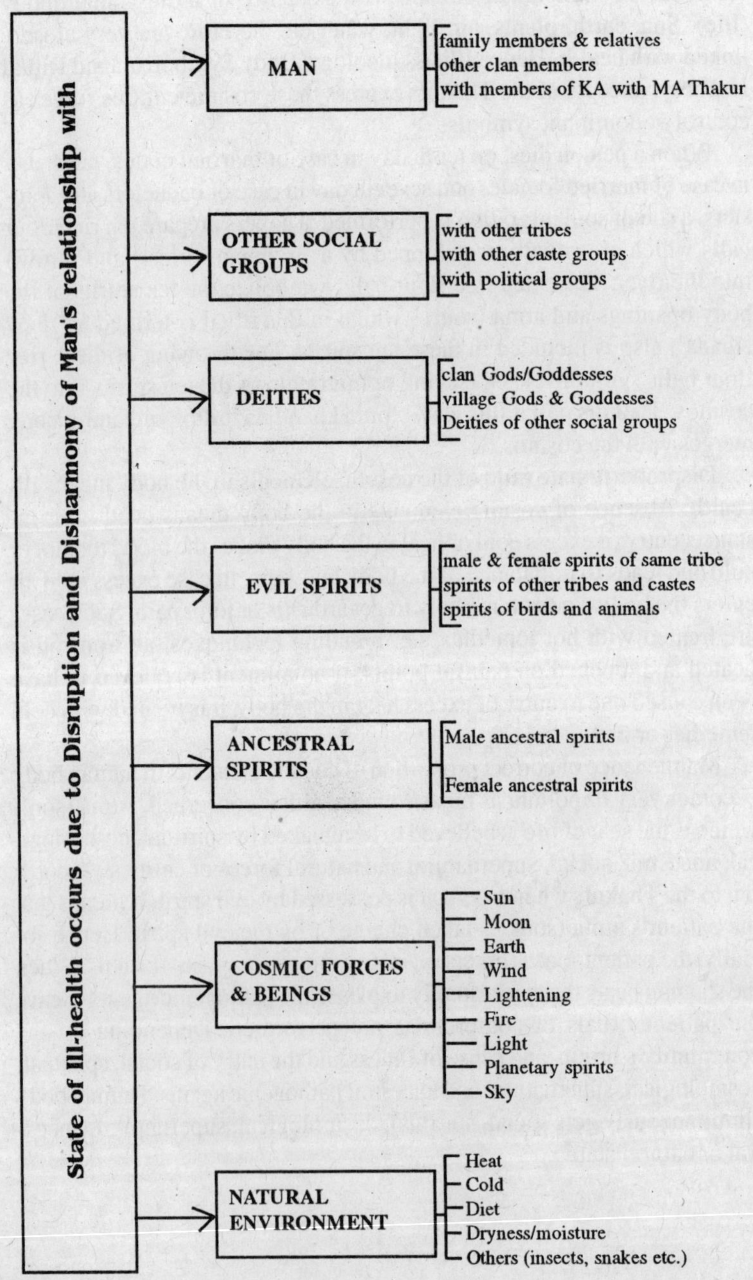

The state of ill-health according to the Thakurs is an intermediate stage between life and death. It occurs due to an imbalanced co-ordination and disharmony between body, mind and soul. Illness occurs due to the disruption of man's relationship with his fellowmen (tribesmen), other social groups (castes and tribes), deities, evil spirits, cosmic forces and entities, and the natural agents.

Illness experiences of the Thakurs documented in the form of illness episodes have provided the following definition of the state of ill-health. 'The state of ill-health is not merely a malfunctioning of biological and psychological processes, but a symbolic and meaningful expression of human conflicts, social indifferences, grudge, jealousy, deviance, hatred, cultural disorder etc. that exists at social level. It is a condition which signals the disruption of culturally ordered man's harmonious relationship with his family, clan members, members of other social groups, with spiritual, supernatural, ancestral, natural and cosmological forces and beings. In other words a state of ill-health depicts man's disrupted natural and socio-cultural order.

The conceptual model of ill-health presents the Thakur conception of their relationships or bonds with nature, with their tribesmen, with their deities, cosmic forces/entities, ancestral spirits, with members of other tribes and caste groups with deities of other caste and tribal groups. Illness episodes reported in the thesis support the above statement. To cite examples, illness is caused due to wrath of village Gods if they are not offered sacrifices regularly by the Thakurs. Diseases such as chicken pox, measles, body sores, boils etc. are believed to be caused due to visitation of "Mothya Baya" (the planetary spirits). They bring about these diseases because man forgets his duty towards divine beings and deviates from cultural norms. Witchcraft and sorcery are expressions of disruptions at social level. It projects jealousy, hatred, social conflict, grudge etc that exists at social level which is solved at spirit level through ritual healing.

The symbolic aspects associated with Thakur illness ideology cross-cuts into other spheres of social life. For instance concepts of the origin and cause of albinism and congenitally deformed children cross-cuts into other domains of social life of Thakurs such as marriage, sex, family life, concepts of evil spirits, types of evil spirits, concepts of soul, jati (caste) concepts, social conflicts, death, child birth ceremonies etc. Albino and congenitally deformed children are killed right after their birth. It is believed that these children are born as a result of sexual intercourse a woman has with munja or khais (male evil spirits). What is produced from an evil source is evil. It's bodily form and order does not resemble thecosmos. It is therefore killed and buried with its back facing the sun. It is not allowed to grow in the human society as it belongs to the world of evil spirits. The entire set of actions and normative albinos and congenitally deformed children is very much meaningful to Thakurs.

Turners (1967 : 50) has emphasized the polysemic nature of ritual symbols with different meanings of the same symbol becoming paramount in different contexts. the polysemy is an obvious quality of symbols used in situations in which a particular symbol has number of meanings in only one situation or context. For example albinism is a symbol of evil spirit, body deformity, cosmic disorder, sexual frustration of bachelors who die and turn into troublesome souls. There are many other instances where a symbol has many meanings in a single context.

The symbolic aspects of illness experience are interrelated to many groups of meanings which are finally interwoven into a symbolic system. Illness episode no. 5 in illness ideology chapter, for instance highlights how a person's health is disturbed on shifting into a house, which does not resemble the culturally designed houses of the Thakurs. The Thakurs have culturally specified ways of finding a suitable place for building a house, rituals of cleansing the land, rituals of building it, the directional symbolism involved in building a house, the meanings of symbols (objects, actions, relationships, ideas) associated with the house. The Thakur house is built in such a way that it symbolizes the cosmos. Living in the cosmos means living in a world of good spirits. Living in a house which does not resemble their culturally prescribed design means living in a world of evil spirits and inviting trouble.

Episode no. 5 shows how illness experience helps an anthropologists to understand other spheres of social life such as material culture, religion, ideas regarding cosmos, directional symbolism, concept of evil spirits, preventive rituals, symbolic aspects related to child birth, various conceptions involved in building a house, social deviance and so on.

While other episodes have shown how social conflicts are solved ritually at spirit level. Casting of evil spells or evil eye is predominantly prevailing practice among the tribal and even the caste groups of pathraj and kashale. Episodes have highlighted that there are two main division of jatis (castes and tribal groups together) namely the Dev jatis and Davan jatis. Dev jatis (God like jatis) include the Brahman (priests), Marathas and kunbis (agriculturalists), Gujratis (business people), Agris (agricultural caste), Malis (gardener), sutars (Carpenters), Lohars (blacksmith), Sonars (Goldsmiths), Dhangars (shepherds), Mahadev kolis (tribe), Kannada (Nomadic caste group). The Davan jatis include Thakurs (tribe), Mahars, Mangs, Chamars, Muslims (untouchables caste groups) and kathkaris (Tribe).

The concept of witchcraft, sorcery and evil eye is an expression of social conflict that exists among the social groups due to jealousy, hatred, grudge, social status, social hierarchy and purity and pollution concepts that exist at social level are reconciled at spirit level. Episodes have highlighted that black magical spells have been caste on a Thakur by kathkari or a Thakur woman has been sexually mishandled by a Muslim evil spirit, or a Thakur child has become a victim of evil eye of Mahar caste, or a Thakur sterile woman used umbilical chord of a new born to hurt the child. All these things point towards a greater social system that exists among the tribals and caste groups of Pathraj and Kashale. The members of davan jatis usually prefer to go to the practitioners of davan jatis for treatment. For example most of the members of Thakurwadi, Borwadi, Kautewadi visit the Mahar caste bhagatins (female shaman) of Kotimbe village. While the members of dev jatis prefer their own medical practitioners and modern medicine. The members of dev jatis always blame the members of davan jatis for practising witch craft, sorcery and casting evil eye. Thus the symbolic aspects of ethnomedicine have not only uncovered the Thakur cultural system but also a greater system (Dev and Davan jati system) of which the Thakurs are a part.

Presentation and Interpretation of Illness :

The first and foremost step in presentation and interpretation of the origin and cause of illness is the process of initial diagnosis. This is done at the family level. Elderly members of the family first contribute their suggestions regarding the originators of illness after studying the context in which illness might have occurred. Their suggestions are cross checked with elderly members of the village, friends or relatives. It is the Bhagat who diagnoses the cause ritually and confirms the pathogenic agent. Decision to choose a therapy also depends on the family and village elders.

Symptoms of illness are studied before interpreting the cause. Duration of illness is also another criterion where contributions of suggestions regarding origin and cause of illness fluctuate. Stomach ache initially could be interpreted as imbalance of bodily equilibrium. If it persists for a longer duration then a suggestion regarding the origin and cause starts flowing in from the village elders, friends, relatives, They advice the patient's parents that the cause of illness could be due to witch craft, sorcery, evil eye, spirit possession, warth of God and Goddesses and so on. As Chilivumbo A.B. (1977:70) states that diagnosis and therapeutic measures acquiring meanings through subjective perceptions and the defined symbolic world view in which irrationalities assume meanings. Illness experience is shaped by cultural symbols and meanings in a defined cultural context or situation.

The state of ill-health according to the Thakurs is an intermediatory stage between life and death. Illness signals the impurity of body, mind and soul, body deformity and order, it signals the disharmony of man's relationship with natural, social, cosmological, ancestral, spiritual and supernatural world. Where as when the human body resembles the cosmos and that its atma (mind), is pure, has form and is ordered, it is said to be healthy.

Ritual Healing :

The process of ritual healing here is defined as culturally prescribed normative actions or ritualized forms of behaviour of medical practitioners, patients and other participants historically designed in order to compromise with the pathogenic agents (social, natural, spiritual, ancestral, cosmological, supernatural) so as to recreate the disrupted cultural order in order to restore the health of the patient.

The normative behaviour of medical specialists falls more within the sphere of rituals than that of therapeutic actions. Ethnomedicinal therapy, may it be herbal/chemo, mechanical or magico-religious is combined with culturally prescribed health rituals. Even to treat natural causes such as sprains, fractures, cuts, fever etc. the medicinal herbs are administered. The normative behaviour of medical specialists, patients and other participants assumes meanings with in the healing context.

Outstanding characteristics of the shamanistic concepts of healing is the belief that human beings are an integral part of an ordered system and that illness is a consequence of some disharmony of man with social, natural, supernatural, ancestral, spiritual beings. Accordingly shamanistic therapies emphasize the restoration of health by patching up relationships or recreating the disrupted cultural order.

Besides patching up man's relationships with social, cosmological, spiritual, supernatural, ancestral and natural forces and beings, the Thakur ritual healing has also shown how desires, demands and expectations of the above said forces/beings is solved by human beings through the process of ritual healing. For instance, episode no. 28 highlights how human beings satisfy the Baya (planetary spirits) who desire to have sex with the moon. The ritual of 'pani ghalne' which is performed when a patient suffers from chicken pox. The patient is believed to be visited by Baya, who enter his body in the form of hot air. Hot air here symbolizes the sexual heat or urge for having sex. The heat has to be cooled down by the semen of the moon. Ficus glomerata in this context symbolizes the moon and the sap extracted from its roots symbolizes the semen of the moon. Patient's body symbolizes the Baya. Administration of the sap symbolizes sexual intercourse and the digestion of the sap symbolizes sexual satisfaction of the Baya. Hence illness experiences and ritual healing are also an expression of the problems faced by the cosmic, supernatural,

natural, ancestral beings, which are solved by human beings through the process of ritual healing at spirit level. Healing ritual symbols reveal cultural reality. Meanings of symbols associated with illness ideology, body image, and preventive, promotive, curative and destructive aspects of health are interwoven into a symbolic system of medicine as it were.

The practice of not using 'water' after defecation among these divine and cosmic elements that give and sustain life. Thakurs believe that water, sun and moon are brothers which means in their divine hierarchy these three divine beings are given the highest status. In most healing rituals water is used as a symbol for purifying evil effect, warding off evil, dissolving umbilical chord so that it is not used as a magical device to hurt the new mother and child, as a symbol of absorption and so on. Because of water blood, breast milk, semen, vaginal fluids (fluids of life) are produced. Water has multiple uses in the Thakur community. Is is because of its divine status and preventive, promotive and curative use it is given a higher status. What is divine is used for divine activities and not to clean excreta. The Thakurs therefore do not use water after defecation but make use of stones and leaves.

Healing ritual symbols have highlighted many aspects of Thakur culture. The data has also revealed that the main functions of healing rituals and therapeutic actions are to diagnose the origin and cause of illness and then create a symbolic and clinically meaningful situation or reality so as to meet the needs or make a compromise with the pathogenic agents and at the same time recreate the disrupted cultural order.

Herbal Therapies have highlighted the significance of colour symbolism. Thakurs associate red, orange, white and green colour with sound health. While yellow, black, dark red and blue colour of bodily fluids and secretions are symbolic of ill-health. Yet another aspect as far as medicinal herbs are concerned is that the tribals have their own notions and classification of medicinal plants, their intrinsic qualities and their efficiency.

Healing rituals are performed to :

1. Ward off/neutralize the evil effect.
2. Driving away evil spirits or pathogenic agents.
3. Satisfy the demands of pathogenic agents.
4. Pleasing or worshipping the pathogenic agents.
5. Patching up disrupted cultural order.
6. Recreating the disrupted cultural order.
7. Therapeutic rituals or actions are performed to balance the bodily equilibrium.
8. To excommunicate the soul of a person from the community.
9. To ex-communicate a patient from social circle, temporarily ot per-

manently.

10. Rituals associated with collection, preparation and administration of medicine.
11. Rituals of thanks giving to thank the originator and curer of the cause of illness.

The entire set of actions, objects, ideas, concepts, chants, words, songs, gestures, utterances used in ritual healing are meaningful. The meanings of healing ritual symbols are interwoven into a symbolic systems and represents the cultural whole. The symbolic aspects associated with preventive, curative, promotive and destructive actions or rituals of health create culturally recognized clinically meaningful reality. A conceptual model has been developed to explain the processes through which a person passes.

Ethnomedicine is conceptually defined as a culturally ordered interrelationship of medical symbols and meanings that are associated with the community's notions of illness ideology, body image and the entire set of preventive, promotive, curative and destructive health rituals and/ or therapeutic actions performed by the participant actors in various healing contexts into a symbolic system, thereby representing the cultural whole.

Practical Implications of the Study :

Today if we take a glance at the Indian population, about 80% of the Indians live in rural and tribal areas where only 20% of the health services are rendered. While the 20% of the urban population has an advantage of receiving 80% of health services. An allopathic doctor who spends a huge amount of capital to earn a M.B.B.S. degree aims to recover what he has invested in his education. Most M.B.B.S. graduates prefer to settle in the cities and and small towns. Professional medical practice is centered on Commerce or money making business".

On the other hand the health infrastructure is dominated by the allopathic lobby. Doctors who plan and implement health care programmes for the rural and tribal folks of India do not take into account people's beliefs, customs, values and normative practices regarding health and diseases, while planning and implementing health care and health education programmes.

The primary health workers who are actually in touch with the grass root (i.e. people) hardly find any time to educate the rural and tribal folks, as much their time goes in hunting family planning, cataract, leprosy, T.B., Malaria etc. targets. Moreover maintenance of health records and registers to please the higher authorities and the concerned District Health Officer becomes first priority. The target population to be covered by a health workers is not within his reach. Adding to their workload the number of daily assignments keep increasing and they are unable to give health justice to the tribals who according to 1981 census are about 50 million, or almost 7.76% of the total Indian population.

Health is no more the responsibility of an individual or family. It is the responsibility of the nation. Given this background it is necessary to draft out strategies to reach the tribal people, understand them, understand their belief system, motivate them, using culturally accepted media of education such as Bhajans, dramas, folk songs, kirtans, folk dances, etc. and finally build on what they (tribal) have through community participation.

The present study has shown the significance of understanding health as understood by the tribals. It has shown that the beliefs and practices regarding health and disease are meaningful to the tribals. It pointed out how there is marked resistance by tribal cultures to the government health care and health education programmes as well as to the programmes in their spheres of social life and this resistance does not stem out of ignorance, illiteracy and superstitions as erroneously thought.

The study emphasizes that deep and radically different categorization which arises from the meaning systems prevents the meshing of forms, other than their own into their own meaning structures.

Such in depth studies have tremendous potential in the field of application to provide symbolic information on indigenous health beliefs regarding illness, body image, ritual healing, maternal and child health are beliefs and practices, nature and role of ethnomedical specialists, ethnophysiology, food habits and health behaviour.

This information will serve the purpose of planning and implementing culturally acceptable health care and health educational programme for the rural and tribal folks of India. The models namely 'Ethnomedical pathway' given in ritual healing chapter and the model of 'Ill- health' given in the concluding chapter will certainly help anthropologists and other social scientists to carry out comparative studies of ethnomedical beliefs and practices. Such knowledge also contributes to an understanding of human behaviour in relation to culture change.

Suggestions For Policy Planning :

1. The study points out that there are urgent practical reasons for quickening the application of social science in planning and implementing and following up culturally acceptable and appropriate health care and health education programmes.

2. Social scientists should be included in planning health care and health education programmes along with medical scientists as they are

equipped with the knowledge of society. They can help in understanding apathy and resistance of people also contribute to understanding of health behaviour.

3. The present study suggests that traditional medical practitioners are a valuable resource for providing primary care to communities. They stand in between the community and the divine beings. They are respected by the members of their community. They are more readily accepted by their own people than the health workers and allopathic doctors. health services can be strengthened so as to prevent illness if traditional practitioners are properly trained and utilized. Traditional practitioners can help their own people to improve their quality of life.

4. The use of folk media i.e. health education through Bhajan, dramas, folk songs, folk dances, kirtans, puppet shows etc. should be made popular.

5. Principles of preventive, promotive and curative health should be introduced in schools to lay the foundation of health in the student's mind at a very early age. This is the age where ideas of positive health should be introduced as part of socialization process. It is difficult to introduce these ideas among the older folks.

6. Encourage primary health centre staff to work with traditional medical practitioners, school teachers, gram panchayat members, mahila mandals (women association), bhajan mandals (meric association), farmers clubs, youth clubs and voluntary organizations to work out strategies for the tribals.

7. Health education programmes must be based on sacred values so as to make them culturally acceptable. For example the Academy of Development Science - a voluntary organization is co-ordinating training for the herbalists and midwives. Their meetings are held under a banyan tree on poornima (full moon) of Amosha (new moon) days. Before the meeting starts all the herbalists sing the traditional song. Even during the discussion the participants sit informally and share their experiences of treatments with other. Poornima and Amosha is better understood by the herbalists and midwives than the English calendar.

8. Encouraging cultivation of medicinal plants and kitchen gardens.

9. It has been observed that while study ethnomedical beliefs and practices of the Thakurs the tribals get convinced of the efficiency of allopathic treatment by witnessing cured cases. For example successful cataract operation, treatment of T.B. and leprosy cures have convinced them of the efficiency of modern medicine. Demonstration of cured case must be promoted in health education classes.

10. Health educators or health care providers whether from government or non-government organizations must establish a very close rap-

port with the target group. This is done by accepting local foods and drinks, mixing with people, participating in their cultural activities, encouraging them to organize their programmes. In doing so the health educators will win the minds of tribals as well as their confidence. It is only when the tribals accept the health educator as friend only then they will accept the ideas of health education. Thus creating a friendly image of health education and the worker is very significant. (Tribhuwan Robin and Tribhuwan Preeti, 1993).

11. The health team working with and for tribals must survey the health problems and health needs of the tribals before planning any health programme for them. At times what may seems to be a problem to a health worker may not necessarily be a health problem to the tribals. Therefore it is very necessary that the tribals themselves define their needs and problems related to health. It is absolutely wrong to conduct health education classes for a tribal group which is hand to mouth. Efforts should be made to meet their basic needs first.

12. The programmes planned should fit into the cultural frame work of the people. It is very necessary to understand people's cultural beliefs and practices regarding health and disease.

13. The personal working in the field of health education and health care should be well equipped with skills to approach and motivate the tribals. Motivation should be such that it will induce a change among the people. Motivating the younger generation is more easier than the older generation is more receptive to new ideas and changes.

14. Motivation of people should be followed with community participation. Without people participating in health programmes the action of implementation becomes a one way traffic. People value new programmes when they are involved in the programmes.

15. Finally, I would like to stress the importance of planning, implementing and following up health care and health education programmes. Whatever is planned should be implemented and what is implemented should be followed up to know the success and the failure of the programme. Most of the times programmes are only planned but not implemented and even if implemented not followed up. Thus health programmes should be planned along with people, implemented with people and followed up with people so as to promote community participation.

Further Research Needed :

Health is an aspect of culture and as such the health attitudes and practices of the people also the prejudices are integrated with aspects of culture. The importance of research carried out by anthropologists on the relationship of customs and practices., beliefs and ideas regarding health and disease lies in furthering the programme of health education because such research can provide basic information to health providers and health educators on 'what to educate' and search out ways and means of 'how to educate'. Given below are some topics where further research is needed.

1. An investigation of the socio-cultural barriers that hinder health care and health education programmes.
2. A comparative study of ethnophysiology i.e. the way the tribals perceive the functioning of their bodily processes.
3. An in depth study of medicinal plants and animal extracts which are medicinal in nature to further develop their efficacy 4. An investigation of the problems of accepting modern health care services and health education programmes.
5. An anthropological study of maternal and child health care beliefs and practices of the tribals.
6. Scientific assessment of the objects, gestures, songs, music, utterances etc. used in ritual healing.
7. A scientific study that highlights the relationship of human health with cosmos.
8. An anthropological study of tribal health expenditure patterns.
9. A survey study of water problems faced in rural and tribal areas.
10. An assessment of the work load of the primary health centre staff and the actual time they devote for health education and health service of the tribals.

GLOSSARY

Ajya - great grandfather
Amosha - No moon night
Ai - mother, father's brother's wife
Agni - fire
Aba - father is addressed as Aba
Atma - soul
Aada - a jamun (Engenia jambolina) plank, placed center of the roof. It is a symbol of the sky in house construction text.
Agris - an agricultural (criminal) caste group.
Aatadi - Intestines
Aangat vara yene - getting into trance.
Akshar lihine - a ritual during which (it is believed) Satvai (Mother Earth) comes and writes the fortune on the forehead of the newborn on the fifth day.
Arshi - migraine.
Athvar - an unmarried boy/girl.
Aag - pain, fire, chilly hot food.
Bandi - a male garment resembling a waistcoat.
Bhagat - Male Shaman.
Bhagatin - Female Shaman.
Bhutala - Sorcerer.
Bhutali - witch
Bukka - a black powder used in rituals also known as Abir.
Baya - A band of planetary spirits.
Bhakar - a bread made of nagli (Eluane coracana) Bhajan - prayers sung in a chorus by a group of devotees.
Bhut - the spirit of a deceased person, a figure of lead representing this.
Bhakti - the esoteric art of a bhagat.
Bhavani - deity of lower caste.
Badi Saunf - seeds of Foenicum vulgare.
Brahmins - highest caste in the caste system.
Bembi - naval.
Badva - local term used by the Bhil tribe for a Shaman.
Bhairi - village God of the Thakurs.

Badam - Almond.
Bai - woman.
Bhagwana - God
Beldari - A nomadic community.
Chandra grahan - lunar eclipse.
Chul - hearth.
Chocha dene - branding on a painful spot.
Chandra - moon.
Chamars - shoe maker caste
Chokhya Baya - band of planetary spirits which take the form of non-vegetarian caste groups.
Chedoba - A village god symbolizing the cobra.
Copra - dry coconut.
Chatni - a pungent paste made out of chillies.
Dithmani - a chain of blackyellow beads used to ward off evil effects.
Devjati - higher social groups (castes/tribes) given a divine status in certain rituals.Dantari - mother Earth.
Dir - husband's brother.
Daha darawaze - tenbodily openings of the body symbolic of the ten planets in the universe.
Devi mandal - band of planetary spirits.
Daru - liquor.
Dudh kandh - corm (Diascorea indica).
Dhangars - a nomadic shepherds caste group.
Dholki - a small drum, musical instrument.
Deha bhangache gane - songs related to the body.
Dil - heart.
Dole - eyes.
Divas -a special day to perform the soul migration ritual, seventh day in case of bachelors and spinsters, ninth day in case of married females and tenth day in case of married males.
Dith bhut - spirit of the evil eye.
Devmantra - ritual performed by the bhagat to gain divine power to diagnose the cause and heal their patients.
Drishti phodne - rituals performed to ward off evil eye effect.
Dagadi pala - leaves of Tridax procubens used to heal wounds.
Drishti lagne - evil eye.
Dassera - a Hindu festival.
Dhakti - mother's sister.
Dhamdi - A dance performed by elderly people during Pitra Amosha.
Fodya Baya - disease classificatory term used for diseases such as

body sores, small pox, chicken pox etc.

Fatya - firewood.Gawli - milk man.

Ghat - a specific arrangement in which a coconut is placed on a metal pot around which Plumeria rubra flowers are scattered in a ritual context. Thus arrangement is symbolic of the planetary spirits and the cosmos.

Ghorpad - monitor.

Gala patta - necklace.

Gupta darwaza - Secret opening (anal opening)

Gorej - a type of social referred in the myth creation of man.

Gham - sweat.

Ghas - morsel.

Gulal - a red powder used in rituals.

Gomtir - cow's urine.

Gonda - an ornament worn by women in the hair.

Gandhicha tap - measels.

Germany Baya - planetary spirits taking the form of Britishers and causing trouble to the Thakurs.

Gupit Bhut - secret evil spirit.

Guru - teacher.

Guy - cow.

Garbha padne - abortion.

Gaon dev - village God.

Halad - Turmeric.

Hadeli - a female evil spirit.

Hatachi nadi - wrist pulse.

Holi - a festival of fire also the Thakur Goddess of fire.

Hava - air.

Had vaidu - Bone setter.

Ibut - charmed ask taken from a hearth used by the bhagat to apply on the forehead of the planets.

Ilkat bhut - evil spirit of wealth.

Inchu chavane - scorpian sting.

Ibut mantra - Therapeutic ritual.

Jantu - germs

Jant - worms

Janmacha rog - a disease which is genetical in nature. Leucoderma (kode) according to Thakurs is a disease which occurs right from birth.

Jeev - life.

Jeevkhada - a stone picked up from the grave of a dead person and used in the ritual of soul migration. The stone in the ritual symbol-

izes soul.
Jholi - a swing for infants.
Jamun - Eugenia jambolina.
Jagran - A healing ritual of planetary spirits (Baya) which is participated by the villagers by keeping awake and singing praises to Baya.
Khaisache por - a congenital deformed child, believed to be the off spring of a evil spirit known as khais. There children are killed by the Thakurs.
Kharik - Date.
Khota bolne - speaking lies.
Kurud - a pinkish white wild flower.
Khambya - village God.
Kharuj - scabies.
Kilkachya Devi - Goddesses that reside on the peth fort
Khais - A male evil spirit.
Kuldev - clan Gods.
Karanj - pongamia pinnata.
Kunku - pink powder applied on the forehead as an auspicious mark.
Kanji - porridge
Kaka - mother's sister's husband.
Kushta Rog - Leprosy.
Khanda Sarkha pind - Human body is an image of the cosmos.
Kalij - Liver.
Kan - Ear.
Kanir Dev - God of Ear.
Kannadi Baya - Planetary spirits that take the form of a nomadic caste group namely kannadis.
Kirtankar - a person who composes religious songs and is also a singer.
Kolha bhut - an evil spirit of the fox.
Kode - Leucoderma.
Kidas - Referred to as the two worms present in the forehead just above the fronto-nasal suture. These two worms release sperms in males and egg in females.
Kid lagne - to rot.
Karla - Bitter gourd.
Kunbis - an agricultural caste group.
Khekada - Crab.
Lambavaleli koni - Delayed delivery.
Lohan Baya - The term is used to refer the female planetary spirits which take form of human caste annd tribal groups. eg. Brahmani Baya, Kolani Baya.
Lugade - a garment worn by Thakur women.

Lugna - Wedding.Lohar - blacksmith caste.

Mamadev - pathogenic agent (moon)which cause boils.

Mantra - chant.

Mavalat baju - West direction where sets the sun.

Mothur med - A wooden pole which is situated on the south- east direction of every Thakur house. This pole symbolizes sun duriing the construction rite and hence is worshipped first before constructing the house.

Munja - is a white skinned male evil spirit. It is believed that Munja forcefully has sex with a woman and hence an albino children and hence killed at birth by the midwives.

Mantrik - an herbalist who is specialized in curing scorpian stings and snake bites using herbal and magico- ritual therapy.

Mang - untouchable caste.

Mahar - untouchable caste.

Mahadev koli - A tribe which enjoys a hiigher social status than the Thakurs.

Marai - A female deity of lower caste and tribal groups.

Manav - human beings.

Mothya Baya - Female planetary spirits.

Mali - Garner caste group.

Mala varcha chedha - Cobra's spirit that protects wealth.

Mun - mind.

Manushya Avtar - Incarnation of man.

Mogra - A wild flower (Jasminum SP)

Mauha - Bacia latefolia.

Maruti - Mankey God also known as Hanuman. The deity of Hindus. He is the God of Medicine for Thakurs.

Munjache por - An albino child believed to be an offspring of Munja a white skinned male evil spirit.

Mehuni - wife's sister.

Mothi ai - grandmother.

Mutlani - urinary bladder.

Malai - Fishing aparatus.

Nag chavne - cobra bite.

Nada - string.

Nadi - pulse.

Nadi parikasha - a method of diagnosis by checking wirst pulse.

Nagli - Eleucine coracana.

Naru - Local name for guinea worms.

Navin pani - Fresh water from the well.

Nhavi - Barber.

Naska dudh - Cholostrom milk is believed to be spoilt milk.

Nadya - veins.

Nal - Umbilical chord.

Nak - nose.

Navnath - The nine planets.

Naraj - a type soil referred in the myth. This soil was used to create human life.

Navaratra - Nine days of training a Shamans.

Oti - symbol of a woman womb.

Oti bharane - is a rite wherein fruits (symbolize of spring) are put in the sari of a married woman during the wedding ceremony. Its a fertility rite which aims to bless a woman's woman for being productive.

Pani - water.pani ghalne - a ritual which symbolically aims at satisfying the sexual desires of Baya, by giving a patient sap of Ficus glomerata. This sap symbolizes the moon's sperms and the patient's body as Baya who get sexually satisfied.

Pornima - Full moon night.

Pachvi punjan - A ritual performed to worship mother earth (satvai) of the fifth day after a woman's delivery.

Punjarin - A woman who performs the pachvi punjan rite.

Pitra amosha - Festival of Ancestral spirits.

Pipal tree - Ficus religiosa.

Phirta mela - Bond of planetary spirits who move in the form of wild honey bees.

Paush - one of the months in Thakurs calender.

Potali - stomach.

Phupus - lungs.

Pitta - bile.

Pitha - spleen.

Pinjara - cage.

Phool - flower, an egg cell released by a woman is believed to be as flower by the Thakurs which on getting fertilized by a sperm becomes a fruit (offspring).

Palas leaf - Butea Frondosa leaf.

Parmatma - God, super soul.

Panch Amrut - five holy fluids namely milk, water, honey, cow's urine and coconut milk.

Pita - father.

Potdhari - Assistant midwife.

Pisha - An evil spirit which moves in the jungle.

Panch mukhee chedha - The five hooded cobra God.
Pashu - Animals.
Pakshi - Birds.
Phasva-phasvi - cheating.
Paisa - coin or money.
Pani marne - A ritual performed by a mantrik to cure snake bites.
Pitrya - Bert man.
Pitari - Brides maid.
Payachi nadi - pulse of the feet.
Rakta - Blood.
Rakta vahane - blood flow.
Rui - calotropis gigantia.
Rama - Deity of hindus, for Thakurs, Sun is their Rama.
Rakshas Jati - The lower castes and tribes who do evil deeds such as black magic, sorcery etc. and have a low social profile.
Ratya baya - Planetary spirits taking the form of non- vegetarian castes and tribes to trouble Thakurs.
Rog - Disease.
Ras - Fluid.
Rakshas - Giants.
Sadguru - spiritual teacher.
Surya dev - Sun God.
Surya Rakhad - ash from the hearth, used during ritual healing.
Swarg - heaven.
Sasu - mother in law.
Supali - female ancestor spirit.
Suine - mid-wife.
Supari - Arecnut.
Shelbhut - Evil spirit of goat.
Surya Grihan - solar eclipse.
Swachha atma - Pure soul.
Sag - Tectona grandis.
Suj - swelling.
Satvai - Goddess of fertility and fortune (Mother Earth).
Suvasini - A woman married by the first marriage rites.
Sali - sister in law (wife's sister).
Shendur - orange coloured paste mixed with oil to put on shrines.
Sonar - Goldsmith caste.
Tej - light.
Tond - Mouth and/or Face.
Tambya - Small metal pot, used in diagnosis ritual. Tambya symbolizes the soul of a person.

Thakurwadi - A hamlet exclusively or mainly occupied by Thakurs.
Umbari - The female functionary at a wedding who associates with umbarya, her husband in his work.
Ungvat baju - East direction.
Ukhali - A hollow place of pounding rice.
Vaidu - Herbalist.
Virya - Sperms.
Vara - Wind.
Var - Placental waste.
Vat - Wick.
Vat vaghul - Bat.
Virdev - Male ancestral spirit.
Vetal - An evil spirit.
Vadi - A hamlet.
Vaghoba - The tiger God.
Vad-vadil - Ancestors.
Veetal - Menstrual blood.
Vari - Panicum sp.
Vanachi baju - Evil forces of the jungle.
Vara yene - To get into trance.
Vanjuti - Barren woman.
Yiv - neck.
Zendu - Tagitus sp.
Zokhachya devi - The Goddesses that swing.
Zakham - wound.
Zadya - viper.
Zadu - broom.

BIBLIOGRAPHY

Ackernecht, Erwin H.
1942 "Problems of primitive Medicine" in Bulle tin of the History of Medicine XI - 503 - 21.

Ackernecht, E.H.
1946 "Natural Disease and Rational Treatment Primi tive Medicine",inBulletin of the History of Medicine 19 (May 1946) : 467 - 97.

Adams, Richard N.
1951 "Un Analisis de les enfernedadesy sus. curacioneseneuna poblacion indegena de Gautemala "(con sugerencious relacion adas conla practica de medicina en el axa maya)". Institute de Nutricion de centro America y Panama Gautemala.

Adams, Richard N.
1955 A Nutritional Research Programme in Gautemala in Health Culture and Community B.D. Paul (ed) pp. 435 - 58. New York Russel Sage Foundation.

Adams, R and A. Rubel
1967 Handbook of Middle American Indians Robert Wanchope and Manning Nash eds. Austin : University of Texas Press.

Adams, Richard N.
1963 An Analysis of Medical Beliefs and Practices in a Gauteman Indian Town : Gautemala city Pan American Sanitary Bureau.

Alland, Alexander R.
1970 Adaptation in Cultural Evolution : An ap proach to Medical Anthropology, New York, London, Columbia University.

Arikiev, M.D. (ed).
1964 Magic, Faith and Healing; (Studies in Primi tive Psychology Today. The Free Press of Glencoc Collies. Mc Millian Hd, London.

Atkibson, Jane Monnig
1987 The Effectiveness of Shamans in a Indone- sian Ritual in Social Science & Medicine 89, 2, June 1987, pages 342 - 355. U.S.A.

Barth, Frederick.
1956 Nomads of South Persia, London; Allen and Unwin.

Bhatnagar, G.S.
1975 Community Response to Health, Dept. of Sociology, Punjab University, Patiala.

Bharara, S.S.
1961 "Public Attitudes in Relation to Small Pox Eradication", Health Education Bureau, Lucknow (U.P.)

Banerjee, D.
1961 Social Aspects of Tuberculosis Problems in India, in Rao K.N. (ed) Text book of Tuber culosis, Vikas Publication. New Delhi.

Bauwens, Eleaner E
1978 The Anthropology of Health, The C.V. Mosby Co. St. Louis, Toronto

Caudil, William
1955 Applied Anthropology in Medicine in Kroeber A.R. (Ed.) Anthro Today, The Uni versity of Chicago Press, Chicago.

Cavendish, Richard
1985 Man, Myth and Magic. The illustrated ency clopedia of Mythology, Religion and the Unknown. Vol 10, Marshal Cavendish, New York

Clements, Forrest E.
1932 "Primitive Concepts of Disease", University of California Publications in American Archaelogy and Ethnology XXXII 185-252.

Camaroff, J.
1978 Medicine and Culture : Some Anthropologi cal perspectives, in *Social Science & Medi cine* 12, 4 B, Oct. 1978, pages 247-254. U.S.A.

Camaroff, Jean
1981 Healing and Cultural Transformation; "The Tswana of Southern Africa" in *Soccial Sci ence & Medicine*. Vol 15B pp 367-378.

Csordos, Thomas J.
1988 Elements of Charismatic Persuation and Healing in *'Medical Anthropology Quarterly'* 2,2, June p.p. 121-142 U.S.A.

Carpa, Fritjof
1991 Healing Tradition and the Universe in *'Health for Millions.'* February Vol XVII No.1.

Clark, Margaret
1959 Health in the Mexican-American Culture. Berkeley: University of California Press.

Crombie, Aliston
1969 Discussion in Medicine and Culture ed. F.N.L. Poynter London :. Welcome Institute of Medicine.

Carstairs, G.M.
1985 Medicine & Faith in Rural Rajasthan, in Paul BD (ed) Health, Culture & Community, Russel Sage Foundation, New York.

Chaphekar, L.N.
1960 The Thakurs of Sahyadri Oxford University Press, Amen House, London EC 4.

Chaudhari, B. (Ed)
1986 Tribal Health : Socio-cultural dimension Inter-India Publications, D-17 Raja Garden Extn. New Delhi.

Cohen, Milton
1984 The Ethnomedicine of the Garifuna of Rio Tinto, in Anthropology Quaterly 57, 1 Jan. 1984, Pages 16 - 27, U.S.A.

David, Lotz
1987 "Ritual" in The Encyclopaedia of Religion Vol. 12 (ed) by Mircea Eliade, Macmillan Publishing Company, New York.

Devish, Renaat
1985 'Polluting and Healing among the Northern Yaka of Zaire.' in *Soc. & Sci. and Medicine* 21,16,693-700 U.S.A.

Douglas, Mary
1963 The Lele of Kasal London Oxford University Press, for International African Institute.

Douglas, Mary
1966 Purity and Danger : An analysis of the concepts of pollution and taboo Routledge and Kegan Paul, London.

Douglas, Mary
1970 Natural Symbols (Exploration in Cosmology) Pantheon Books, A Div. of Random House, New York.

Douglas, Mary
1975 Implicit Meanings (Essays in Anthropology) Routledge & Kegan Paul, London, Boston, Melbourne.

Durkhiem, Emile
1954 Elementary Forms of the Religious Life. London : Allen & Unwin.

Dhillon, H.S. and Karim, S.E.
1961 Investigation of Cultural Patterns & Beliefs among tribal population in Orissa with regard to Malaria eradication. CHEB, New Delhi.

Dfurfeldt, G and Lindberg, S.
1975 Pills against Poverty - A study of the Introduction of Western Medicine in a Tamil Village. Oxford and IBH publishers, New Delhi.

Early, Evelyn
1982 'The Logic of Wellbeing. Therapeutic Narratives in Cairo, Egypt.' in *Soc. Sci. & Med.* Vol 16 No : 15, July-Sept pp 1491-1497.

Elworthy, Fredrick
1895 The Evil Eye Reprint, New York Machmillan 1958.

Field, M.J.
1937 Religion and Medicine of the Ga People. Oxford University Press, London.

Foster, George
1962 Traditional Cultures and Impact of Technological change. New York, Harper & Row.

Foster, George M.
1965 "Peasent Society and the Image of Limited Good" American Anthropologist 67, No 2 293-315.

Foster, George M.
1972 A Study of Symbolic Behaviour Current Anthropology 13 (1972) 165-202.

Foster, G.M.; Anderson; Barbara
1978 Medical Anthropology Johnwilly & Sons, New York.

Foster, George
1983 An Introduction to Ethnomedicine in Traditional Medicine and Health Coverage. A reader for Health Administration and Practitioners ed. Bannerman & others. WHO Geneva.

Fabrega, Horacio Jr.
1977 Group Differences in the structure of Illness, in *Culture, Medicine and Psychiatry* 1, 4, 379-394. Netherlands.

Fabrega, Horacio Jr.
1977 The scope of Ethnomedical Science, in *Culture, Medicine and Psychiatry.* 1, 2, 201 -228.

Foster, George M.
1953 'Relationship between Spanish and Spanish-American Folk Medicine.' in *Journal of American Folklore* 60, 201-17.

Foster, George M.
1967 Tzintzuntzan : Mexican peasant in a changing World. Boston : Little Brown.

Frank, Lawrence K.
1948 Society as the patient. New Brunswick : Rutgers University Press.

Gillin, John
1948 "Magical Fright" *Psychiatry*, XI 387-400

Gifford, Edwards S.
1958 The Evil Eye : Studies in the folklore of vision. New York, Macmillian.

Glick, Deborah
1988 Symbolic, Ritual and Social Dynamics of Spiritual Healing in Social Sceince & Medicine 27, 11, Pages 1197 - 1206. U.S.A.

Glick, Leonard B.
1967 'Medicine as an Ethnographic category.' The Gini of the New Guinea Highlands in Ethnology 6 : 31-56.

Gennep, Arnold Van
1960 The Rites Passage. Chicago.

Geertz, Clifford
1957 Ritual and Social Change : A Javanese example, in *American Anthropologist* 59 : 32-54.

Harley, George W.
1941 Native African Medicine. Harvard University Press, Cambridge.

Hastings, J. ed.
1908 Encyclopedia of Religion and Ethics Edinburgh : Clark.

Hall, Oswald
1951 "Sociological Research in the field of Medicine: Progress and Prospects", in *American Sociological Review* XVI, 639-44.

Honigman, J.J.
1959 The World of Man. New York, Harper.

Honigman, J.J.
1973 Handbook of Social & Cultural Anthropology Chicago : Rand Mcnally and Company.

Halowell, Irving A.
1934 "Sin, Sex and Sickness in Saulteaux Belief", in *British Journal of Medical Psychology* XVIII, 191-99.

Halowell, Irving A.
1942 The role of conjuring in the Saulteaux Society University of Pennysylvania Press, Phila delphia.

Halowell, Irving A.
1950 "Values, Acculturation and Mental Health", in *American Journal of Orthopsychiatry* XX, 732-43.

Halowell, Irving A.
1958 Cultural factors in spatial organisations in culture and experience. Philadelphia, University of Pennysylvania Press.

Halowell, Irving A.
1963 Ojibwa World View and Disease in Man's Image in Medicine and Anthropology. ed. I. Gladstone, pp 258-315, New York : International Universities Press.

Hart, Donn V.
1969 Bisayan Fillipino and Malayan Humoral Pathologies : Folk Medicine and Ethnohistory in Southeast Asia. South Asia program, data paper no. 76, Ithaca : Dept. of Asian Studies, Cornell University.

Haurd, Pierre
1969 Western Medicine and Afro-Asian Ethnic Medicine in Medicine and Culture. ed. F.N.L. poynter pp 211-37 London : Wellcome Institute of History of Medicine.

Hasan, K.A.
1967 The Cultural Frontiers & Health in a village of India, Manaktalas, Bombay. Hahn, Robert and Kleinman, Arthur 1983 Belief as pathogen, Belief as Medicine : "Voodoo Death" and the "placebo phenomena" in Anthropological perspective. In *Medical Anthropology Quaterly* Vol 14 No 4, Aug. 3, 16-19.

Harner, Michael
1973 Shamanism & Hallucinogens Oxford University Press, New York.

Hasan, K.A. and Prasad, B.G.
1959 A note on the contributions of Anthropology to Medical science, in *Journal of Indian Medical Association*, 33, 182-190.

Joshi, O.P.
1992 Marks and Meanings Anthropology of Symbols, BSA Publishers, Jaipur.

Jelliffe, D.B.
1956 Cultural Variation and the Practical Pediatrician. in *Journal of Pediatrics*, 49 : 661-71.

Joshi, Vibha
1986 "Health, Disease and Social Structure : Their Relationship in a Nagaland Village" In *Indian Anthropologist*, Vol 16, No 2, pp 125 137.

Kakar, Sudhir
1982 Shamans; Mystics and Doctors (A Psychological Inquiry into India and its healing - tradiditions) Oxford University Press, Delhi, Bombay.

Kluckholn, Clyde
1944 Navaho Witchcraft (Papers of the Peabody Museum of Harvard University Vol XXII, No 2.) Cambridge, Mass

Kurian, J.C. and Bhanu, B.V.
1980 "Ethnomedicine : A Study of Nomadic Vaidus of Maharashtra" In *The Eastern Anthropologist* Vol 33, No. 1, Jan-Mar pp 71-78.

Kurian, J.C. and Tribhuwan, Robin

1990 Traditional Medical Practitioners of the Sahyadri, in *TheEasternAnthropologist*Vol 43(3), July-Sept Issue 1990 pp 251-258. Published by Ethnographic and folk culture Society.Kakar,

D.N. et.al

1976 People's Perceptions of Illness and their Use of Medical care in Punjab.

Khare, R.S.

1963 Folk Medicine in a North Indian village, in *Human Organization*, Vol 22, No. 1.Khan,

Hussain & Ali, Arif

1992 "Relevance of Ethnomedicine" in *Man & Life*Vol 18 Nos 1 & 2, Calcutta

Kleinman, Arthur

1980 Patients and Healers in the Contact of Culture. (An exploration of the borderland between Anthropology, Medicine and Psychiatry) University of California Press, Berkley, Los Angles.Kark, Sidney & Emily Kark 1962 A Practice of Social Medicine, S.L. Kark and G.E. Steuart (ed) pp 3-40 Edinburgh & London : E & S Livingstone.

Knight, Chris

1985 Menstruation as Medicine, in Social Science & Medicine 21, 6, pages 671-683, U.S.A.

Langer, Susane K.

1956 The World of Man Menter Book Publishers, New York.

Lee, Dorothy

1950 Nonlineal condification of reality in *Psycho somatic Medicine*, Vol. 12, pp 87-89.

Leighton, A.H. and D.C.
1941 "Elements of Psychotherapy in Navaho Religion", in *Psychiatry* IV 515-23.

Lieban, Richard
1973 Medical Anthropology in Honingman, J.J. ed Handbook of Social and Cultural Anthropology Rand Mcnally and Company, Chicago.

Linton, Ralph
1940 Acculuration in seven American Indian tribes R Linton ed. Appleton-Century Crafts, New York.

Leach, Edmund R.
1968 "Ritual", in International Encyclopedia of the Social Sciences, Vol 13, New York.

Leighton, A.H.
1944 The Navaho Door Cambridge : Harvard University Press.

Levi-strauss, Claude
1966 The Savage Mind.

London.Lieban, Richard
1962 The Dangerous Ingkantos : Illness and So cial control in a Philippine community, in *American Anthropologist* 64 : 306 12.

Lieban, Richard
1967 Cebuana Sorcery Berkley : University of California Press.

Lieban, Richard
1962 Qualifications for Folk Medical Practice in Sibulan Negros Oriental, Philippines, in *Journal of Science* 91 : 511-21.

Marwick, Max
1952 "The Social Context of Cewa Witch Beliefs", in *Africa* XXII No. 2 and 3.

Maclagan, R.C.
1902 Evil Eye in the Western Highlands London.

McCraknes
1971 Lactose Deficiency An example of Dietary Evolution, in *Current Anthropology* 12 : 479-517.

McGuire, Meredith B.
1987 Ritual, Symbolism and Healing in Social Compass, 34, 4 pages 365-379 Belgium.

Meerloo, Joost A.M.
1971 Institution and the Evil Eye Wasenaar (Netherlands).

Mead and Henry
1949 "Anthropology and Psychosometrics", in *Psychosomatic Medicine* XI pp 216-22.

Middletten, John and Winter, E.H. ed.
1963 Witchcraft and Sorcery in East Africa London, Routledge and Kegan Paul.

Munn, Nancy
1973 Symbolism in a ritual. context. Aspects of symbolic action in Handbook of Social and Cultural Anthropology ed. Honingman J.J. Rand Mcnally and Company, Chicago.

Murray, David
1977 Ritual Communication: Novajo Ceremonials in Symbolic Anthropology : A reader in the study of symbols and weanings ed. Dolgin J. and others. Columbia University Press. Guildford pp 195-220.

Maclean, Catherine M.V.
1969 Traditional Healers and their female clients : An aspect of Nigerian sickness behaviour,

in *Journal of Health and Social behaviour* 10 : 172-86.

Messing, Simmon D.
1968 Interdigitation of Mystical and Physical Healing in Ethiopia. Behaviour Science Notes 3 : 87-104.

Metzger, Duane and Gerald, Williams
1963 Tenejapa Medicine I : The Curer South West *Journal of Anthropology* 19 : 216-34.

Marriot, M.
1955 "Western Medicine in a village of Northern India". In Paul B.D. (ed) Health, Culture and Community, Russel Sage Foundation pp 239-268, New York.

Mutatkar, R.K.
1979 Society and Leprosy Shubhada, Saraswati Publishers, Pune.

Nitcher and Nitcher
1981 An Anthropological approach to Nutrition Education International Nutrition Commu nication Service Education Development Centre, 55 Chapel Street, Newton U.S.A.

Newell, Kenneth
1975 Health by people Geneva World Health Organization.

Needham, Rodney (ed)
1973 Right and Left : Essays on Dual Symbolic classification. Chicago.

Nash, Manning
1965 The Golden Road to Modernity New York, Wiley.

Nurge, Ethel
1958 'Etiology of Illness in Guinhangdan', in *American Anthropologist* 60 : 1158-72.

Opler, Morris
1936 "Some points of Comparison and contrast between the treatment of Functional Disorrders by Apache Shamans and Modern Psychaitric Practice", in *American Journal of Psychiatry* XCII 1371-87.

Opler, Morris E.
1941 An Apache Life-way University of Chicago Press, Chicago.

Ozturk, Orhan M.
1964 Folk treatment of Mental Illness in Turkey. In Magic, Faith and Healing, ed. Ari Kiev pp 343-63 New York : Free Press, Macmillan.

Opler, M.E.
1963 "Cultural Definition of Illness in village In dia" in *Human Organization* VOL 22, No. 4, 32-35.

Paul, B.D.
1955 Health Culture and Community Case Studies of Public Reactions to Health Programmes. New York : Russel Sage Foundation.

Pelto and Pelto
1978 Anthropological Research Cambridge University Press, Cambridge, London, New York.

Pritchard, Evans
1937 Witchcraft Oracles and Magic among the Agande Clarondon Press, Oxford.

Parsons, Talcott
1951 The Social System Glencoe Ill : Free Press.

Parsons, Talcott
1953 Illness and the role of the Physician in per

sonality in Nature, Society and Culture. ed. C Kluckholm and H.A. Murray, 2nd ed. pp 607-17. New York : Knopy.

Parsons, Talcott
1958 Definitions of Health and Illness in the light of American values and Social Structure in patients, Physicians and Illness. ed. E.G. Jaco, pp 165-87. Glencoe, Ill : Free Press.

Parsons, Talcott and Renee, Fox
1952 Illness, Therapy, and the American Family. in *Journal of Social Issues* 8 : 2-3, 31-44.

Parsons, Talcott
1964 Social Structure and Personality. New York : Free Press, Macmillan.

Paul, Benjamin D.
1963 Anthropological Perspective on Medicine and Public Health Annuals of the American Academy of Political and Social Science. 346 : 34-43.

Polgar, Steven
1962 Health and Human Behaviour of Interest common to the Medical Sciences, in *Current Anthropology* 3 : 159-205.

Polgar, Steven
1968 Health : International Encyclopaedia of Social Sciences. 6 : 330-36.

Pathan, B.R.
1986 Stigma In Leprosy. Unpublished, PhD Thesis, Dept. of Anthropology. University of Poona, Pune 7.

Quisumbing, Euardo
1951 Medicinal Plants of the Philippes. Dept. of Agricultural and Natural Sources, Technical Bulletin No, Manila : Republic of Philippes, Bureau of Printing.

Redfield, R. and M.P.
1940 Disease and its Treatment in Dzitas, Yucatan Carnergie Institution of Washington. Publications No 523, Vol VI No. 32, Washington.

Reynolds, Barrie
1963 Magic, Divination and Witchcraft aomong the Barotse of Northern Rhodesia. (Robins series, Rhodes-Livingstone Museum). London : Chath and Windus.

Rivers, W.H.R.
1924 Medicine, Magic and Religion Harcourt and Brace Company, New York.Roseman,

Marina
1988 The Pragmatics of Aesthetics : The Performana of Healing among Senoi Teniar, in Social Science & Medicine 27, 8, pages 811-818. U.S.A.

Rubel, Arthur
1977 The epidiomology of Folk Illness, Susto in Hispanic America. In Culture, Disease and Healing (ed) David Landy. Mcmillan Publishing Corporation Inc. New York.

Rizvi, S.N.H.
1991 Medical Anthropology of the Jaunsaris Northern Book Centre, New Delhi.

Schock, Helmut
1966 Envy : A Theory of Social behaviour Micheal Glenny and Betty Ross trans New York, Harcourt, Brace.

Schneider, David
1976 Notes towards a theory of culture in Meaning in Anthropology. (ed) K. Basso and H.Selby Albuquerque, University of New Mexico Press.

Schneider, David
1969 Kinship Nationality and Religion in Ameri can Culture : Towards a definition of kinship in forms of symbolic actions. (ed) V. Turner New Orleans LA : American Ethno logical Society.Tulane University.

Seligmann, Sigfried
1910 Der Bos Blick 2 Vols. Berlin.

Sigerist, Henry
1951 A History of Medicine. Oxford University Press, New York.

Shutler, Mary
1979 Disease and Curing in a Vaqui Community in Ethnic Medicine of the South West. pp 169-237 (ed) Spicer E. The University of Amazon Press, Tuscon.

Simon, G.
1973 The Evil Eye in Guetemalan Village Ethnomedicine 2, No. 3, 437-41.

Spooner, Brain
1970 "The Evil Eye in the Middle East" in witchcraft confessions and Accusations, M. Douglas ed.Association of Social Anthropologists,Monograph No 9 London, Tavistock.

Scarpa, Antonio
1967 Introduction : *Ethnoiatria* Vol. 1 : 2-4.

Shilloh, Ailon
1961 The system of Medicine in the Middle East Culture. *Middle East Journal* Vol. 15 : 277 - 88.

Simmon, Ozzie G.
1955 Popular and Modern Medicine in Mestizo Communities of Coastal Peru and Chile. *Journal of American Folklore* Vol. 68 : 57-71.

Shukla, K.
1980 Traditional Healers in Community Health Gomati Krishna Publications, Varanasi.

Singh, I.P.
1988 "Anthropological Strategies of Tribal Health" In *Indian Anthropologist* Vol 18, No. 1, pp 69-79.

Sutherland, Anne
1977 The Body As A Social Symbol, in The Anthropology of the Body (ed) John Blacking Academic Press, New York, ASA Monograph No. 15.

Turner, Victor
1967 The Forest of Symbols Ithaca : Cornell University Press.

Turner, Victor
A Ndembu Doctor in Practice, in Practice, in Magic, Faith and Healing (ed) by Arkiev The Free Press Glenco, Colher-Mcmillan Ltd. London, pp 230-263.

Tribhuwan, Robin and Gambhir, R.D.
1990 Ethnomedical Pathway III International Congress on Traditional Asian Medicine Abstracts. Bombay.

Tribhuwan, Robin and Peters, Preeti
1992 Medico-Ethnobiology of the Kathkaris and Thakurs *Tribal Research Bulletin* Vol XIV No 1, March Issue, TRTI, Pune.

Tribhuwan, Robin, Khatri and Ganguly
1993 Maternal Child Health care Beliefs and practices of the Mavchis *Tribal Research Bulletin*, Vol XV No. 2, Sept. Issue, TRTI, Pune.

Tribhuwan, Robin
1988 Ethnomedicine : A Comparative study Unpublished fieldwork Report, Dept. of Anthropology, University of Poona, Pune7.

Tribhuwan, Robin
1989 Ethnomedicine of the Thakurs Unpublished field work Report, Dept. of Anthropology, University of Poona, Pune 7.

Tribhuwan, Robin and Tribhuvan, Preeti
1993 Community Development : An Integrated effort to enable people help themselves in Tribal Research Bulletin Vol XV No. 1, March Issue, TRI, Pune.

Vidyarthi, L.P. and Rai, B.K.
1985 The Tribal Cultures of India Concept Publishing Company, H-13, Bali Nagar New Delhi.

Vuorela, Turvo
1967 Der bose Blick in Lichte der finnische Uberlieferung, Helsinki.

Warner, W. Lloyd
1939 A Black Civilization Harper and Brothers, New York.

Warren, Dennis M.
1978 The interpretation of Change in a Ghanian Ethnomedical study, in Human Organization 37, 1, Spring, Pages 73 - 77, U.S.A.

Wintrob, Ronald
1973 "The influence of others : Witchcraft and Rootwork as explanation of behaviour

disturbancees" in *The Journal of Nervous and Mental Disease* Vol. 156 No. 5. The Wilhiams and Wilkins Co., U.S.A.

Young, Allan
1982 The Anthropology of Illness and sickness in An-nual Reviews of Anthropology, No 11,pp 257- 85.

Zurbeig, S.
1984 Rakkas Story : Structure of Health and Source of Change. V.H.A.I., New Delhi.

❋❋❋